Suggested Citation

Sunshine, J. H., and Dicker, M.: Family Out-of-Pocket Expenditures for Health Care, United States, 1980. *National Medical Care Utilization and Expenditure Survey.* Series B, Descriptive Report No. 11. DHHS Pub. No. 87–20211. National Center for Health Statistics, Public Health Service. Washington. U.S. Government Printing Office, Aug. 1987.

Library of Congress Cataloging-in-Publication Data

Sunshine, Jonathan N.
   Family out-of-pocket expenditures for health care, United States, 1980.
   (Series B, Descriptive report ; no. 11) (DHHS publication ; no. 87–20211)
   Contract no. 282–84–2108, prepared for National Center for Health Statistics.
   Author: Jonathan H. Sunshine, Marvin Dicker.
   "May 1987."
   Bibliography: p.
   1. Medical care, Cost of—United States—Statistics.
2. Family—United States—Statistics (U.S.) I. Dicker, Marvin.
II. National Center for Health Statistics (U.S.) III. Title.
IV. National Medical Care Utilization and Expenditure Survey (Series). Series B, Descriptive report. V. Series: DHHS publication ; no. 87–20211. [DNLM: 1. Expenditures, Health—United States—statistics. 2. Financing, Personal—United States—statistics. W 74 S958f]
RA410.53.S94   1987   338.4'33621'0973   87–7721
ISBN 0–8406–0372–X

National Medical Care Utilization and Expenditure Survey

The National Medical Care Utilization and Expenditure Survey (NMCUES) is a unique source of detailed national estimates on the utilization of and expenditures for various types of medical care. NMCUES is designed to be directly responsive to the continuing need for statistical information on health care expenditures associated with health services utilization for the entire U.S. population.

NMCUES will produce comparable estimates over time for evaluation of the impact of legislation and programs on health status, costs, utilization, and illness-related behavior in the medical care delivery system. In addition to national estimates for the civilian noninstitutionalized population, it will also provide separate estimates for the Medicaid-eligible populations in four States.

The first cycle of NMCUES, which covers calendar year 1980, was designed and conducted as a collaborative effort between the National Center for Health Statistics, Public Health Service, and the Office of Research and Demonstrations, Health Care Financing Administration. Data were obtained from three survey components. The first was a national household survey and the second was a survey of Medicaid enrollees in four States (California, Michigan, Texas, and New York). Both of these components involved five interviews over a period of 15 months to obtain information on medical care utilization and expenditures and other health-related information. The third component was an administrative records survey that verified the eligibility status of respondents for the Medicare and Medicaid programs and supplemented the household data with claims data for the Medicare and Medicaid populations.

Data collection was accomplished by Research Triangle Institute, Research Triangle Park, N.C., and its subcontractors, the National Opinion Research Center of the University of Chicago, Ill., and SysteMetrics, Inc., Berkeley, Calif., under Contract No. 233–79–2032.

Co-Project Officers for the Survey were Robert R. Fuchsberg of the National Center for Health Statistics (NCHS) and Allen Dobson of the Health Care Financing Administration (HCFA). Robert A. Wright of NCHS and Larry Corder of HCFA also had major responsibilities. Daniel G. Horvitz of Research Triangle Institute was the Project Director primarily responsible for data collection, along with Associate Project Directors Esther Fleishman of the National Opinion Research Center, Robert H. Thornton of Research Triangle Institute, and James S. Lubalin of SysteMetrics, Inc. Barbara Moser of Research Triangle Institute was the Project Director primarily responsible for data processing.

Contents

List of Text Tables

Symbols

\-   No families with these characteristics in sample

*   Potential reliability problem; statistic is based on sample size of fewer than 50 or has relative standard error greater than 30 percent

...   Category not applicable

Family Out-of-Pocket Expenditures For Health Care: United States, 1980

By Jonathan H. Sunshine, Ph.D.,
Applied Management Sciences, Inc.
and Marvin Dicker, Ph.D.,
National Center for Health Statistics

Executive Summary

Information on out-of-pocket health care expenditures for families in 1980 is presented in this report. The data discussed here were gathered through the national household sample of the National Medical Care Utilization and Expenditure Survey (NMCUES). Information for the year 1980 was collected on health problems, health care received, expenditures for care, health insurance, and related topics from approximately 6,800 families in the U.S. civilian, noninstitutionalized population. All individuals who are in institutions or in the military are excluded from this analysis as are all families with military heads of family, even if they have civilian members.

For this report, a family was initially defined as: two or more persons living together who were related either by blood, marriage, adoption, or a formal foster care relationship; or as a single person living outside such relationships. Because these data were collected throughout an entire year, the important concept of "longitudinal family" was developed. This concept was necessary to deal with the fact that the composition of a family could change over time, and that families could come into existence and go out of existence over time. As the data are based on this dynamic concept of families, all measures of health care expenditures are calculated in terms of annual rates.

Family data are important for understanding the health care system because decisions to seek and use health care are usually family decisions, health care

is usually paid for out of family resources, and family distributions for health-related variables differ from the distributions found for individuals.

General Findings

The mean amount paid out of pocket in 1980 by all U.S. multiple-person families for all health care services examined in NMCUES was $575 per family. (The term "multiple-person families" refers to families with an average size of 1.5 persons or more during the survey year.) Major components of the $575 total, and the mean out-of-pocket expenditure per family for each service, include: dental care, $159; ambulatory physician care, $126; inpatient hospital care, $79; and prescription medications, $68. It should be noted that NMCUES did not include information on long-term care, and that out-of-pocket expenditures for health insurance premiums are also not discussed in this report or included in the calculations. If multiple-person families that did not use any health care services (1.2 percent of all multiple-person families) are removed from the analysis, the mean out-of-pocket amount spent per care-using family in 1980 was $582. The median, however, was lower— $350 per care-using family—an indication that 50 percent of all care-using multiple-person families had out-of-pocket expenditures that fell below this amount. Nevertheless, at the high end of the distribution of out-of-pocket expenditures, 10 percent of all care-using multiple-person families had out-of-pocket expenditures for health care of $1,310 or more.

The mean out-of-pocket expenditure in 1980 by all U.S. one-person families for the health care services examined in NMCUES was estimated to have been $287 per family. ("One-person families" refer to families with an average size of less than 1.5 persons during the survey year.) When one-person families that did not use health care services (9.6 percent of all one-person families) were removed from the analysis, the mean expenditure per care-using family was estimated to have been $317.

Data on both multiple-person families and one-person families are presented in this report. In the remainder

NOTE: The authors are grateful for the support received during all stages of the preparation of this report from our colleagues at both the National Center for Health Statistics and Applied Management Sciences, Inc. At the National Center for Health Statistics, Gretchen K. Jones did special and innovative programming, Robert J. Casady consulted and advised on difficult problems of weighting and estimation, and Rolf Larson and Margot Brown were exceptionally helpful as table editors and text consultants. Robert A. Wright and Mary Grace Kovar also made important contributions to this report.

At Applied Management Sciences, Inc., Alfred J. Meltzer and Colleen Goodman provided executive management, skillfully making the firm's resources available to meet the changing needs of the project. Alan Cohen provided a unique combination of programming skills and statistical knowledge as the staff member principally responsible for data processing. Dr. Robert Clickner acted as statistical consultant for most of the project, and Jan Edelmon served as research assistant for most of the project. Celestine Darby gave yeoman service in word processing, including the demanding work of table preparation.

of this section, however, only findings for multiple-person families will be addressed as it is multiple-person families that are usually referred to in discussions of families by both the general public and professional social scientists.

Out-of-Pocket Expenditure and Total Expenditure

Although the tables in this report do not contain information on total health care expenditures, a better understanding of the role of out-of-pocket expenditures among family health care expenditures is gained by a comparison with total expenditures. (The data on total health care expenditures is from Sunshine and Dicker, 1987).

Whereas the mean out-of-pocket health care expenditure per family for all multiple-person families using any form of health care was $582, for total health care expenditure it was $2,111. This was more than three and a half times the out-of-pocket amount.

Not only did the means for out-of-pocket health care expenditures and total health care expenditures for all care-using families differ by a large amount when expenditure for all health care was examined, but when family socioeconomic, demographic, and health status characteristics were independently examined, the differences by these characteristics in mean expenditures for all health care never exceeded $550 in out-of-pocket expenditures compared with more than $4,000 for total expenditures.

Therefore, by comparison with total health care expenditures for all health care, out-of-pocket health care expenditures for all health care tend to be small and not to vary a great deal by family characteristics. In all likelihood, this lessening and smoothing of health care expenditures found for out-of-pocket expenditures as compared with total expenditures is the result of the combined effect on family health expenditures of the availability in the U.S. of private health insurance and public health care programs.

Out-of-Pocket Expenditure and Family Characteristics

Turning from statistics on the out-of-pocket expenditures of all U.S. families to statistics on different types of families defined by socioeconomic, demographic, and health status characteristics, the overall finding is that in 1980 there was great variation in both the strength and direction of the association found among family type, type of health service used, and out-of-pocket expenditures. For example, among care-using multiple-person families with no member 65 years and over, mean out-of-pocket expenditures for most types of health care were generally higher in 1980, the poorer the health

status rating of a family. However, the reverse pattern was found for dental care. The poorer the health status rating of a family, the lower were the expenditures.

If family age (measured by the presence or absence of a family member 65 years and over) and other family characteristics are examined simultaneously, interesting patterns also emerge. For example, when care-using multiple-person families were classified simultaneously by family age and family health status, it was found that significant differences in mean out-of-pocket health care expenditures were associated with differences in health status. However, no significant differences in mean expenditures were associated with age differences. This finding indicates that differences in health status, not age, underlie the differences in out-of-pocket health care expenditures that occur when families are classified solely by age.

Extremely High Out-of-Pocket Expenditures

The following family categories listed as having extremely high out-of-pocket expenditures are those for which the 90th percentile of family out-of-pocket spending by care-using multiple-person families was highest in 1980. (Categories for which the sample size was too small—fewer than 50 care-using families—are not included.) The expenditure given for each category is among the highest 10 percent of families with expenditures using the particular service.

- For all *health care combined*, the 1980 out-of-pocket spending by care-using multiple-person families was extremely high for the following: families whose members spent more than 20 days in bed ($2,136 or more in expenditures); families with a member rated as being in poor health ($1,797 or more in expenditures); and families with an unstable head-and-spouse structure ($1,745 or more in expenditures).

- For *inpatient hospital care*, the 1980 out-of-pocket spending by care-using multiple-person families was extremely high for the following: families with some members completely lacking health care coverage (expenditures of $1,549 or more); families with an unstable head-and-spouse structure ($1,292 or more in expenditures); and families with income of 150 to 199 percent of the poverty level ($1,280 or more in expenditures).

- For *inpatient physician care*, the 1980 out-of-pocket spending by care-using multiple-person families was extremely high for the following: families with some members completely lacking health care coverage (expenditures of $755 or more); families with a head, but no spouse or child ($747 or more in expenditures); and families with a member rated as being in poor health ($715 or more in expenditures).

- For *ambulatory physician care,* the 1980 out-of-pocket spending by care-using multiple-person families was extremely high for the following: families whose members in total spent more than 20 days in bed (expenditures of $386 or more); families whose head had a college degree or more education ($377 or more in expenditures); and families with income of $35,000 or more (also $377 or more in expenditures).

- For *hospital outpatient and emergency room care,* the 1980 out-of-pocket spending by care-using multiple-person families was extremely high for the following: families with some members completely lacking health care coverage (expenditures of $343 or more); families with a member rated as being in poor health ($264 or more in expenditures); and families with an unstable head-and-spouse structure ($259 or more in expenditures).

- For *dental care,* the 1980 out-of-pocket spending by care-using multiple-person families was extremely high for the following: families with an income of $35,000 or more (expenditures of $849 or more); families with five or more members ($779 or more in expenditures); and families with a head of "other" (neither black nor white) race ($772 or more in expenditures).

- For *prescription medicines,* the 1980 out-of-pocket spending by care-using multiple-person families was extremely high for the following: families with a member rated as being in poor health (expenditures of $386 or more); families with a member who could not perform his or her usual major activity ($367 or more in expenditures); and families with all members having full year health care coverage and the family's coverage coming from Medicare and from private insurance ($347 or more in expenditures).

Introduction

This is the second in a series of descriptive reports dealing with families' use of and expenses for health care in the United States during 1980. Data are presented on family out-of-pocket expenditures for seven major types of health care: inpatient hospital care, inpatient physician care, ambulatory physician care, hospital outpatient and emergency room care, dental care, prescription medicines, and all health care combined. The last category, all health care combined, includes the other six listed types of care plus: care by other independent health practitioners (such as psychologists); and the use of other health supplies (such as eyeglasses and orthopedic items). Additional types of health care, such as long-term care, were not surveyed or are not discussed in this report. In other descriptive reports from this series, data will be presented on families' use of and total expenditures for health care.

The data in this report are from the National Medical Care Utilization and Expenditure Survey (NMCUES). In NMCUES, information was collected during 1980 from a sample of the U.S. civilian noninstitutionalized population on health problems, health care received, expenditures for care, health insurance, and related topics. NMCUES included both a national household sample, which encompassed approximately 6,800 families, and four State Medicaid samples. All information in this report is based on the national household sample. Detailed technical information on the sample, and on estimation and measurement procedures can be found in Appendixes I and II.

NMCUES differs from most surveys of health in that it was a panel (or longitudinal) survey. Altogether, either four or five interviews, approximately 3 months apart, were conducted with each family in the sample from early 1980 to early 1981. In each interview, information on all family members was gathered, usually from a single family respondent.

Definition of the Family

Because NMCUES is a longitudinal survey that covers an entire year, the important concept of *"longitudinal family"* was developed to deal with the facts that the composition of a family can change over time, and that families come into and go out of existence over time. The concept of longitudinal family used in this report is presented in detail in Appendix I. Simplified, it is as follows:

At a point in time, a family is defined as a group of persons sharing a common housing unit and related by blood, marriage, adoption, or a formal foster care relationship. An unmarried student 17–22 years of age who lives away from home is also considered part of a family.

When an initially sampled family had a change in membership during 1980, the prechange and postchange groups were considered the same family if and only if the "majority" of members of the prechange group became members of the postchange group, and the "majority" of members of the postchange group had previously been members of the prechange group. For the purpose of counting a "majority," persons moving into or out of the sample universe—namely, the universe of civilian noninstitutionalized persons residing in the United States—were omitted from the count. For example, persons born, dying, or moving into or out of institutions, and those in the military were omitted from the count.

Only those families with civilian heads are included in this report. Data on families with military heads, even though they may have had civilian members, were omitted. Complete data were not collected on the health care expenditures of the military head-of-family, and inclusion of these families would have led to other anomalies as well. This omission eliminates approximately 0.7 percent of families in the NMCUES sample.

Purpose of Report

This report supplements the more familiar reports published by the National Center for Health Statistics on *individuals'* expenditures for health care. It is published under the assumption that an examination of the U.S. health system from the perspective of the *family* will add to our understanding of that system. There are several reasons why focusing on families can improve our understanding of the U.S. health care system.

First, the family is the social unit that consumes and pays for health care. Decisions to seek and use health care (except in certain emergencies) are usually family decisions. They involve family decisionmaking processes and the allocation of family resources.

Second, focusing on families eliminates the covariance problems that arise when several members of the same family are treated as independent actors but, in fact, are responding to a common stimulus. Covariance problems arise when, as in NMCUES and most other surveys of persons, the basic sampling unit is the household, not the individual, and all household members are included in the survey. The behavior and experience of household members, and also of family members, are often not independent of each other or of the environmental conditions and social situations within which the household or family exists. For example, similar behavior by a number of individuals below the poverty level may not reflect several independent acts, but rather the response of a single family to its economic situation. Also, family members may have similar propensities for disease conditions.

Third, the distribution of health-related phenomena among families may be quite different from the distribution of these phenomena among individuals. For example, during the first 6 months of 1980, 33 percent of all families had at least some public health insurance coverage, compared with only 21 percent of all individuals (Dicker, 1983a, Table 1).

Fourth, families are often heterogeneous in nature; that is, they tend to contain different types of individuals (typically males and females, old and young). As a result, differences in behavior and experience at the individual level may cancel each other out both as determinants of decisionmaking, and in statistical distributions at the family level. For example, almost all families with two members or more have both male and female members. (In NMCUES, only 2 percent of all multiple-person families did not include members of both sexes.) Therefore, the well-documented finding that females generally use more health care and have higher health care expenditures than males (Feldstein, 1983, p. 3) is less relevant for assessing the burden of illness on the family than for assessing the burden on individuals.

To summarize, the heterogeneity or homogeneity of family membership, the associated canceling out or clustering of statistical effects, and the fact that the family rather than the individual is the unit of health care decisionmaking and payment may have consequences for the U.S. health system that cannot be understood from the study of individuals.

Analytical Procedures

Strategy

A longitudinal panel survey like NMCUES, in which the same subjects are interviewed more than once, has at least two advantages over a cross-sectional survey or a conventional time-series survey in which subjects are not reinterviewed. First, because of repeated interviews, a relatively more accurate count of health events can be acquired. For example, a panel survey can provide an accurate count of both incidence and prevalence; something a cross-sectional survey cannot do. Second, through a panel survey, change can be measured both in the unit of analysis (in this case, the family), and in the health events associated with this unit. Thus, changes in health events can be associated with changes in the unit of analysis.

Two general strategies can be used to conduct analyses of this type of data. One involves change-over-time research designs. In these designs, measurements of the unit of analysis are taken at different points in time and then compared with one another. (See Campbell and Julian, 1980.) Another strategy is to treat the data as referencing an extended point estimate (in this case, the year 1980). In this design, repeated measurements are aggregated or combined to give a single total measurement that characterizes the time period in question. (See Dicker, 1983b). The total measurement is a summary of the overall health experience of a family and the overall experience of its members during a time period. As a result, single summary measures incorporate the time-related change experience of a family. This second approach is the one followed in this report.

Quantitative measures of families are reported here as average values for families during the time they were eligible for the survey. For example, family size was measured as the average number of family members during the period the family was eligible for the survey. This measure thus takes into account variability in family size over time. Qualitative measures of families used in the report include a category for families that changed, as well as categories for families in which there was no change. For example, the measure of family head-spouse structure includes a category for families that changed their head-spouse structure during their period of survey eligibility (labeled "other" in the tables), as

well as a category for head-and-spouse families and a category for head-only families. This set of categories again takes into account variability over time.

Standardization for Part-Year Families

One problem with analyzing data from a longitudinal survey is that some families enter and leave the survey universe during the time covered by the survey. This has two consequences. First, the number of different families in the longitudinal universe is larger than the number of families that would be found in a cross-sectional survey. Second, a fair number of families (about 12 percent in NMCUES) did not exist for the full survey year (Dicker and Casady, 1984).

If each family that ever existed during the year were treated equally as one unit, the count of families, which would be equal to the gross total number of distinct families that ever existed during the year, would be larger than the average number of families that existed at a single point in time (the average cross-sectional estimate). Also, if each family that ever existed during the year were treated as one unit, measures of the health behavior of families would not be comparable, for some counts of family behavior would be for a whole year and some for less than a whole year.

Consequently, the following standardizing procedures were chosen. The population of families was time adjusted so that, for example, half-year families counted as only one-half of a unit. Therefore, in this report the total number of families in any category represents the total number of family years for that category. (Alternatively, this can be considered the average daily number of families in that category during the year 1980.) Moreover, the counts for any health behavior event were adjusted to represent annual rates for that event. For example, a family in the survey for one-half of the year with $30 spent out of pocket on physician ambulatory care is represented as one-half of a family year unit with out-of-pocket spending on physician ambulatory care at an annual rate of $60 per year. Because these concepts are awkward to use in writing, families will be generally discussed in the following text as if they represented one unit each, and the expenditures will be discussed as if they were actual expenditures rather than rates. It should be noted, however, that the term, "family," as used in the text, means *family years* and that all health expenditures are rates per family year.

This standardizing scheme readily allows for the calculation of estimates of total out-of-pocket expenditures for a family category in 1980. The mean expenditure per family year multiplied by the total number of family years for the category gives the estimated actual out-of-pocket expenditures for that family category during the year. For example, black multiple-person families had a mean annual rate of out-of-pocket expenditures for inpatient hospital care of $106 per family year (Table 1). This rate, multiplied by the number of family years for the category ($106 × 6,090,000), gives an estimate of approximately $645.5 million spent out of pocket in 1980 for inpatient hospital care by the population of black multiple-person families that ever existed in 1980. (For more details on the weighting procedures, see Appendix I.)

Sampling Error

Because the statistics shown in this report are based on a sample of families rather than on information from all families, they are subject to sampling error. The standard error is a statistic that measures such errors. Standard errors for mean out-of-pocket expenditures and for percents of families with use of care are reported in Tables I to XXX in the Appendix. Because NMCUES is a survey with a complex design, the usual, simple formulas for computing standard errors are not applicable, and reported standard errors were computed with a special software package for estimating standard errors (Shah, 1981).

To alert the reader to potential reliability problems resulting from sampling errors, an asterisk has been placed before estimates whose reliability is problematic because of a sample size of fewer than 50 families, or a relative standard error (standard error divided by the estimate) of greater than 30 percent.

Nonsampling Error

Estimates presented in this report are also subject to nonsampling errors, such as biased interviewing and reporting, misrecording of responses, undercoverage, and nonresponse. Extensive efforts were made to minimize these errors in the data collection and processing for the survey (Bonham, 1983).

For nonsampling error, it should be noted that data in this report are derived from information furnished by a survey of households—that is, "consumers" of health care. Data reported by providers of care· (for example, in surveys of physicians, hospitals, and nursing homes) are generally different from those reported by households. Such differences result in part from differences in the definitions of covered events and the scope of surveys. Other differences may result from nonsampling errors. For example, Sunshine (1984) presented evidence of differences in the reporting of health care coverage by families, compared with information from administrative record sources. Anderson and Thorne (1985) specifically compared use of health care and expenditures on health care as reported by families in NMCUES with estimates underlying the national health accounts, which are generally provider-based. They reported good agreement in total United States use of health care and out-of-pocket expenditures on health care, once coverage differences—such as the omission of military and institutionalized persons in NMCUES—were taken into account. However, Anderson and Thorne found approximately a 10-percent difference between the national health accounts and NMCUES in total expenditures on health care. (A more detailed discussion of sampling and nonsampling error is found in Appendix I.)

Other Limitations of the Data

The population totals in this report were adjusted to accord with totals from the March Supplement to the 1980 Current Population Survey, which is based on an updating of the 1970 census. Thus, population totals will be found to differ somewhat from those of the 1980 census. Totals for expenditures will also differ somewhat from those found in reports in which population statistics were based on the 1980 Census.

Data on institutionalized and noncivilian individuals and all families with military heads, even those with civilian members, are omitted from this report. Although institutionalized persons are relatively few in number, they are heavy users of health care and contribute significantly to expenditures for care. As a result of exclusions, total out-of-pocket expenditures for health care, as presented in this report, are less than actual totals for the United States.

Out-of-pocket health expenditure variables generally are not distributed normally. Rather, the typical distribution involves a substantial percent of families with no expenditures and a small percent of families with very high expenditures in the right-hand "tail" of the distribution. Thus, the mean is a less informative statistic than it is for normally distributed data. To be more informative, tables in this report generally provide not only means but also information on the percent of families using care, and on medians and other percentiles of the distribution of out-of-pocket expenditures for these care-using families. Because of the right-skewed distribution of out-of-pocket expenditures, the mean expenditure among families that used care is generally well above the median (50th percentile) expenditure.

For convenience of presentation, all estimates in the detailed tables of this report have been rounded to the nearest whole integer for dollar amounts, to the nearest single decimal place for percents, and to the nearest thousand for numbers of families. As a consequence, estimates for subcategories may not aggregate to precisely the same estimate as is presented for larger categories. Because of rounding, data in text tables also may not precisely add to totals.

Tests of Significance

All tests of significance discussed in this text, unless otherwise stated, are multiple t-tests at the 0.05 level of significance based on the Bonferroni inequality. (See Levy and Lemeshow, 1980, p. 296.) This report, however, is primarily descriptive. Relationships among variables that are identified here by tests of significance indicate statistical associations, and should not be taken to imply causality. In some studies of causal relationships in the health care field, it is stressed that certain procedures are required to assure that causal relationships have been properly identified. It is necessary both to use multivariate analysis involving several variables simultaneously, and to conduct intensive analyses of specific patterns of relationships. (See, for example, Andersen and Benham, 1970, and Hershey, Luft, and Gianaris, 1975.)

Variables and Organization of Report

Health Care Services

As previously noted, data are presented here on family out-of-pocket expenditures for seven types of health care services: inpatient hospital care, inpatient physician care, ambulatory physician care, hospital outpatient and emergency room care, dental care, prescription medicines, and all health care combined. The statistics for all health care combined include the preceding six forms of care plus: care by other independent practitioners (such as psychologists); and use of other health supplies (such as eyeglasses and orthopedic items). Long-term care was omitted from NMCUES and is not included in the "all health care" category. These seven types of expenditures are the dependent variables in the report. More details on the seven types of health care can be found in Appendix II.

Family Characteristics

For each type of health care, the relationship between out-of-pocket expenditures for that form of care and a set of 18 selected family characteristics was examined. These family characteristics were generally treated as independent variables that account for variations in family out-of-pocket expenditures. This is the logical structure of Tables 1–70, which constitute the bulk of the data presented here. All 18 family characteristics are found in the stub (row label) of each table (except where not pertinent or where redundant). They can be grouped into five general categories as follows:

- Demographic characteristics.
    Family size.
    Age of family head.
    Age structure of family (presence of members under 65 years of age and 65 years and over)
    Sex of family head.
    Race of family head.
    Ethnicity (Hispanic or non-Hispanic) of family head.
- Structure and stability characteristics.
    Head-spouse structure.
    Child-adult structure (combined with head-spouse structure).
    Family dynamics.

- Socioeconomic and educational characteristics.
    Total family income.
    Family poverty status.
    Education of family head.
    Family employment status.
- Health status characteristics.
    Worst perceived health status of any family member.
    Most severe limitation in usual activity of any family member.
    Total bed days for all family members.
- Health care coverage characteristics.
    Completeness of family health care coverage.
    Source(s) of family health care coverage.

Definitions of the above family characteristics are presented in Appendix II.

Three family characteristics have been suggested as being particularly important for understanding family and/or individual health care expenditures. These are family size, the age structure of the family, and the completeness of health care coverage. Because of the importance of these characteristics, the detailed tables include tables that "partial," or control, for these family characteristics as follows:

- *Family size*—Data are presented either on multiple-person families (average family size 1.5 persons or more), or on one-person families (average family size less than 1.5 persons). (As stated previously, because of variability in family membership over time, family size is an average size over time.)

- *Family age structure*—Families are divided into those with no members 65 years of age and over ("younger families") and those with at least one member 65 years of age and over ("older families"). Tables are presented that cover younger families only, older families only, and both age categories combined.

- *Completeness of family health care coverage*—Health care coverage refers to the situation in which a public health care coverage program (such as Medicare or Medicaid) or private health insurance can be used to pay all or part of the health care expenditures of a family's members. Families are divided into those in which all members had health care coverage for their entire period of survey eligibility ("complete coverage"), and those in which some or all members did not have health care coverage during their entire period of survey eligibility ("incomplete coverage"). Tables are presented that cover only families with complete coverage, only families with incomplete coverage, and both coverage categories combined.

Table Order

A knowledge of the sequence of the 70 detailed tables makes it easier to find and use particular sets of data. First, the tables are arranged in sets of 10 according to health care services:

- Family out-of-pocket expenditures for inpatient hospital care, Tables 1–10.
- Family out-of-pocket expenditures for inpatient physician care, Tables 11–20.
- Family out-of-pocket expenditures for ambulatory physician care, Tables 21–30.
- Family out-of-pocket expenditures for hospital outpatient clinics and hospital emergency rooms, Tables 31–40.
- Family out-of-pocket expenditures for dental care, Tables 41–50.
- Family out-of-pocket expenditures for prescription medicines, Tables 51–60.
- Family out-of-pocket expenditures for all health care, Tables 61–70.

Tables are arranged in the same order within each set of 10, according to the partialling (or control) variables. The arrangement is as follows:

Last digit of table number	Families included in table
1	Multiple-person families—all.
2	Multiple-person families—all younger families.
3	Multiple-person families—younger families with complete health care coverage only.
4	Multiple-person families—younger families with incomplete health care coverage only.
5	Multiple-person families—all older families.
6	One-person families—all.
7	One-person families—all younger families.
8	One-person families—younger families with complete health care coverage only.
9	One-person families—younger families with incomplete health care coverage only.
0	One-person families—all older families.

For example, suppose information is desired about out-of-pocket expenditures on hospital outpatient or emergency room care for multiple-person families with all members under 65 years of age that have members with part-year or no health care coverage. Because hospital outpatient and emergency room care is found in Tables 31–40, it would be necessary to examine that set of 10 tables. The multiple-person family tables end in numbers 1 to 5. The table that ends in 4 is for families with all members under 65 years of age and with some members who have part-year or no health care coverage. Therefore, for this particular example, the information is shown in Table 34.

Interpreting the Findings: Important Considerations

The Two-Part Model

In the following discussion one statistic is highlighted: the mean out-of-pocket expenditure for those families that used a given form of health care. This statistic is found in the fourth column of each detailed table, and constitutes one part of a two-part description of family out-of-pocket expenditures. The second part is provided by statistics on the percent of families in each family category that used health care. This two-part description of health care expenditures follows a model recommended by the Rand Corporation that was found to be superior to other approaches (Duan, et al., 1982).

The second part of the description, the percent of families in each category that used health care, is shown in the third column of each detailed table. For an extensive discussion of findings on this percent, see the companion Series Report, *Family Use of Health Care: United States, 1980* (Dicker and Sunshine, 1987).

It is worth noting here, however, that the percent of families that used care varied substantially by family category and by type of care. In Table A, this fact is illustrated for multiple-person families. The percent of multiple-person families using a given form of care in 1980 ranged from 30 percent for inpatient hospital care and 24 percent for inpatient physician care, to 93 percent for both ambulatory physician care and prescription medications.

Table A also shows that patterns of out-of-pocket expenditures are different when viewed from the perspective of care-using families than when viewed from the perspective of all U.S. families. For example, the mean out-of-pocket expenditure in 1980 for inpatient hospital care was $259 per care-using family for multiple-person families that used this form of care. This was much larger than the mean for ambulatory physician care of $136 per care-using multiple-person family. However, when these same two means are calculated on the base of all multiple-person families in the United States, the relationship is reversed. The mean out-of-pocket expenditure for inpatient hospital care per U.S. family (including nonusers) is only $79 compared with a mean of $126 for ambulatory physician care per U.S. family (including nonusers).

The difference between the two perspectives results from the fact that, as noted, the percent of care-using families varied by type of care. Because relatively few multiple-person families (30 percent) used inpatient hospital care, the mean out-of-pocket expenditure for all U.S. multiple-person families for this form of care diverged a lot from the mean for the smaller population of care-using families. By contrast, because ambulatory physician care was used by almost all multiple-person families (93 percent), the mean expenditure for all U.S. families for this form of care compared closely with the mean for care-using families.

Table A

Out-of-pocket expenditures and percent of multiple-person families using health care, by type of health care: United States, 1980

Expenditures and percent using care	Inpatient hospital care	Inpatient physician care	Ambulatory physician care	Hospital outpatient and emergency room care	Dental care	Prescription medications	All health care combined
Mean out-of-pocket expenditures for families using this type of care	$259	$167	$136	$53	$223	$74	$582
Percent of families using this type of care	30.4	23.8	93.1	60.0	71.3	92.6	98.8
Mean out-of-pocket expenditures for all U.S. families, whether or not using care	$79	$40	$126	$32	$159	$68	$575
Relative standard error in percent of mean expenditures for user families	10%	8%	2%	5%	4%	3%	2%
Percent of total expenditures that are paid out-of-pocket	8%	20%	44%	21%	63%	65%	28%

NOTE: Statistics for "all health care combined" refer to families using any one or more types of care. "All health care combined" includes the six types of care listed in the first six columns of the table plus: care by other independent health practitioners (such as psychologists); and other health supplies (such as eyeglasses and orthopedic items).

SOURCES: Tables 1, 11, 21, 31, 41, 51, 61, I, and XI.

Arithmetically, the mean for all U.S. families is equal to the mean for care-using families times the percent of families using care. Thus, both components of the two-part description of expenditures are figured into the calculation of mean expenditures for all U.S. families. The mean for all U.S. families may be calculated by multiplying the user-family mean and the percent of families using care. Alternatively, the mean for all U.S. families may be read from the detailed tables, where it appears as the second column.

Large Standard Errors

Throughout this report, two related difficulties recur in the data on care-using families' mean out-of-pocket expenditures for inpatient hospital and physician care. First, the sample size is often small—sometimes too small (under 50)—to permit comparisons. Second, the relative standard error (standard error divided by the mean) is large. Large relative standard errors seriously impair the ability to make comparisons.

Because of large relative standard errors, differences in estimates that are numerically large are found to be unreliable differences when tests of statistical significance are applied. In other words, when relative standard errors were large, family out-of-pocket expenditures were so varied that it was impossible to demonstrate that the estimates of means being compared were different estimates. An example of relatively large standard errors is found in the fourth row of Table A. Among all care-using families, the relative standard errors for inpatient physician care and inpatient hospital care were generally twice as large, or even more than twice as large, as the relative standard errors for other health care services.

Large relative standard errors for care-using families' mean out-of-pocket expenditures for inpatient hospital care and inpatient physican care are endemic to statistical distributions of expenditures for these types of health care. In this report, these large relative standard errors are the result of three simultaneously occurring conditions:

1. A small proportion of families used these two forms of care. (See the second row of Table A; only 30 percent and 24 percent, respectively.) This low proportion also gives rise directly to the problem of small sample size.

2. A large proportion of care-using families had zero out-of-pocket expenditures. More than 50 percent of multiple-person families using hospital inpatient care had no out-of-pocket expenditures for this form of care, and the same was true for more than 25 percent of families using inpatient physician care. (See Tables 1 and 11.)

3. Long right-hand tails existed in the distribution of expenditures. (This problem was also reported for

inpatient expenditures in the Rand Corporation study by Duan et al., 1982.)

Because of these problems, any comparisons presented here of mean out-of-pocket expenditures that involve inpatient hospital care and inpatient physician care can provide only relatively limited information.

The Health Care Coverage Effect

A primary objective of health care coverage (both private insurance and public programs) is to spare families from large out-of-pocket expenses, even when the total cost of their health care is high. Therefore, to the extent that health care coverage is effective, families' out-of-pocket spending for health care will vary much less than will the total cost of their health care (Aday, Fleming, and Andersen, 1984; Sunshine, 1982).

In this report, differences noted in out-of-pocket expenditures between categories of families are often not statistically significant; moreover, sometimes this is true even when there are statistically significant differences among the same family categories in their use of care. This finding seems due, in substantial part, to the effect of health care coverage. Approximately 96 percent of multiple-person families had members with some health care coverage in 1980, and 73 percent of multiple-person families had all members covered all year. Given this extent of coverage, health care coverage would be expected to diminish differences in out-of-pocket expenditures among these families.

The absence of significant differences in out-of-pocket expenses among various categories of families was particularly common for the three forms of hospital-based care included in this study: inpatient hospital care; inpatient physician care; and hospital outpatient and emergency room care. As the last row of Table A shows, these are also the forms of care for which health care coverage was particularly prominent. Only 8 percent, 20 percent, and 21 percent, respectively, of multiple-person family expenses for these three forms of care was paid out of pocket in 1980. The remainder was paid by health care coverage. In comparison, the next most fully covered type of care was ambulatory physician care, where out-of-pocket payments covered more than twice as much—44 percent—of this category of expenditure. Hence, the frequent absence of statistically significant differences among family categories in out-of-pocket spending for the three forms of hospital-based care was, in large part, an effect of health care coverage.

Health care coverage may also be responsible, in part, for the large standard errors in out-of-pocket expenditures for inpatient hospital and physician care that was discussed previously. One statistical reason for the problem is the large proportion of care-using families with zero out-of-pocket expenditures for these types of care. These zero expenditures result when health care coverage pays the entire bill for the family.

Focus of Report

The focus of this report is on presenting a large amount of data on family out-of-pocket expenditures for health care, rather than on testing hypotheses or developing a detailed analysis of particular variables. Consequently, the extensive descriptive data in the detailed tables are far too voluminous to be discussed completely in the text. Therefore, only selected findings are presented.

The detailed tables are far from exhausting the full range of information that can be found in the NMCUES family data. A public use tape of family data from NMCUES will be available from the National Technical Information Service at approximately the time that this report is published. Many variables and relationships not covered in this report, or in companion reports on health care use and on total expenditures for health care, can be investigated through use of the tape. Data users are invited to obtain a copy.

Younger Multiple-Person Families: Selected Findings

In this section, out-of-pocket health care expenditures of multiple-person families with no members age 65 and over ("younger families") are examined. As noted earlier, the statistic featured in this report is the mean out-of-pocket expenditure among those families that used a given form of care in 1980.

Health Care Coverage

Findings

Table B presents statistics on the relationship between completeness of health care coverage and family out-of-pocket expenditures for seven types of health care. When families with all members having full-year health care coverage (complete coverage) are compared with families with some or all members not having full-year coverage (incomplete coverage), all possible patterns exist. For both inpatient hospital care and hospital outpatient and emergency room care, the mean out-of-pocket expenditure per care-using family was much greater for families with incomplete coverage than for those with complete coverage. Also, families with incomplete coverage averaged at least twice as much in out-of-pocket expenditure for these services as did families with complete coverage ($362 to $181 and $88 to $38, respectively). For dental care, the reverse was true. Families

with complete coverage had a higher mean out-of-pocket expenditure than families with incomplete coverage—$240 compared with $182. Finally, similar mean out-of-pocket expenditures were found for several forms of care: ambulatory physician care, prescription medicines, and all health care combined.

The subcategories into which incomplete coverage is divided are also important considerations. These include: no coverage ("all family members not covered [at all]"); and two categories of partial coverage ("all members covered, some [only] part year," and "some members not covered [at all]"). (See Table B.) The companion Series Report on family use of care (Dicker and Sunshine, 1987) found that families with partial coverage were generally similar in use of care to families with complete coverage. Only families with no coverage reported using significantly less care.

It is instructive to determine whether the same pattern exists for out-of-pocket expenditures. The first question that must be answered is: "Do families with partial coverage have similar out-of-pocket expenditures to those with full coverage?" Relevant data are found in Table B. For hospital outpatient and emergency room care, the coverage categories were not similar in out-of-pocket expenditures. Mean out-of-pocket expenditures for this form of care were larger for families with partial coverage than for families with complete coverage ($63 or $135

Table B

Completeness of health care coverage and out-of-pocket health care expenditures for multiple-person, health-care-using families with all members under 65 years of age: United States, 1980

Completeness of health care coverage	Inpatient hospital care	Inpatient physician care	Ambulatory physician care	Hospital outpatient and emergency room care	Dental care	Prescription medications	All health care combined
	Mean out-of-pocket expenditures						
All members covered full year	$181	$145	$135	$38	$240	$58	$557
Some or all members without							
full year coverage	362	195	133	88	182	61	553
All members covered, some part year . . .	211	152	132	63	198	61	513
Some members not covered	*601	251	141	135	171	66	690
All members not covered	*863	*423	115	100	128	49	449

NOTE: Statistics for "all health care combined" refer to families using any one or more types of care. "All health care combined" includes the six types of care listed in the first six columns of the table plus: care by other independent health practitioners (such as psychologists); and other health supplies (such as eyeglasses and orthopedic items).

SOURCES: Tables 2, 4, 12, 14, 22, 24, 32, 34, 42, 44, 52, 54, 62, and 64.

compared with $38). A statistically significant difference also existed for dental care, however, in the reverse direction. One partial coverage category ("some members not covered") had significantly lower expenses than fully covered families ($171 compared with $240). Families with some members not covered also appear to have larger expenses for inpatient hospital and physician care than families with full coverage. However, these apparent differences, although large, are not statistically significant because of the large relative standard errors discussed previously.

A second question to determine whether patterns for family out-of-pocket expenditures are similar to those for family use of care is: "Do families without coverage differ from those with full coverage?" Again, the relevant data are found in Table B. For inpatient hospital and physician care, this question cannot be answered because few families with no coverage (less than 50) used these forms of care. For hospital outpatient and emergency room care, noncovered families had much higher expenses than fully covered families ($100 compared with $38); for dental care, the relationship was the reverse, with noncovered families having much lower expenses ($128) than fully covered families had ($240). Finally, for ambulatory physician care, prescription medications, and all health care combined, no statistically significant difference in out-of-pocket expenditures existed between families with full coverage and families with no coverage.

Discussion

Table B illustrates clearly that the relationship between completeness of health care coverage and the mean out-of-pocket expenditures of care-using families is complex, and that it differs according to the type of health care used. No single, simple explanation for the patterns will suffice.

Nonetheless, dental expenses are perhaps easiest to explain. Dental care was covered only infrequently by insurance in the study period (Farley, 1985), and the relationship between out-of-pocket expenditures and health care coverage is almost certainly not a direct causal one. Instead, use of dental care is strongly related to income (Dicker and Sunshine, 1987) as is health care coverage. The apparent relationship between coverage and dental expenditures is probably merely a consequence of both the positive association of dental care use and income, and of income and insurance coverage.

For other forms of care, higher out-of-pocket expenditures for families with less-than-full coverage might generally be expected. Limited health care coverage has been associated with lower use of care, presumably because of the greater out-of-pocket expenditures that less coverage requires (Newhouse, et al., 1981). (This pattern of expenditure and use was found for hospital inpatient care and hospital outpatient and emergency room care.)

Another explanation for the association between

lower use of care and little insurance could be that persons without coverage disproportionately tend to be young adults in good health (by certain measures), who are thus innately unlikely to use much care. Families composed of such persons may have decided to risk going without coverage because they expect low health care expenses (Kaspar, Walden, and Wilensky, 1980; Wilensky and Walden, 1981). To the extent this latter phenomenon takes place, an association of low out-of-pocket expenditures and limited health care coverage might be expected. However, it is not found in Table B. Perhaps the absence of a relationship between completeness of coverage and out-of-pocket expenditures—as is found, for example, for all health care expenditures combined and several other types of care—occurs because these two opposite phenomena have offsetting effects.

If there were one dominant pattern of difference in out-of-pocket expenditures associated with completeness of health care coverage, then it would clearly be helpful to base the following discussion of the relationship between out-of-pocket expenditures and other family characteristics on data for families that all have the same health care coverage. However, no one pattern exists. Thus, limiting the data only to families with the same completeness of coverage reduces the sample size without any offsetting gain. A smaller sample size would particularly create problems for any comparisons that involved inpatient hospital and physician care. Therefore, the following discussion of out-of-pocket expenditures and family characteristics includes all younger multiple-person families, regardless of their health insurance coverage.

Family Health Status

In 1980, out-of-pocket expenditures for health care differed not only by family health care coverage, but also according to the health status of family members. This report presents data on three measures of family health status: (1) a scale ranking families by the worst perceived health status of any family member; (2) a scale of limitations in activity in which families are ranked by the most severe limitation of any family member in performing a usual activity; and (3) a scale of families ranked by the total number of bed days of all family members. Only the relationship between out-of-pocket expenditures and the first two of these health status measures will be examined.

Perceived health status

Table C presents statistics on mean out-of-pocket expenditures made by younger multiple-person families that used each form of care, with families categorized according to the worst perceived health status of any family member. With the exception of dental care, mean out-of-pocket expenditures for each form of care were

15

Table C

Health and economic status and out-of-pocket health care expenditures for multiple-person, health-care-using families with all members under 65 years of age: United States, 1980

Health and economic status	Inpatient hospital care	Inpatient physician care	Ambulatory physician care	Hospital outpatient and emergency room care	Dental care	Prescription medications	All health care combined
Worst perceived health status of any family member			Mean out-of pocket expenditures				
Excellent	$138	$102	$121	$36	$257	$41	$486
Good	207	143	138	48	224	54	540
Fair	310	216	139	73	195	73	614
Poor	372	233	153	79	171	117	794
Most severe limitation in usual activity of any family member							
None	216	144	134	49	229	53	529
Cannot perform	316	238	137	76	191	103	735
Family income relative to poverty level							
Below 150 percent	235	114	85	45	124	44	372
150–199 percent	*563	238	144	97	195	62	677
200–299 percent	196	145	135	53	222	67	543
300–499 percent	169	174	146	44	255	60	581
500 percent or more	*177	147	156	49	275	61	639

NOTES: Statistics for "all health care combined" refer to families using any one or more types of care. "All health care combined" includes the six types of care listed in the first six columns of the table plus: care by other independent health practitioners (such as psychologists); and other health supplies (such as eyeglasses and orthopedic items).
Scale for limitations in activity is abbreviated.

SOURCES: Tables 2, 12, 22, 32, 42, 52, and 62.

generally higher the poorer a family's health status. This overall finding is not surprising, as it suggests that families with poor health spend more on care.

Often, expenditure differences associated with health status were large. For example, the mean out-of-pocket expenditure per family for inpatient physician care was more than twice as large for families with a member perceived to be in either fair or poor health as it was for families with all members perceived to be in excellent health. Large, inverse differences associated with health status in mean out-of-pocket expenditure were also found for hospital outpatient and emergency room care, prescription medicines, and all health care combined. However, the apparent large, inverse differences associated with health status for inpatient hospital care were not statistically significant because of large standard errors. The small, inverse differences for ambulatory physician care were also not statistically significant.

Because the standard error of the mean for out-of-pocket expenditure for families rated in poor health tended to be large, the statistically significant findings upon which the above discussion were based were between families rated in excellent health and those rated in fair health.

For dental care, mean out-of-pocket expenditures per family were generally lower the worse a family's health status. A similar pattern was reported for use of dental care (Dicker and Sunshine, 1987), and the finding for out-of-pocket expenditures may indicate that

families in poor health direct their energy and resources to health care concerns they judge to be more important or more pressing than dental care. The finding may also stem from the association between low family income and low out-of-pocket expenditures for dental care. Families in poor health generally have lower incomes than those in better health, and thus would be expected to have relatively low out-of-pocket expenditures for dental care.

Limitations in activity

The person health indicator of limitation in activity was converted to a family health indicator by classifying families according to the most severe limitation in performing a usual activity (play, school, or work, depending on age) reported for any family member. This health status indicator is of interest because it has been used as a proxy for locating chronically ill persons (Newacheck, 1985a, 1985b). Moreover, using person-level data, the activity limited population has previously been found to represent a more severe subset of all persons with chronic illnesses (Newacheck, 1985a). By analogy, families with members limited in activity should represent a more severe subset of all families with chronically ill members because not all families that have members with chronic illnesses have members who have long-term limitations in usual activities.

Table C presents data on mean out-of-pocket expenditures for younger multiple-person families that used each form of care, with the families classified according to the indicator of limitations in activity. This indicator demonstrates much the same pattern as the perceived health status indicator. Again, with the exception of dental care, mean out-of-pocket expenditures are generally higher for families in worse health—that is, for families with a member unable to perform his or her usual activity. For example, mean out-of-pocket expenditures for prescriptions were nearly twice as high for these families as for families with no members limited in usual activity ($103 compared with $53). However, ambulatory physician care again showed a different pattern, with mean out-of-pocket expenditures quite similar regardless of limitation in activity. Also, although the apparent differences between limitation-in-activity categories in mean out-of-pocket expenditures for inpatient hospital and inpatient physician care were large, these differences were not statistically significant because of large standard errors. For dental care, apparent differences were again "backward"; that is, families in poorer health apparently had lower expenditures. However, the differences were not statistically significant.

Family Income

A useful measure of family income that takes family size into account is the relationship of a family's income to the poverty level. Table C shows the relationship between this measure and the mean amounts paid out of pocket by younger multiple-person families that used each form of care in 1980. Three different patterns were found. In one, a threshold effect was found for ambulatory physician care, prescription medicines, and all health care combined. Out-of-pocket expenditures by families below 150 percent of the poverty level were smaller than those for higher income families; however, differences among the various higher income categories were not significant. For example, the mean out-of-pocket expenditure for ambulatory physician care for families that used this form of care and who had incomes below 150 percent of poverty was $85 in 1980. The corresponding mean among families with higher incomes was $135 to $156, depending on the income category.

A plausible explanation for this first pattern is that income of families below 150 percent of poverty was often so low that these families could not afford to pay for their care. Thus, when an out-of-pocket payment was due, some or all of the expenses quite possibly were never paid, and care providers had to treat the expenditure as a charity or bad debt. Another possible explanation is that those families with members on Medicaid would have almost all health care expenses covered for these members.

Dental care showed a different pattern, as was often the case. Out-of-pocket expenditures were generally greater the higher a family was above the poverty level.

For example, mean out-of-pocket expenditures were $124 for care-using families below 150 percent of the poverty level, compared with $275 for families at or above 500 percent of the poverty level. This pattern for dentistry concurs with the widespread finding that use of dental care is associated positively with income (Dicker and Sunshine, 1987). Families generally treat dental care as a discretionary expenditure, spending more for it if their incomes are higher.

A third income-related pattern found that for three forms of care—inpatient hospital, inpatient physician, and hospital outpatient and emergency room—no statistically significant differences occurred among families based on income relative to the poverty level. Health care coverage for these three forms of care was particularly extensive. Such extensive health care coverage tends to reduce differences among family categories in out-of-pocket expenditures.

Family Size

Large family size, although generally associated with a greater percent of families using care in 1980, was not found to be consistently associated with a greater *quantity* of care used among those families. For families who used care, only ambulatory physician care and dental visits showed positive associations between family size and the quantity of care used (Dicker and Sunshine, 1987). Given these findings, a varied pattern might be expected for out-of-pocket expenditures by care-using families, with only some forms of care showing larger expenditures associated with larger family size.

In Table D, data are presented on the relationship between family size and mean out-of-pocket spending by younger care-using multiple-person families in 1980. These data support the above expectation. For three types of care—inpatient physician, hospital outpatient and emergency room, and prescription medicines—there were no statistically significant differences according to family size in mean out-of-pocket expenditure.

For another three types of care—ambulatory physician care, dental care, and all health care combined—larger family size was associated positively with higher mean out-of-pocket expenditure. For example, the mean out-of-pocket expenditure for dental care by care-using families was $183 for two-person families as compared with $310 for families with five or more members. In general, for these three forms of care, the increase in expenditure was not continuous with family size. Two- and three-person families tended to have rather similar out-of-pocket expenditures, and four-person and five-or-more person families also tended to have fairly similar expenditures. However, on the whole, the latter categories (that is, four-person or larger families) tended to have higher expenditures than the two- or three-person families. In other words, there seems to have been a threshold effect, with four-member families being the

Table D

Family structure and dynamics and out-of-pocket health care expenditures for multiple-person, health-care-using families with all members under 65 years of age: United States, 1980

Family structure and dynamics	Inpatient hospital care	Inpatient physician care	Ambulatory physician care	Hospital outpatient and emergency room care	Dental care	Prescription medications	All health care combined
Family size				Mean out-of-pocket expenditures			
2 persons	$388	$192	$115	$51	$183	$62	$494
3 persons	126	142	127	49	173	54	472
4 persons	156	149	153	52	246	62	591
5 persons or more	273	151	149	57	310	56	705
Head-spouse structure							
Head and spouse present whole time	200	154	150	51	253	64	597
Head only, no spouse at any time	*345	187	83	55	138	42	420
Other	*231	*113	152	68	161	69	608
Family head-spouse-child structure							
Head and spouse							
Child under 17	194	150	162	48	280	58	642
No child under 17	214	162	128	57	203	73	522
Head only							
Child under 17	*335	150	79	54	131	35	414
No child under 17	*403	*310	95	60	164	62	437
Stability							
Unchanging, full year	215	157	134	46	234	60	539
Changed in composition or existed less than full year	275	163	137	73	193	56	620

NOTE: Statistics for "all health care combined" refer to families using any one or more types of care. "All health care combined" includes the six types of care listed in the first six columns of the table plus: care by other independent health practitioners (such as psychologists); and other health supplies (such as eyeglasses and orthopedic items).

SOURCES: Tables 2, 12, 22, 32, 42, 52, and 62.

threshold at which higher out-of-pocket expenditures appeared. Finally, for inpatient hospital care, the mean out-of-pocket expenditure by care-using families was significantly higher for two-person families ($388) than for three- or four-person families ($126 and $156, respectively).

The relationships found between family size and mean out-of-pocket expenditure were generally consistent with the relationships found between family size and mean quantity of care used. The principal exception was inpatient hospital care, for which mean quantity of care used did not depend on family size, but mean out-of-pocket expenditures did.

Head-Spouse Structure

Because of the longitudinal nature of the survey, it was possible for families to have changes in head-spouse structure during the time the family was eligible for the survey. As a consequence, multiple-person families were divided into three categories: those families in which a head and spouse were present the whole time (73 percent of all families); those families in which a head only was present the whole time (24 percent); and those families that experienced a change in head-

spouse structure (3 percent). This last aggregate is labeled as having an "other" type of family structure in the detailed and Appendix tables. These families may be considered as having an unstable head-spouse structure.

Table D shows the mean out-of-pocket expenditure for younger care-using families in the three head-spouse structure categories. No significant difference is revealed between head-spouse structure categories in mean out-of-pocket expenditures in 1980 for hospital-based care (inpatient hospital care, inpatient physician care, and outpatient and emergency room care). This finding may again reflect the great extent of health care coverage for these services.

For other forms of care, head-and-spouse families had significantly higher mean out-of-pocket expenditures in 1980 than head-only families. This pattern was found for ambulatory physician care ($150 to $83), dental care ($253 to $138), prescription medications ($64 to $42), and all health care combined ($597 to $420). To some extent, these differences may reflect differences in size.

Head-and-spouse families also had a significantly higher mean expenditure than families with an unstable head-spouse structure ("other" families) for dental care ($253 as compared with $161). Otherwise, mean out-of-pocket expenditures for families with an unstable head-spouse structure ("other" families) did not differ significantly in 1980 from expenditures by head-and-spouse families. Families with an unstable head-and-spouse structure also generally did not differ significantly in mean out-of-pocket expenditures from head-only families in 1980. Ambulatory physician care was the only exception. Families with an unstable head-and-spouse structure spent more on average for this type of care ($152 compared with $83).

Children

One of the more important characteristics distinguishing families from one another is the presence or absence of children. When the use of care by families was examined according to the presence of children in the family, a varied pattern emerged. Among all younger head-and-spouse care-using families, when families with children under age 17 were compared with families with no children, those with children were found to use a greater quantity of ambulatory physician visits and dental care, fewer inpatient hospital days, and no significantly different quantity of prescription medications or hospital outpatient and emergency room visits (Dicker and Sunshine, 1987). For head-only families, no statistically significant differences were found. A similar mixed pattern might be expected for out-of-pocket expenditures by care-using families. Mean out-of-pocket expenses are presented in Table D for younger families that used each type of care, according to whether or not they had children under age 17 in 1980.

For families with a head and spouse throughout the year, there were no statistically significant differences in mean out-of-pocket expenditures for the three forms of hospital-based care (inpatient hospital care, inpatient physician care, and hospital outpatient and emergency room care). Compared with head-and-spouse childless families, head-and-spouse families with children spent significantly more out of pocket on ambulatory physician care (a mean of $162 compared with $128), dental care (a mean of $280 compared with $203) and all health care combined (a mean of $642 compared with $522). However, families with children spent less on prescription medicines (a mean of $58 compared with $73).

Among families with a head but no spouse throughout the year, significant differences generally were not found. Prescription medicines were the exception, with families that had children again having lower mean out-of-pocket expenses than families without children ($35 compared with $62).

The pattern for mean out-of-pocket expenditures in large part parallels that for mean use of care, and the pattern of care used probably partly explains that for out-of-pocket expenditures. This use pattern in turn may reflect age differences in the types of families compared. Another likely explanation for the pattern of out-of-pocket expenditures is the relatively great extent to which hospital-based care is covered by health care coverage. The absence of significant differences in mean out-of-pocket expenditures for the three types of hospital-based care probably reflects the large portion of these expenses that is subsidized by health care coverage.

Family Dynamics

Table D shows the relationship between family stability and mean out-of-pocket expenditures for younger families that used each form of care in 1980. Families were divided into two stability categories: static families, or those that existed for the entire survey year and experienced no change in composition; and dynamic families, or those that changed in composition during 1980 or did not exist for the full year. For four types of care (inpatient hospital, inpatient physician, ambulatory physician, and prescription medicines), no statistically significant differences in mean out-of-pocket expenditures were found when static and dynamic families were compared. However, as reflected in Table D, dynamic families had a higher mean expenditure for hospital outpatient and emergency room care ($73 compared with $46) and for all health care ($620 compared with $539); yet, they had a lower mean expenditure for dental care ($193 compared with $234). This pattern is similar to that found for the quantity of care used (Dicker and Sunshine, 1987).

Older Multiple-Person Families: Selected Findings

In this section, out-of-pocket expenditures for health care made by multiple-person families with members age 65 and over ("older families") are examined. Again, this discussion is focused on the mean out-of-pocket expenditure among those families that used a given form of care in 1980.

Because some family patterns are atypical among older families, and few examples of these patterns are in the NMCUES sample, somewhat fewer relationships are discussed here for older families than were discussed previously for younger families. For example, only about 4 percent of older families were single parent families. Only 25 such older families were in the NMCUES sample, too small a number to permit reliable estimates. In contrast, close to 20 percent of younger families had this pattern and 522 such families were in the sample.

Health Care Coverage

Data are presented in Table E on the relationship between the health care coverage of older families that used each form of care and their mean out-of-pocket expenditures for health care in 1980. The table includes only a comparison between families with all members having full-year health care coverage (complete coverage) and families with some or all members not having full-year coverage (incomplete coverage). (Additional data are presented in the detailed tables, including information on subcategories of the incomplete coverage cate-

gory. As these subcategories are generally too small to determine statistically significant differences, they are not discussed in the text.)

According to Table E, mean out-of-pocket expense per family for inpatient hospital care was much larger for user families with incomplete health care coverage than for user families that had complete coverage ($874 compared with $219). This pattern corresponds with that found for younger families discussed earlier. In contrast, user families with incomplete coverage had a smaller mean expenditure for ambulatory physician care than did user families with complete coverage ($105 compared with $148). Differences in mean out-of-pocket spending for other forms of health care were not statistically significant.

Family Health Status

Data are presented on the following measures of family health status: families ranked by the worst perceived health status of any family member, and families ranked by the most severe limitation of any family member in performing a usual activity.

Perceived health status

Table F presents statistics on mean amounts paid out of pocket by older multiple-person families that used each form of care in 1980, with families categorized

Table E

Completeness of health care coverage and out-of-pocket health care expenditures for multiple-person, health-care-using families with members 65 years and over: United States, 1980

Completeness of health care coverage	Inpatient hospital care	Inpatient physician care	Ambulatory physician care	Hospital outpatient and emergency room care	Dental care	Prescription medications	All health care combined
	Mean out-of-pocket expenditures						
All members covered full year	$219	$174	$148	$50	$220	$142	$659
Some or all members without full year coverage	874	284	105	*87	154	116	894

NOTE: Statistics for "all health care combined" refer to families using any one or more types of care. "All health care combined" includes the six types of care listed in the first six columns of the table plus: care by other independent health practitioners (such as psychologists); and other health supplies (such as eyeglasses and orthopedic items).

SOURCES: Tables 5, 15, 25, 35, 45, 55, 65, and unpublished NMCUES data.

Health and economic status and out-of-pocket health care expenditures for multiple-person, health-care-using families with members 65 years and over: United States, 1980

Health and economic status	Inpatient hospital care	Inpatient physician care	Ambulatory physician care	Hospital outpatient and emergency room care	Dental care	Prescription medications	All health care combined
Worst perceived health status of any family member			Mean out-of pocket expenditures				
Excellent	*$492	*$172	$113	*$110	$212	$71	$559
Good	152	211	152	39	205	124	617
Fair	155	139	142	41	206	145	603
Poor	624	229	139	78	216	178	1,004
Most severe limitation in usual activity of any family member							
None	191	179	132	59	244	100	551
Cannot perform	383	201	146	51	179	166	800
Family income relative to the poverty level							
Below 150 percent	*384	*174	102	*59	71	135	530
150–199 percent	*605	*220	121	*54	172	168	754
200–299 percent	257	191	159	46	162	141	678
300–499 percent	*338	221	151	53	242	128	745
500 percent or more	*176	*153	163	78	329	124	831

NOTE: Statistics for "all health care combined" refer to families using any one or more types of care. "All health care combined" includes the six types of care listed in the first six columns of the table plus: care by other independent health practitioners (such as psychologists); and other health supplies (such as eyeglasses and orthopedic items).

SOURCES: Tables 5, 15, 25, 35, 45, 55, and 65.

according to the worst perceived health status of any family member. For four types of care—inpatient physician care, ambulatory physician care, hospital outpatient and emergency room care, and dental care—no statistically significant differences in expense were associated with differences in perceived health status.

For the remaining three types of care, mean out-of-pocket expenditures in 1980 were, in varying ways, higher among families with members in poorer health. For prescription medicines, expenditures generally were higher the worse the perceived health status of any family member. Mean spending was $71 for families with all members perceived to be in excellent health, as compared with $178 for families with a member perceived to be in poor health. For all health care expenditures combined, families with a member perceived to be in poor health had much higher mean out-of-pocket spending ($1,004) than families with other perceived health status ratings for whom mean expenditures clustered around $600. Moreover, for the families with other ratings, no statistically significant differences in mean expenditure were found. Similarly, families using inpatient hospital care also had a much higher mean out-of-pocket expenditure if they included a member in poor health ($624) than families with other perceived health status ratings that used this type of care. Again, there were no statistically significant differences among mean expenditures for the families with other ratings. Therefore, all health care

combined and inpatient hospital care apparently show a threshold effect associated with perceived health status in contrast to the generally linear effect found for expenditures for prescription medications.

These findings for older families contrast somewhat with those for younger families, where an increase in out-of-pocket expenditures with poorer health was more common.

Limitations in Activity

For older families, differences related to the limitations in activity measure of family health status paralleled those related to the measure based on worst perceived status of any family member (Table F). Care-using families with a member unable to perform his or her usual activity spent an average of $383 out of pocket for inpatient hospital care compared with $191 for families with no members limited in their usual activities. For prescription medicines, mean expenditures were $166 and $100, respectively, and for all health care combined, $800 and $551. For the other four types of care—inpatient physician care, ambulatory physician care, hospital outpatient and emergency room care, and dental care—there were again no statistically significant differences in mean out-of-pocket spending according to health status when families with different limitations in activity statuses were compared.

Family Income

A measure of family income that takes family size into account is the relationship of a family's income to the poverty level. The relationship between this measure and mean amounts paid out of pocket by older multiple-person families that used each form of care in 1980 is shown in Table F. In one distinguishable pattern, mean spending generally increased with higher income for some forms of care (ambulatory physician care, dental care, and all health care combined). For example, older families that used ambulatory physician care had an average out-of-pocket expenditure of $102 if they had an income below 150 percent of the poverty level, compared with $163 if they had an income of 500 percent of the poverty level or above. For dental care, the corresponding means were $71 for the lowest income category compared with $329 for the highest income category; for all health care combined the corresponding means were $530 and $831, respectively. Because health care coverage is greater among higher income families, these differences presumably reflect more use of care and greater total and out-of-pocket spending among higher income families. Lower income families may have to spend less for health care, as they do for most things.

Expenditure for prescription medicines represented another pattern, where expenses were relatively similar across income categories. Finally, for the three forms of hospital-based care (inpatient hospital, inpatient physician, and hospital outpatient and emergency room care), large standard errors in the data preclude recognition of any statistical patterns.

Family Size

Data is presented in Table G on the relationship between family size and mean out-of-pocket expenditures for older multiple-person families that used each form of care in 1980. Because more than 85 percent of older multiple-person families had either two or three members in 1980, the relatively rare larger sized families will be omitted from this discussion. Mean out-of-pocket expenditures for three-person families were larger than those for two-person families for ambulatory physician care ($169 compared with $132) and for all health care combined ($899 compared with $623). For other health care categories, mean expenditure differences were not statistically significant.

Family Structure

Also in Table G are the mean 1980 out-of-pocket expenditures for older care-using families for various family structure categories. In this table, families that had both a head and spouse throughout the year are compared with families that had a head throughout the year but no spouse at any time. (The third category—families with an unstable head-spouse structure—is omitted from Table G because it was too small.)

For most forms of care, families with a head and spouse throughout the year had a higher mean out-of-pocket expenditure per family than those with a head only. For example, mean out-of-pocket expenditures for

Table G

Family structure and dynamics and out-of-pocket health care expenditures for multiple-person, health-care-using families with members 65 years and over: United States, 1980

Family structure and dynamics	Inpatient hospital care	Inpatient physician care	Ambulatory physician care	Hospital outpatient and emergency room care	Dental care	Prescription medications	All health care combined
Family size			Mean out-of-pocket expenditures				
2 persons	$317	$194	$132	$55	$176	$135	$623
3 persons	395	*238	169	*62	247	148	899
4 persons	*422	*129	195	*78	*383	136	939
5 persons or more	*363	*167	133	*45	224	152	904
Family structure							
Head and spouse present whole time	334	170	151	57	237	144	724
Child under 17	*396	*215	195	66	337	136	971
No child under 17	326	164	146	55	221	145	696
Head only, no spouse at any time	*265	198	110	43	112	114	518
No child under 17	*286	*224	107	43	122	110	523
Stability							
Unchanging, full year	297	154	142	45	194	139	633
Changed in composition or existed less than full year	487	333	138	102	286	132	1,095

NOTE: Statistics for "all health care combined" refer to families using any one or more types of care. "All health care combined" includes the six types of care listed in the first six columns of the table plus: care by other independent health practitioners (such as psychologists); and other health supplies (such as eyeglasses and orthopedic items).

SOURCES: Tables 5, 15, 25, 35, 45, 55, and 65.

all health care combined for the two categories were $724 and $518, respectively. Quite possibly these differences in mean expenditures between the two categories reflect the fact that in head-and-spouse families there are generally two elderly adults for whom care must be paid. In head only families, the presence of two elderly adults is probably rare.

An exception to the pattern of higher out-of-pocket expenditures for head-and-spouse families occurs only for the three forms of hospital-based care: inpatient hospital, inpatient physician, and hospital outpatient and emergency room care. For these forms of care, there were no significant differences in mean out-of-pocket expenditure. This finding may reflect the relatively great extent of health care coverage for such care, as described earlier.

Children

Another important aspect of family structure is whether or not families include children. In 1980, only about 11 percent of older families had children under 17, compared with more than 60 percent of younger families. As a consequence, only among older families headed by both a head and spouse were there enough families with children to make meaningful comparisons feasible. Older head-and-spouse families with children had a higher mean out-of-pocket expenditure for all health care combined than similar families with no children ($971 compared with $696). This difference may reflect families with children having more members.

For other forms of care, estimated mean expenditures for families with children generally were higher but not statistically significant in 1980. Thus, the presence of children apparently added a relatively small amount to out-of-pocket expenditures for older families, but an amount that was only statistically significant when the expenses for all forms of care were combined.

Family Dynamics

Table G shows the relationship between family stability and the mean out-of-pocket expenditures for older multiple-person families that used each form of care in 1980. Families were divided into two stability categories: static families, or those that existed for the entire survey year and experienced no change in composition; and dynamic families, or those that changed in composition during 1980 or did not exist for the full year. Dynamic families had higher mean out-of-pocket expenditures for inpatient physician care, hospital outpatient and emergency room care, and all health care combined. For the other forms of care, no statistically significant differences in mean out-of-pocket expenditures could be attributed to the dynamic character of families. The relatively high mean expenditure, for dynamic older families compared with static older families when all out-of-pocket health care expenditures are combined (almost twice as high), may result from the fact that death—a type of event that causes families to be characterized as dynamic—is associated typically with both large health expenditures and older families.

Comparison of Younger and Older Multiple-Person Families: Selected Findings

Out-of-pocket health care expenditures by multiple-person families with no members age 65 or older ("younger families") are compared here with corresponding expenditures for families that included a member age 65 or older ("older families"). Again, the focus of the report is on the mean out-of-pocket expenditures among those families that used a given form of care in 1980.

Basic Comparison

Data is presented in Table H on mean 1980 out-of-pocket expenditures for younger and older care-using families by type of care. Based on patterns for use of care (see Dicker and Sunshine, 1987) various patterns in out-of-pocket expenditures might be expected. In 1980, older care-using families reported much higher quantities of inpatient hospital care and prescription medicines than younger families, but these age categories did not differ substantially in use of other forms of care. To a great extent, a similar pattern is shown in Table H for out-of-pocket expenditures by care-using families. Older families' mean out-of-pocket expenditure for prescription medicines were much higher per family than those for younger families ($138 compared with $59). On the average, older families also spent significantly more than younger families for all health care combined. Mean out-of-pocket expenditures per family for all care combined were $700 and $556, respectively, for older and younger care-using families in 1980. Older families seem to have spent substantially more out of

pocket for inpatient hospital care, but the difference between family age categories was not statistically significant because of large relative standard errors. For other types of care, no large or statistically significant spending differences existed among family age categories.

Age, Health Status, and Out-of-Pocket Expenditures

An important question is the extent to which differences—or lack of differences—between age categories in out-of-pocket spending reflect differences attributed to age alone or to other factors associated with age. For example, older families are, on the average, in poorer health than younger families. Over one-half of older families report having a member in fair or poor health compared with less than one-fourth of younger families. Because greater out-of-pocket expenditures are often associated with poorer health, a greater mean out-of-pocket expenditure for all health care combined by older families might be caused by their poorer health rather than their greater age.

In Table J, the mean 1980 out-of-pocket expenditures by care-using older and younger families on all health care combined are classified according to health status. Two scales are used to measure health status: the worst perceived health status of any family member; and the most severe limitation in usual activity of any family member.

Both scales show the same phenomenon: First, with health status held constant, statistically significant differ-

Table H

Family age and out-of-pocket health care expenditures for multiple-person, health-care-using families: United States, 1980

Family age	Inpatient hospital care	Inpatient physician care	Ambulatory physician care	Hospital outpatient and emergency room care	Dental care	Prescription medications	All health care combined
	Mean out-of-pocket expenditures						
All members under 65	$234	$159	$135	$52	$226	$59	$556
Some member(s) 65 or older	341	193	141	56	209	138	700

NOTE: Statistics for "all health care combined" refer to families using any one or more types of care. "All health care combined" includes the six types of care listed in the first six columns of the table plus: care by other independent health practitioners (such as psychologists); and other health supplies (such as eyeglasses and orthopedic items).

SOURCES: Tables 2, 5, 12, 15, 22, 25, 32, 35, 42, 45, 52, 55, 62, and 65.

Table J

Comparison of out-of-pocket health care expenditures for multiple-person, health-care-using families by family age and other characteristics: United States, 1980

Characteristic	Younger families	Older families	Difference
Worst perceived health status of any family member	Mean out-of-pocket expenditures for all health care combined		
Excellent	$486	$559	$73
Good	540	617	77
Fair	614	603	−11
Poor	794	1,004	210
Difference between excellent and poor family health status	#308	#445	...
Most severe limitation in usual activity of any family member			
None	529	551	22
Cannot perform	735	800	65
Difference	#206	#249	...
Family size			
2 persons	494	623	#129
3 persons	472	899	#427
4 persons	591	939	#348
5 persons or more	705	904	199
Difference between 2-person and 5-person-or-more families	#211	#281	...

NOTES: # is difference significant at 0.05 level.
See also Tables C, D, F, and G.

ences were not found between younger and older families in their mean out-of-pocket expenditure for all health care combined. Thus the relationship between the age of a family's members and the family's out-of-pocket expenditures for all health care tends to disappear when the health status of the family's members is taken into account. Second, with family age held constant, statistically significant differences were found between families with better and poorer health statuses in their mean out-of-pocket health expenditure for all health care combined. This means that, in contrast to the finding for age, the relationship between the health status of a family's members and the family's out-of-pocket expenditures for all health care remains even after the age of the family's members is taken into account.

Moreover, these differences in mean out-of-pocket spending attributable to differences in health status could be large. For example, among older families, those rated as having all members in excellent health had a mean out-of-pocket expenditure of $559. Families in the same age category, however, with one or more members rated as having poor health had a mean out-of-pocket expendi-

ture of $1,004. This is almost twice the amount spent by the families with all members in excellent health. The findings in Table J suggest that the health status of a family's members is more strongly associated with a family's level of out-of-pocket spending for all health care than the age of a family's members. However, it should be noted that out-of-pocket expenditures in this report do not include out-of-pocket premium payments for health care coverage and that both health status and family age are only measured in a limited way.

Age, Family Size, and Out-of-Pocket Expenditures

As older families are generally smaller than younger families, family size is another important variable to examine. In 1980, only 14 percent of older multiple-person families were composed of four or more members compared with 45 percent of younger multiple-person families. Mean out-of-pocket expenditures were sometimes lower for smaller families. Thus, differences in family size may mask expenditure differences associated with age unless these family charcteristics are considered separately. Note that this is the opposite of the situation with health status. These differences tend to exaggerate differences due to age rather than mask them.

Again, Table J contains the relevant statistics on mean 1980 out-of-pocket expenditures by care-using families on all health care combined. For any given family size category, older families generally spent significantly more than younger families. For example, the difference for three-person families was $427 ($899 for older families compared with $472 for younger families). Moreover, the data in the table also indicate that for younger and older families, larger size was associated with significantly higher out-of-pocket expenditures in 1980. Thus, when family age and size are considered simultaneously, both are found to be associated with significant differences in mean out-of-pocket expenditures for all health care combined.

In summary, the statistical associations between mean out-of-pocket expenditures and family age that are found when family age is considered alone sometimes change when other variables are considered simultaneously. Therefore, it is important to note that because this report is primarily descriptive and does not enter into extensive analyses involving a large number of variables simultaneously, care must be taken not to assume that the statistical associations revealed are necessarily causal relationships.

One-Person Families: Selected Findings

The term "family" is often used to denote multiple-person families only; nonetheless, the report also contains extensive data on one-person families. In the following discussion, some basic findings on one-person families are presented. The brevity of this section reflects the greater general interest in multiple-person families, as well as the lesser variety of structural forms the one-person family may assume. Again, this analysis is based on the mean amount spent out-of-pocket for each form of care by care-using families in 1980.

Comparing One-Person and Multiple-Person Families

Data on mean out-of-pocket expenditures by one-person care-using families in 1980 are shown in Table K. The first line of this table includes all one-person care-using families, and can be compared with the first line of Table A, in which all multiple-person care-using families are covered.

Mean out-of-pocket expenditures for inpatient hospital care were higher for one-person families that used this form of care in 1980 than they were for corresponding multiple-person families ($444 compared with $259). The reverse might have been expected because of the larger family size of multiple-person families. Also, in both family categories, approximately 60 percent of user

families had only one episode of hospitalization in 1980, and a larger percent of multiple-person families compared with one-person families lacked complete health care coverage. An explanation for the difference may be that the mean number of hospital days for one-person families that used inpatient hospital care in 1980 was 14, compared with 11 days for multiple-person families (Dicker and Sunshine, 1987). That is, one-person families spent more time in the hospital, and longer hospital stays are more expensive than shorter stays. Longer hospital stays for one-person families may result from more severe illnesses in these families, compared with multiple-person families, or from the absence of family support for recovery at home. Note that these possibilities are not mutually exclusive. In contrast, mean out-of-pocket expenditure for inpatient physician care did not differ significantly between one-person and multiple-person care-using families in 1980.

For all other forms of care, out-of-pocket expenditures for one-person care-using families were smaller than those for multiple-person user families. Indeed, expenses for one-person families were sometimes only about one-half as large. For example, mean out-of-pocket expenditures for ambulatory physician care in 1980 were $77 for one-person user families, compared with $136 for multiple-person user families. For all health care combined, the respective means were $317 and $582. The larger means for multiple-person families probably

Table K
Out-of-pocket health care expenditures for one-person health-care-using families: United States, 1980

Family age and health care coverage	Inpatient hospital care	Inpatient physician care	Ambulatory physician care	Hospital outpatient and emergency room care	Dental care	Prescription medications	All health care combined
	Mean out-of-pocket expenditures						
All one-person families	$444	$201	$77	$33	$132	$54	$317
Under 65 years of age	494	175	68	33	133	41	280
With full-year health care coverage	*218	*132	68	28	124	40	247
Without full-year health care coverage	*1,336	*319	70	49	162	42	364
65 years of age or older	388	228	94	32	127	81	401

NOTE: Statistics for "all health care combined" refer to families using any one or more types of care. "All health care combined" includes the six types of care listed in the first six columns of the table plus: care by other independent health practitioners (such as psychologists); and other health supplies (such as eyeglasses and orthopedic items).

SOURCES: Tables 6–10, 16–20, 26–30, 36–40, 46–50, 56–60, and 66–70.

reflect their larger family size and a correspondingly greater number of episodes of care.

Age

One-person families under age 65 ("younger families") are compared in Table K with those age 65 and over ("older families"). Mean out-of-pocket expenditures for user families were similar in the two age categories for dental care and for hospital outpatient and emergency room care. Those out-of-pocket expenditures on ambulatory physician care, prescription medications, and all health care combined, were higher for the older families. For example, mean out-of-pocket expenditures for prescriptions were $81 for older families compared with $41 for younger families, and mean out-of-pocket expenditures for all health care combined were $401 for older families compared with $280 for younger families. These differences probably reflect greater use of health care by older one-person families compared with younger one-person families (see Dicker and Sunshine, 1987).

For inpatient physician care and inpatient hospital care, differences in out-of-pocket spending between the two age categories were not statistically significant. This finding possibly reflects the problem of large standard errors discussed above.

Health Care Coverage

Also in Table K, statistics are presented on mean out-of-pocket health care expenditures in 1980 by younger one-person user families according to whether or not the families had full-year health care coverage. Because of statistical difficulties, comparisons were precluded for inpatient hospital care and inpatient physician care. Among the other five forms of care, only hospital outpatient and emergency room care had statistically significant differences in coverage categories. Mean out-of-pocket expenditures were $49 for families without complete coverage, compared with $28 for those with complete coverage.

Final Note on Family Data

Only one measure of family out-of-pocket expenditures has been discussed in the text of this report—the mean expenditure for those families in a family category that used a given form of care in 1980. Data on this measure occupy only one of the eight columns found in the detailed tables; in other columns, additional measures of out-of-pocket expenditures are available. These measures include: mean out-of-pocket expenditures for all families in a category, not merely those families that used care; and percentiles of the distribution of out-of-pocket expenditures for care-using families. Thus, the detailed tables can be consulted for further information on expenditures that is not included in the text.

References

Aday, L. A., Fleming, G. V., and Andersen, R.: Access to medical care in the U.S.: Who has it, who doesn't. *Research Series.* No. 32. Center for Health Administration Studies, University of Chicago. Chicago. Pluribus Press, 1984.

Andersen, R., and Benham, L.: Factors Affecting the Relationship Between Family Income and Medical Care Consumption, in H. E. Klarman, ed., *Empirical Studies in Health Economics.* Baltimore. The Johns Hopkins Press, 1970.

Anderson, J. M., and Thorne, E.: Estimates of Aggregate Personal Health Care Expenditures in 1980, Comparison of the National Health Accounts and the National Medical Care Utilization and Expenditure Survey Data. Working Paper No. 30, Division of Health Interview Statistics, The National Center for Health Statistics, Hyattsville, Md., 1985.

Bonham, G. S.: Procedures and questionnaires of the National Medical Care Utilization and Expenditure Survey. *National Medical Care Utilization and Expenditure Survey.* Series A, Methodological Report No. 1. DHHS Pub. No. 83–20001. Public Health Service. Washington. U.S. Government Printing Office, Mar. 1983.

Campbell, D. T., and Julian, C. S.: *Experimental and Quasi-Experimental Designs for Research.* Chicago. Rand McNally College Publishing Co., 1980.

Cox, G., Parker, A. E., Sweetland, S. S., et al.: *Imputation of Missing Item Data for the National Medical Care Utilization and Expenditure Survey.* Prepared for the National Center for Health Statistics under Contract No. HRA–233–79–2032. Research Triangle Park, N.C. Research Triangle Institute, 1982.

Cox, G., and Sweetland, S. S.: *Imputation of Attribution-Related Missing Data for the National Medical Care Utilization and Expenditure Survey.* Prepared for the National Center for Health Statistics under Contract No. HRA–233–79–2032. Research Triangle Park, N.C. Research Triangle Institute, 1982.

Dicker, M.: Health care coverage and insurance premiums of families, United States, 1980. *National Medical Care Utilization and Expenditure Survey.* Preliminary Data Report No. 3. DHHS Pub. No. 83–20000. Public Health Service. Washington. U.S. Government Printing Office, May 1983a.

Dicker, M.: Panel Surveys and Family Level Measures, Problems and Solutions, in *1983 Proceedings of the American Statistical Association*, Social Statistics Volume. Washington. American Statistical Association, 1983b.

Dicker, M.: Demographic Analysis and a General Theory for Measuring Social Change in Organizations, The Case of the Family. Paper presented at the Annual Meeting of the Southern Regional Demographic Group. Orlando, Fla., Oct. 19, 1984.

Dicker, M., and Casady, R. J.: A Reciprocal Rule Model for Defining Longitudinal Families for the Analysis of Panel Survey Data, in *1982 Proceedings of the American Statistical Association*, Social Statistics Volume. Washington. American Statistical Association, 1982.

Dicker, M. and Casady, R. J.: Empirical Findings on the Distribution and Construction of Longitudinal Families, Part I, Modeling the Universe, Inscope Changes, and Static and Dynamic Families, in *1984 Proceedings of the American Statistical Association*, Survey Research Methods Volume. Washington. American Statistical Association, 1984.

Dicker, M., and Sunshine, J. H.: Family use of health care, United States, 1980. *National Medical Care Utilization and Expenditure Survey.* Series B, Descriptive Report No. 10. DHHS Pub. No. 87–20210. National Center for Health Statistics, Public Health Service. Washington. U.S. Government Printing Office, Feb. 1987.

Duan, N., Manning, W. G., Jr., Morris, C. N., et al.: *A Comparison of Alternative Models for the Demand for Medical Care.* Contract No. R–2754–HHS. Santa Monica, Calif. Rand Corporation, Jan. 1982.

Farley, P. J.: Private insurance and public programs, Coverage of health services. *National Health Care Expenditures Study.* Data Preview 20. DHHS Pub. No. (PHS) 85–3374. Rockville, Md. National Center for Health Services Research and Health Care Technology Assessment, Mar. 1985.

Feldstein, P. J.: *Health Care Economics.* New York. John Wiley and Sons, 1979.

Feldstein, P. J.: *Health Care Economics*, 2d ed. New York. John Wiley and Sons, 1983.

Hershey, J. C., Luft, H. S., and Gianaris, J. M.: Making sense out of utilization data. *Med. Care* 13(10):838–852, Oct. 1975.

Kaspar, J. A., Walden, D. C., and Wilensky, G. C.: Who are the uninsured? *National Health Care Expenditures Study.* Data Preview 1. Hyattsville, Md. National Center for Health Services Research, Public Health Service, 1980.

Landis, J. R., Lepkowski, J. M., Eklund, S. A., and Stehouwer, S. A.: A statistical methodology for analyzing data from a complex survey, the first National Health and Nutrition Examination Survey. *Vital and Health Statistics.* Series 2, No. 92. DHHS Pub. No. (PHS) 82–1366. National Center for Health Statistics, Public Health Service. Washington, U.S. Government Printing Office, Sept. 1982.

Levy, P. S., and Lemeshow, S.: *Sampling for Health Professionals.* Belmont, Calif. Lifetime Learning Publications, 1980.

McCarthy, P. J.: Replication, an approach to the analysis of data from complex surveys. *Vital and Health Statistics.* Series 2, No. 14. DHEW Pub. No. (PHS) 79–1269. National Center for Health Statistics, Public Health Service. Washington. U.S. Government Printing Office, Apr. 1966.

McMillen, D. B., and Herriot, R.: Towards a Longitudinal Definition of Households. SIPP Working Paper Series No. 8402. U.S. Bureau of the Census. Washington, D.C., 1984.

Moser, B., Whitmore, R., Frick, G. G., et al.: *National Medical Care Utilization and Expenditure Survey: Analytic Family File Construction Methodology Report*. RTI Project No. 251U–1898–14. Research Triangle Park, N.C. Research Triangle Institute, Oct. 1983.

Newacheck, P. W.: *Utilization and Expenditures for Medical Care Services Provided to Children with Activity Limitations*. Grant MCJ–063468–01–0. Prepared for National Maternal and Child Health Resource Center. Institute for Health Policy Studies, University of California, San Francisco, 1985a.

Newacheck, P. W.: *Prevalence and Severity of Chronic Conditions Among Children*. Prepared for National Maternal and Child Health Resource Center. Institute for Health Policy Studies, University of California, San Francisco, 1985b.

Newhouse, J. P., Manning, W. G., Morris, C. N., et al.: Some interim results from a controlled trial of cost sharing in health insurance. *N. Engl. J. Med.* 305:1501–1507, 1981.

SAS Institute, Inc.: *SAS Users Guide, Basics*, 1982 ed. Cary, N.C. SAS Institute, Inc., 1982.

Shah, B. V.: *SESUDAAN, Standard Errors Program for Computing Standardized Rates From Sample Survey Data*. Research Triangle Park, N.C. Research Triangle Institute, Apr. 1981.

Sunshine, J. H.: Medicare, past, present, and future. *National Journal* 14(23):1030–1033, June 5, 1982.

Sunshine, J. H.: How many Americans lack outside sources of payment for major health care costs? *Journal of the Health and Human Resources Administration*. 6(3):341–360, Winter 1984.

Whitmore, R. W., Cox, B. G., and Folsom, R. E.: *Family Unit Weighting Methodology for the National Household Survey Component of the National Medical Care Utilization and Expenditure Survey*. Contract No. HRA–233–79–2032. Prepared for National Center for Health Statistics. Research Triangle Park, N.C. Research Triangle Institute, 1982.

Wilensky, G. R., and Walden, D. C.: Minorities, Poverty, and the Uninsured. Paper presented at the 109th Annual Meeting of the American Public Health Association. Los Angeles, Nov. 1981.

List of Detailed Tables

Inpatient Hospital Care

Inpatient Physician Care

Ambulatory Physician Visits

Hospital Emergency Room and Outpatient Visits

Dental Visits

Prescription Acquisitions

All Health Care Services

Table 1

Out-of-pocket expenditures for inpatient hospital care for multiple-person families, by selected characteristics: United States, 1980

[Rate per family year. Civilian noninstitutionalized population with civilian family head]

Characteristic	All families		Families with discharges					
	Number in thousands	Mean expenditures	Percent	Mean expenditures	Expenditures at selected percentiles			
					25th	50th	75th	90th
Total....................	58,135	$79	30.4	$259	$0	$0	$159	$658
Family size[1]								
2 persons................	22,916	93	26.2	354	0	0	183	724
3 persons................	12,567	52	30.6	172	0	0	149	520
4 persons................	12,269	56	32.0	175	0	0	129	564
5 or more persons........	10,383	107	37.7	283	0	0	130	761
Age of head								
Under 25 years...........	4,308	85	33.0	258	0	0	119	673
25-44 years..............	25,173	69	29.5	233	0	0	100	531
45-64 years..............	20,129	65	28.6	228	0	0	175	630
65 years and over........	8,525	137	36.2	379	0	2	201	800
Sex of head								
Male.....................	44,874	83	30.2	273	0	0	180	676
Female...................	13,262	66	31.1	213	0	0	62	502
Race and ethnicity[2] of head								
White....................	51,015	76	30.3	251	0	0	171	665
Hispanic.................	3,403	95	33.6	284	0	0	210	1,001
Non-Hispanic.............	47,613	75	30.1	249	0	0	171	636
Black....................	6,090	106	31.1	339	0	0	86	644
Other....................	1,030	*49	29.7	*166	*0	*0	*220	*270
Family structure								
Head and spouse present whole time.....	42,556	69	30.0	229	0	0	180	635
Child under 17 years.....	22,442	66	32.5	203	0	0	141	640
No child under 17 years..	20,114	72	27.2	265	0	0	188	616
Head only, no spouse at any time.....	13,977	94	29.1	325	0	0	64	624
Child under 17 years.....	8,643	*104	32.0	*324	0	0	5	777
No child under 17 years..	5,334	*80	24.3	*328	0	18	180	458
Other....................	1,602	209	53.6	390	0	0	298	1,292
Family dynamics								
Unchanging, full year....	46,990	63	26.6	236	0	0	130	550
Change in composition or existed less than full year....	11,145	147	46.7	315	0	0	269	777

34

Family poverty status in 1980

Below 150 percent poverty level	10,938	95	35.6	266	0	0	102	763
Below poverty level	6,047	51	33.7	152	0	0	0	557
Poverty level to 149 percent	4,892	148	37.8	392	0	0	175	911
150-199 percent	6,355	187	32.5	575	0	1	257	1,280
200-299 percent	12,860	69	32.6	213	0	0	186	630
300-499 percent	17,047	57	27.6	205	0	0	119	516
500 percent or more	10,935	46	26.0	177	0	0	120	344

Family income in 1980[3]

Less than $10,000	10,629	113	34.1	333	0	0	159	763
$10,000-$19,999	16,728	96	31.1	310	0	0	201	777
$20,000-$34,999	19,706	57	28.4	201	0	0	140	520
$35,000 or more	11,073	58	29.5	198	0	0	125	465

Education of head[4]

None or elementary school	10,491	104	35.0	298	18	0	264	912
Some high school	9,267	*71	33.2	*214	0	0	45	500
High school graduate	20,605	86	30.2	284	0	0	149	644
Some college	8,651	45	27.3	164	0	0	98	520
College graduate or more	9,099	*75	25.8	*289	5	0	145	476

Family employment status[5]

2 or more persons worked full year	14,607	44	24.7	176	0	0	105	411
Only 1 person worked full year	24,549	81	28.5	284	0	0	175	748
Some part-year work	11,303	95	37.9	249	0	0	170	624
No person worked	7,676	117	36.5	319	0	0	180	724

Worst perceived health status of any family member[6]

Excellent	16,200	36	21.5	170	0	0	100	421
Good	24,467	56	28.5	198	0	0	130	450
Fair	11,131	94	35.9	262	0	0	154	777
Poor	6,318	248	51.2	485	0	0	298	1,065

Most severe limitation in usual activity of any family member

None	43,941	55	25.7	214	0	0	133	509
Some limitation	3,679	*99	35.3	*282	0	0	105	448
Cannot perform usual activity	10,515	172	48.4	354	0	0	207	926

Family's bed days[3]

0	11,173	*5	1.6	*298	*0	*57	*289	*1,200
1-5	14,527	31	16.7	186	0	0	194	421
6-10	8,834	39	33.2	117	0	0	113	336
11-20	9,982	76	40.4	188	0	0	60	404
More than 20	13,619	219	59.6	367	0	0	207	911

Table 1—continued

Out-of-pocket expenditures for inpatient hospital care for multiple-person families, by selected characteristics: United States, 1980

[Rate per family year. Civilian noninstitutionalized population with civilian family head]

Characteristic	All families			Families with discharges				
	Number in thousands	Mean expenditures	Percent	Mean expenditures	Expenditures at selected percentiles			
					25th	50th	75th	90th
Family health care coverage								
All members covered full year...........	42,453	$58	30.5	$191	$0	$0	$113	$406
Private insurance only.................	25,759	52	26.6	196	0	0	105	411
Medicaid only.........................	1,621	*3	35.8	*8	*0	*0	*0	*0
Medicare only........................	*574	*61	*23.5	*260	*3	*185	*264	*724
Medicare and other public programs.....	*471	*49	*40.9	*119	*0	*0	*1	*675
Medicare and private insurance.........	7,475	89	38.3	234	0	0	188	708
Other public and private mixes.........	5,853	61	34.6	*176	0	0	40	243
Other mixes of public programs.........	*135	*7	*16.8	*41	*40	*41	*41	*41
Source unknown.....................	*564	*78	*52.0	*151	*0	*0	*45	*351
All members covered, some part year.....	8,669	80	32.9	241	0	0	130	747
Some members not covered.............	4,963	234	32.9	710	0	145	703	1,549
All members not covered..............	2,051	*125	11.2	*1,121	*0	*893	*1,133	*2,271

[1]Average size during period of family's existence rounded to nearest integer; exactly half an integer rounded upward.
[2]There were too few Hispanic families of races other than white for separate tabulation.
[3]Annual rate.
[4]Includes only families with heads 17 years of age and over.
[5]Excludes families with all members under 14 years of age.
[6]Excludes families with all members with health status unknown.

NOTE: Multiple-person families are families with average size 1.5 or greater.

Table 2

Out-of-pocket expenditures for inpatient hospital care for multiple-person families with all members under 65 years of age, by selected characteristics: United States, 1980

[Rate per family year. Civilian noninstitutionalized population with civilian family head]

Characteristic	All families		Families with discharges					
	Number in thousands	Mean expenditures	Percent	Mean expenditures	Expenditures at selected percentiles			
					25th	50th	75th	90th
Total..........	47,327	$67	28.5	$234	$0	$0	$120	$564
Family size[1]								
2 persons.......	14,958	83	21.3	388	0	0	175	761
3 persons.......	11,228	36	28.4	126	0	0	106	498
4 persons.......	11,546	49	31.4	156	0	0	90	476
5 or more persons....	9,595	99	36.2	273	0	0	113	520
Age of head								
Under 25 years.......	4,283	86	33.2	258	0	0	119	673
25–44 years.......	24,783	69	29.2	235	0	0	100	523
45–64 years.......	18,261	59	26.5	224	0	0	168	564
Sex of head								
Male.......	36,477	69	28.3	243	0	0	148	564
Female.......	10,850	*60	29.3	*204	0	0	41	540
Race and ethnicity[2] of head								
White.......	41,444	66	28.1	234	0	0	133	579
Hispanic.......	3,040	103	33.0	311	0	0	211	1,189
Non-Hispanic....	38,405	63	27.7	227	0	0	119	531
Black.......	5,064	*75	32.2	*233	0	0	60	542
Other.......	819	*54	26.9	*199	*0	*0	*102	*270
Family structure								
Head and spouse present whole time......	34,963	57	28.4	200	0	0	144	531
Child under 17 years........	21,668	62	32.1	194	0	0	135	600
No child under 17 years.......	13,295	48	22.5	214	0	0	175	460
Head only, no spouse at any time......	11,169	*94	27.2	*345	0	0	25	700
Child under 17 years.......	8,258	*104	31.2	*335	0	0	25	777
No child under 17 years.......	2,911	*64	15.9	*403	*0	*0	*148	*351
Other.......	1,194	*97	42.1	*231	*0	*0	*243	*574
Family dynamics								
Unchanging, full year........	37,714	53	24.6	215	0	0	95	454
Change in composition or existed less than full year.......	9,613	121	44.0	275	0	0	261	747

37

Table 2—continued

Out-of-pocket expenditures for inpatient hospital care for multiple-person families with all members under 65 years of age, by selected characteristics: United States, 1980

[Rate per family year. Civilian noninstitutionalized population with civilian family head]

| | All families | | Families with discharges | | | | | |
| | | | | | Expenditures at selected percentiles | | | |
Characteristic	Number in thousands	Mean expenditures	Percent	Mean expenditures	25th	50th	75th	90th
Family poverty status in 1980								
Below 150 percent poverty level	8,770	$82	35.1	$235	$0	$0	$53	$747
Below poverty level	5,083	44	34.5	129	0	0	0	542
Poverty level to 149 percent	3,687	*135	35.9	*376	0	0	153	900
150–199 percent	4,825	*170	30.1	*563	0	0	289	1,332
200–299 percent	10,075	58	29.8	196	0	0	141	502
300–499 percent	14,307	44	25.8	169	0	0	102	460
500 percent or more	9,350	*43	24.2	*177	0	0	125	348
Family income in 1980[3]								
Less than $10,000	7,496	*82	33.5	*243	0	0	35	665
$10,000–$19,999	12,555	90	27.6	325	0	0	180	747
$20,000–$34,999	17,279	55	27.3	200	0	0	114	509
$35,000 or more	9,997	47	27.9	169	0	0	125	368
Education of head[4]								
None or elementary school	5,822	74	31.9	233	0	0	220	911
Some high school	7,546	40	31.1	129	0	0	40	351
High school graduate	18,299	84	28.8	291	0	0	135	644
Some college	7,556	39	26.6	146	0	0	95	451
College graduate or more	8,084	*73	24.8	*296	0	10	144	427
Family employment status[5]								
2 or more persons worked full year	13,629	39	23.6	166	0	0	101	355
Only 1 person worked full year	21,782	75	27.8	269	0	0	154	703
Some part-year work	9,021	95	36.9	258	0	0	108	658
No person worked	2,896	*46	30.7	*149	0	0	0	351
Worst perceived health status of any family member[6]								
Excellent	14,771	30	21.4	138	0	0	80	351
Good	20,837	58	27.8	207	0	0	106	476
Fair	8,021	106	34.2	310	0	0	214	900
Poor	3,678	181	48.5	372	0	0	204	911

Most severe limitation in usual activity of any family member								
None	39,751	56	25.9	216	0	0	119	509
Some limitation	2,814	*82	35.0	*233	0	0	50	242
Cannot perform usual activity	4,762	147	46.6	316	0	0	238	833

Family's bed days[3]

0	7,825	*4	1.6	*215	*0	*57	*289	*430
1-5	12,427	30	14.8	202	0	0	148	540
6-10	7,470	34	28.9	118	0	0	98	364
11-20	8,884	*66	38.5	*171	0	0	53	344
More than 20	10,722	179	55.5	322	0	0	183	777

Family health care coverage

All members covered full year	33,575	52	28.5	181	0	0	78	351
Private insurance only	25,502	52	26.3	197	0	*0	106	411
Medicaid only	1,606	*3	35.1	*8	*0	*0	*0	*0
Medicare only	*12	-	-	-	-	-	-	-
Medicare and other public programs	*95	*0	*0.0	-	-	-	-	-
Medicare and private insurance	5,762	*76	*26.3	*287	*180	*180	*401	*401
Other public and private mixes	*135	62	34.5	*179	0	0	37	243
Other mixes of public programs	*463	*7	*16.8	*41	*40	*41	*41	*41
Source unknown		*91	*55.0	*165	*0	*0	*45	*351
All members covered, some part year	7,968	67	32.0	211	0	0	130	722
Some members not covered	3,804	*183	30.4	*601	*0	100	703	1,200
All members not covered	1,980	96	11.1	*863	*0	*804	*1,035	*2,021

[1]Average size during period of family's existence rounded to nearest integer; exactly half an integer rounded upward.
[2]There were too few Hispanic families of races other than white for separate tabulation.
[3]Annual rate.
[4]Includes only families with heads 17 years of age and over.
[5]Excludes families with all members under 14 years of age.
[6]Excludes families with all members with health status unknown.

NOTE: Multiple-person families are families with average size 1.5 or greater.

Table 3

Out-of-pocket expenditures for inpatient hospital care for multiple-person families with all members under 65 years of age and all members with health care coverage all year, by selected characteristics: United States, 1980

[Rate per family year. Civilian noninstitutionalized population with civilian family head]

Characteristic	All families		Families with discharges					
	Number in thousands	Mean expenditures	Percent	Mean expenditures	Expenditures at selected percentiles			
					25th	50th	75th	90th
Total...................	33,575	$52	28.5	$181	$0	$0	$78	$351
Family size[1]								
2 persons................	10,994	*88	22.0	400	0	0	119	460
3 persons................	8,010	25	28.2	88	0	0	60	340
4 persons................	8,464	35	32.5	108	0	0	60	301
5 or more persons........	6,107	43	34.8	124	0	0	61	287
Age of head								
Under 25 years..........	2,585	*73	30.2	*240	0	0	105	455
25–44 years.............	18,256	58	29.7	196	0	0	64	301
45–64 years.............	12,733	38	26.4	143	0	0	80	351
Sex of head								
Male....................	27,351	60	28.6	210	0	0	113	421
Female..................	6,224	*14	27.9	*52	0	0	0	101
Race and ethnicity[2] of head								
White...................	29,902	50	28.6	176	0	*0	95	355
Hispanic................	1,711	*67	36.2	*185	*0	*0	*135	*311
Non-Hispanic............	28,191	49	28.1	175	0	0	90	360
Black...................	3,139	*61	28.1	*216	0	0	25	149
Other...................	533	*67	*26.1	*257	*0	*0	*53	*240
Family structure								
Head and spouse present whole time.....	26,517	44	28.7	154	0	0	105	390
Child under 17 years....	16,251	41	32.3	127	0	0	95	360
No child under 17 years..	10,266	49	22.8	215	0	0	155	421
Head only, no spouse at any time........	6,394	*78	25.8	*301	0	0	0	101
Child under 17 years....	5,051	*69	27.3	*252	0	0	0	50
No child under 17 years..	1,343	*111	20.2	*547	*0	*0	*101	*351
Other...................	663	*98	47.7	*205	*0	*0	*176	*574
Family dynamics								
Unchanging, full year...	28,266	39	25.1	154	0	0	51	289
Change in composition or existed less than full year..........	5,308	*121	46.7	*259	0	0	176	455

Family poverty status in 1980								
Below 150 percent poverty level	4,640	*72	37.5	*191	0	0	35	200
Below poverty level	2,919	*30	33.9	*88	0	0	0	181
Poverty level to 149 percent	1,721	*143	43.6	*328	0	0	50	294
150-199 percent	2,657	*150	33.1	*454	0	0	154	1,280
200-299 percent	7,074	40	30.9	129	0	0	129	425
300-499 percent	11,427	35	25.6	135	0	0	60	351
500 percent or more	7,776	*41	23.6	*176	0	0	113	344
Family income in 1980[3]								
Less than $10,000	4,023	*93	35.4	*263	0	0	0	270
$10,000-$19,999	7,715	68	29.2	*235	0	0	129	430
$20,000-$34,999	13,970	35	27.2	128	0	0	60	305
$35,000 or more	7,867	*43	26.5	*163	0	0	95	344
Education of head[4]								
None or elementary school	3,188	*44	33.6	*131	0	0	70	242
Some high school	4,620	*32	29.3	109	0	0	25	289
High school graduate	13,366	55	28.9	189	0	0	86	360
Some college	5,757	29	26.6	109	0	0	50	399
College graduate or more	6,625	*82	26.3	*312	0	0	137	364
Family employment status[5]								
2 or more persons worked full year	10,347	32	23.4	*136	0	0	60	293
Only 1 person worked full year	16,128	70	28.7	244	0	0	129	430
Some part-year work	4,933	36	38.8	94	0	0	40	289
No person worked	2,167	*42	27.8	*152	0	0	0	351
Worst perceived health status of any family member[6]								
Excellent	11,162	*26	21.9	*117	0	0	50	261
Good	15,029	40	28.0	143	0	0	67	301
Fair	5,209	*96	35.4	*270	0	0	80	559
Poor	2,155	*161	48.8	*330	0	0	181	564
Most severe limitation in usual activity of any family member								
None	28,461	42	25.8	161.	0	0	78	301
Some limitation	2,067	*93	37.3	*250	0	0	60	242
Cannot perform usual activity	3,047	117	47.7	245	0	0	136	523
Family's bed days[3]								
0	5,766	*2	*1.5	*124	*0	*0	*289	*430
1-5	8,806	*21	13.8	*154	0	0	80	220
6-10	5,513	23	29.7	76	0	0	90	275
11-20	6,162	29	38.7	75	0	0	40	236
More than 20	7,328	168	57.9	290	0	0	114	509

Table 3—continued

Out-of-pocket expenditures for inpatient hospital care for multiple-person families with all members under 65 years of age and all members with health care coverage all year, by selected characteristics: United States, 1980

[Rate per family year. Civilian noninstitutionalized population with civilian family head]

Characteristic	All families		Families with discharges					
	Number in thousands	Mean expenditures	Percent	Mean expenditures	Expenditures at selected percentiles			
					25th	50th	75th	90th
Family health care coverage								
Private insurance only...............	25,502	$52	26.3	$197	$0	$0	$106	$411
Medicaid only...............	1,606	*3	35.1	*8	*0	*0	*0	*0
Medicare only...............	—	*0	*0.0	—	—	—	—	—
Medicare and other public programs......	*12	*76	*26.3	*287	*180	*180	*401	*401
Medicare and private insurance...........	*95	62	34.5	*179	0	0	37	243
Other public and private mixes...........	5,762	*7	*16.8	*41	*40	*41	*41	*41
Other mixes of public programs...........	*135	*91	*55.0	*165	*0	*0	*45	*351
Source unknown...............	*463							

1Average size during period of family's existence rounded to nearest integer; exactly half an integer rounded upward.
2There were too few Hispanic families of races other than white for separate tabulation.
3Annual rate.
4Includes only families with heads 17 years of age and over.
5Excludes families with all members under 14 years of age.
6Excludes families with all members with health status unknown.

NOTE: Multiple-person families are families with average size 1.5 or greater.

Table 4

Out-of-pocket expenditures for inpatient hospital care for multiple-person families with all members under 65 years of age and some or all members without health care coverage all year, by selected characteristics: United States, 1980

[Rate per family year. Civilian noninstitutionalized population with civilian family head]

Characteristic	All families		Families with discharges						
					Expenditures at selected percentiles			
	Number in thousands	Mean expenditures	Percent	Mean expenditures	25th	50th	75th	90th
Total.........................	13,752	$103	28.5	$362	$0	$0	$410	$1,001
Family size[1]								
2 persons....................	3,964	68	19.4	348	0	0	700	998
3 persons....................	3,218	63	29.0	218	0	30	238	797
4 persons....................	3,082	87	28.5	305	0	0	453	1,013
5 or more persons...........	3,488	*196	38.6	*507	0	0	379	1,189
Age of head								
Under 25 years...............	1,698	105	37.7	280	0	0	180	825
25-44 years..................	6,527	98	27.6	353	0	0	333	1,189
45-64 years..................	5,528	*110	26.8	*409	0	25	462	911
Sex of head								
Male.........................	9,126	95	27.2	348	0	3	450	1,001
Female.......................	4,627	*121	31.2	*387	0	0	308	1,003
Race and ethnicity[2] of head								
White........................	11,542	106	26.8	396	0	0	*410	1,013
Hispanic.....................	1,328	*148	28.9	*513	*0	*30	1,001	*1,550
Non-Hispanic.................	10,214	101	26.5	379	0	0	308	912
Black........................	1,924	98	38.9	253	0	0	462	911
Other........................	*286	*28	*28.6	*100	*0	*0	*102	*270
Family structure								
Head and spouse present whole time......	8,446	97	27.8	348	0	9	453	998
Child under 17 years.........	5,417	126	31.4	399	0	12	516	1,100
No child under 17 years......	3,029	45	21.2	213	0	0	238	709
Head only, no spouse at any time........	4,775	*116	29.1	*398	0	0	192	1,003
Child under 17 years.........	3,207	*161	37.4	*430	0	0	169	1,013
No child under 17 years......	1,568	*24	12.1	*197	*0	*0	*251	*700
Other........................	*532	*97	*35.0	*277	*0	*0	*368	*1,204
Family dynamics								
Unchanging, full year........	9,448	95	23.0	414	0	0	270	1,013
Change in composition or existed less than full year........	4,304	121	40.7	298	0	0	462	911

Table 4—continued

Out-of-pocket expenditures for inpatient hospital care for multiple-person families with all members under 65 years of age and some or all members without health care coverage all year, by selected characteristics: United States, 1980

[Rate per family year. Civilian noninstitutionalized population with civilian family head]

| Characteristic | All families | | | Families with discharges | | | | | |
| | Number in thousands | Mean expenditures | Percent | Mean expenditures | Expenditures at selected percentiles | | | | |
					25th	50th	75th	90th	
Family poverty status in 1980									
Below 150 percent poverty level......	4,130	$94	32.3	$292	$0	*0	$462	911	
Below poverty level...........	2,164	64	35.2	182	0	0	0	900	
Poverty level to 149 percent.....	1,966	128	29.1	*439	*0	*4	*747	*1,189	
150-199 percent.............	2,168	*193	26.5	*729	*0	*30	*777	*1,549	
200-299 percent.............	3,000	*102	27.3	*374	0	0	379	1,100	
300-499 percent.............	2,880	80	26.6	299	0	33	516	998	
500 percent or more..........	1,574	*49	27.2	*182	*0	*25	*179	*368	
Family income in 1980[3]									
Less than $10,000...........	3,473	68	31.3	218	0	0	169	911	
$10,000-$19,999...........	4,840	*124	25.1	*493	0	0	500	1,013	
$20,000-$34,999...........	3,310	137	27.6	497	0	90	709	1,519	
$35,000 or more...........	2,130	*62	33.4	186	0	4	179	594	
Education of head[4]									
None or elementary school......	2,634	111	29.9	370	0	30	800	1,005	
Some high school...........	2,926	*53	34.1	*156	0	0	62	520	
High school graduate.........	4,934	162	28.3	571	0	0	542	1,332	
Some college.............	1,800	*70	26.7	*264	*0	*0	*333	*724	
College graduate or more......	1,459	*33	17.8	*187	*0	*81	*148	*700	
Family employment status[5]									
2 or more persons worked full year...	3,282	63	24.5	256	0	12	251	851	
Only 1 person worked full year....	5,654	88	25.0	350	0	15	625	1,133	
Some part-year work.........	4,087	*166	34.7	*479	0	*0	462	1,005	
No person worked...........	*729	*57	*39.5	*144	*0	*0	*0	*169	
Worst perceived health status of any family member[6]									
Excellent...............	3,609	42	19.9	211	0	0	251	774	
Good.................	5,808	*103	27.2	*381	0	0	270	851	
Fair.................	2,812	126	31.9	393	0	30	516	1,220	
Poor.................	1,524	*208	48.1	*433	0	0	244	925	

Most severe limitation in usual activity of any family member

None........................	11,290	92	26.1	352	0	0	431	971
Some limitation.............	747	*50	28.7	*175	*0	*0	*3	*1,003
Cannot perform usual activity....	1,715	202	44.7	*453	0	0	520	1,133

Family's bed days[3]

0...........................	2,059	*8	*1.9	*417	*57	*179	*1,200	*1,200
1-5.........................	3,620	*51	17.3	*294	*0	*45	*450	*793
6-10........................	1,957	*66	26.5	250	*0	*0	*190	*1,003
11-20.......................	2,722	*149	38.0	*393	0	0	159	800
More than 20................	3,394	202	50.3	401	0	0	520	1,100

Family health care coverage

All members covered, some part year.....	7,968	67	32.0	211	0	0	130	722
Some members not covered............	3,804	*183	30.4	*601	0	100	703	1,200
All members not covered.............	1,980	96	11.1	*863	*0	*804	*1,035	*2,021

[1]Average size during period of family's existence rounded to nearest integer; exactly half an integer rounded upward.
[2]There were too few Hispanic families of races other than white for separate tabulation.
[3]Annual rate.
[4]Includes only families with heads 17 years of age and over.
[5]Excludes families with all members under 14 years of age.
[6]Excludes families with all members with health status unknown.

NOTE: Multiple-person families are families with average size 1.5 or greater.

Table 5

Out-of-pocket expenditures for inpatient hospital care for multiple-person families with members 65 years of age and over, by selected characteristics: United States, 1980

[Rate per family year. Civilian noninstitutionalized population with civilian family head]

Characteristic	All families		Families with discharges					
					Expenditures at selected percentiles			
	Number in thousands	Mean expenditures	Percent	Mean expenditures	25th	50th	75th	90th
Total............................	10,809	$132	38.8	$341	$0	$1	$201	$840
Family size[1]								
2 persons........................	7,958	112	35.5	317	0	0	188	724
3 persons........................	1,339	*191	48.4	395	0	10	291	1,192
4 persons........................	724	*170	40.3	*422	*0	*1	*497	*1,445
5 or more persons................	788	*201	55.3	*363	*0	*0	*190	*840
Family age								
All members 65 years and over....	4,141	*137	35.1	*391	0	0	189	724
Some members under 65............	6,668	129	41.2	314	0	10	207	925
Sex of head								
Male.............................	8,397	143	38.7	369	0	0	212	975
Female...........................	2,412	*96	39.3	*244	0	18	181	404
Race and ethnicity[2] of head								
White............................	9,571	121	40.2	302	0	3	200	800
Hispanic.........................	*363	*36	*38.6	*94	*0	*0	*0	*458
Non-Hispanic.....................	9,208	125	40.3	310	0	6	201	840
Black............................	1,027	*256	25.7	*993	*0	*0	*291	*6,571
Other............................	*211	*33	*40.5	*82	*0	*0	*223	*223
Family structure								
Head and spouse present whole time.....	7,593	124	37.1	334	0	0	203	832
Child under 17 years.............	774	167	42.1	*396	*0	*120	*761	*925
No child under 17 years..........	6,819	119	36.5	326	0	0	195	725
Head only, no spouse at any time......	2,808	*97	36.4	*265	0	30	181	550
Child under 17 years.............	*384	*83	*48.4	*171	*0	*0	*2	*1,100
No child under 17 years..........	2,424	*99	34.5	*286	0	50	181	458
Other............................	*408	*536	*87.4	*614	*0	*12	*404	*1,614
Family dynamics								
Unchanging, full year............	9,276	103	34.7	297	0	0	195	724
Change in composition or existed less than full year.................	1,533	310	63.7	487	0	50	319	1,378

Family poverty status in 1980

Below 150 percent poverty level	2,169	*144	37.6	*384	0	0	207	926
Below poverty level	964	*89	29.9	*297	*0	*0	*207	*675
Poverty level to 149 percent	1,205	*189	43.8	*431	*0	*0	*181	*926
150-199 percent	1,530	*243	40.2	*605	0	61	246	1,268
200-299 percent	2,785	109	42.6	257	0	18	296	924
300-499 percent	2,740	*124	36.6	*338	0	0	180	776
500 percent or more	1,585	*64	36.4	*176	*0	*6	*120	*195

Family income in 1980[3]

Less than $10,000	3,133	189	35.4	534	0	3	246	975
$10,000-$19,999	4,173	116	41.8	278	0	0	223	1,182
$20,000-$34,999	2,427	74	36.1	205	0	6	180	761
$35,000 or more	1,076	*161	43.5	*369	*0	*10	*180	*832

Education of head[4]

None or elementary school	4,669	141	38.8	364	0	50	291	926
Some high school	1,721	*206	42.1	*489	0	0	190	1,065
High school graduate	2,306	*102	41.6	*245	0	6	180	696
Some college	1,095	*87	32.4	*267	*0	*0	*105	*925
College graduate or more	1,015	*85	34.2	*248	*0	*0	*154	*840

Family employment status[5]

2 or more persons worked full year	979	*103	39.8	*259	*0	*10	*380	*662
Only 1 person worked full year	2,767	*129	33.9	*381	0	0	212	925
Some part-year work	2,282	92	41.9	221	0	18	203	406
No person worked	4,781	159	40.0	398	0	0	188	926

Worst perceived health status of any family member[6]

Excellent	1,429	*107	21.8	*492	*0	*0	*291	*1,282
Good	3,630	49	32.6	152	0	0	182	370
Fair	3,110	63	40.3	155	0	0	80	504
Poor	2,640	342	54.8	624	0	60	488	1,318

Most severe limitation in usual activity of any family member

None	4,190	46	24.1	191	0	6	195	662
Some limitation	865	*157	36.1	*434	*0	*64	*203	*776
Cannot perform usual activity	5,754	192	50.0	383	0	0	207	1,065

Family's bed days[3]

0	3,349	*7	*1.4	*522	*0	*14	*201	*1,903
1-5	2,100	39	27.9	*139	*0	*38	*203	*317
6-10	1,364	64	57.0	113	0	0	180	291
11-20	1,098	*158	56.1	*282	0	0	76	800
More than 20	2,897	367	74.9	490	6	6	313	1,268

Table 5—continued

Out-of-pocket expenditures for inpatient hospital care for multiple-person families with members 65 years of age and over, by selected characteristics: United States, 1980

[Rate per family year. Civilian noninstitutionalized population with civilian family head]

Characteristic	All families			Families with discharges				
	Number in thousands	Mean expenditures	Percent	Mean expenditures	Expenditures at selected percentiles			
					25th	50th	75th	90th
Family health care coverage								
All members covered full year...........	8,879	$84	38.3	$219	$0	$0	$185	$708
Private insurance only...............	*258	*91	*58.8	*155	*0	*0	*58	*329
Medicaid only......................	*15	$0	*100.0	*0	*0	*0	*0	*0
Medicare only......................	*574	*61	*23.5	*260	*3	*185	*264	*724
Medicare and other public programs....	*459	50	*42.0	*119	*0	*0	*1	*675
Medicare and private insurance........	7,380	90	38.4	233	0	0	188	725
Other public and private mixes........	*91	*16	*38.8	*41	*0	*61	*61	*61
Other mixes of public programs........	–	–	–	–	–	–	–	–
Source unknown....................	*102	*22	*38.0	*57	*0	*0	*146	*146
All members covered, some part year.....	701	*217	43.9	*495	*0	*0	*64	*1,445
Some members not covered............	1,159	*401	41.2	*975	*30	*190	*776	*2,201
All members not covered.............	*71	*953	*13.4	*7,130	*7,130	*7,130	*7,130	*7,130

[1] Average size during period of family's existence rounded to nearest integer; exactly half an integer rounded upward.
[2] There were too few Hispanic families of races other than white for separate tabulation.
[3] Annual rate.
[4] Includes only families with heads 17 years of age and over.
[5] Excludes families with all members under 14 years of age.
[6] Excludes families with all members with health status unknown.

NOTE: Multiple-person families are families with average size 1.5 or greater.

Table 6

Out-of-pocket expenditures for inpatient hospital care for 1-person families, by selected characteristics: United States, 1980

[Rate per family year. Civilian noninstitutionalized population with civilian family head]

| Characteristic | All families | | Families with discharges | | | | | |
| | Number in thousands | Mean expenditures | Percent | Mean expenditures | Expenditures at selected percentiles | | | |
					25th	50th	75th	90th
Total........................	26,233	$66	14.8	$444	$0	$0	$180	$901
Sex								
Male.........................	11,866	*42	12.8	*328	0	0	140	1,409
Female.......................	14,367	86	16.5	519	0	0	188	901
Race and ethnicity[1]								
White........................	22,811	60	14.9	399	0	*0	180	873
Hispanic.....................	818	*180	20.6	*872	*0	*0	*150	*1,800
Non-Hispanic.................	21,993	55	14.7	374	0	0	180	871
Black........................	2,711	*107	15.7	*683	*0	*0	*60	*650
Other........................	*712	*115	*8.9	*1,301	*0	*0	*3,217	*3,217
Family dynamics								
Unchanging, full year........	22,570	45	14.6	308	0	0	175	822
Change in composition or existed less than full year.........	3,662	*195	16.2	*1,199	0	27	295	2,196
Poverty status in 1980								
Below 150 percent poverty level.......	9,379	102	19.4	527	0	0	183	1,354
Below poverty level..........	5,252	*76	17.7	*429	0	0	179	1,265
Poverty level to 149 percent........	4,128	*136	21.7	*628	0	0	225	1,416
150-199 percent..............	2,974	*65	13.2	*492	*0	*15	*180	*800
200-299 percent..............	5,563	*82	11.1	*744	*0	*12	*580	*1,484
300-499 percent..............	5,426	*18	13.6	*129	*0	*0	*50	*333
500 percent or more..........	2,891	*8	11.2	*73	*0	*0	*100	*207
Family income in 1980[2]								
Less than $10,000............	14,468	94	18.2	518	0	0	188	1,384
$10,000-$19,999..............	8,280	*42	10.6	*393	0	*0	140	873
$20,000-$34,999..............	2,664	*7	11.0	*62	*0	*0	*25	*400
$35,000 or more..............	820	*7	*11.5	*64	*0	*0	*102	*207
Education[3]								
None or elementary school....	4,782	*56	21.3	*264	0	0	143	624
Some high school.............	3,996	*149	17.5	*850	*0	*6	*183	*1,868
High school graduate.........	7,413	*79	13.7	*575	0	1	211	1,354
Some college.................	4,842	*28	11.9	*238	*0	*40	*223	*901
College graduate or more.....	5,122	*28	11.3	*251	*0	*0	*18	*400

Table 6—continued

Out-of-pocket expenditures for inpatient hospital care for 1-person families, by selected characteristics: United States, 1980

[Rate per family year. Civilian noninstitutionalized population with civilian family head]

Characteristic	All families		Families with discharges					
	Number in thousands	Mean expenditures	Percent	Mean expenditures	Expenditures at selected percentiles			
					25th	50th	75th	90th
Employment status[4]								
Worked full year................	10,374	*$10	7.7	*$135	*$0	*$0	*$25	*$328
Worked part year................	7,129	*137	14.7	*928	0	18	223	1,800
Never worked....................	8,703	75	23.5	317	0	0	180	873
Perceived health status[5]								
Excellent.......................	11,226	*37	9.5	*389	0	0	73	1,384
Good............................	9,642	*85	13.0	*653	0	0	213	696
Fair............................	3,691	*59	25.5	232	0	0	180	767
Poor............................	1,568	*177	38.9	*456	*0	*0	*188	*1,484
Limitation in usual activity								
None............................	21,977	36	11.2	320	0	0	150	799
Some limitation.................	731	*109	27.1	*403	*0	*172	*822	*1,354
Cannot perform usual activity...	3,525	*244	34.7	*703	0	0	180	873
Bed days[2]								
0...............................	12,629	*1	*1.2	*91	*0	*0	*150	*211
1–5.............................	6,587	*4	9.4	*47	*0	*0	*18	*183
6–10............................	2,671	*95	28.3	*335	0	0	183	1,265
11–20...........................	1,924	*269	42.6	*632	0	15	352	1,416
More than 20....................	2,422	378	63.9	592	0	0	188	1,800
Family health care coverage								
All members covered full year...	20,491	46	16.3	284	0	0	140	696
Private insurance only..........	10,523	*17	9.1	*190	0	0	97	333
Medicaid only...................	*317	*0	*25.1	*0	*0	*0	*0	*0
Medicare only...................	1,262	*114	15.9	*717	*0	*180	*871	*2,668
Medicare and other public programs.....	993	*35	25.7	*137	*0	*0	*0	*180
Medicare and private insurance.....	4,819	*92	25.6	*358	0	0	180	767
Other public and private mixes.....	1,361	*77	19.6	*394	*0	*15	*40	*799
Other mixes of public programs.....	*186	*0	*8.5	*0	*0	*0	*0	*0
Source unknown..................	1,030	*40	32.1	*125	*0	*0	*0	*180

All members covered, some part year.....	3,223	*52	10.9	*475	*0	*0	*432	*1,985
Some members not covered............	*24	*3,222	*100.0	*3,222	*0	*0	*7,144	*7,144
All members not covered..............	2,495	*216	*7.3	*2,966	*150	*394	*1,416	*9,220

1There were too few Hispanic families of races other than white for separate tabulation.
2Annual rate.
3Includes only families with heads 17 years of age and over.
4Excludes families with all members under 14 years of age.
5Excludes families with all members with health status unknown.

NOTE: 1-person families are families with average size less than 1.5. For 1-person families with more than 1 distinct individual, characteristics are those of head or of family as in Table 1.

Table 7

Out-of-pocket expenditures for inpatient hospital care for 1-person families under 65 years of age, by selected characteristics:
United States, 1980

[Rate per family year. Civilian noninstitutionalized population with civilian family head]

Characteristic	All families		Families with discharges					
					Expenditures at selected percentiles			
	Number in thousands	Mean expenditures	Percent	Mean expenditures	25th	50th	75th	90th
Total..............	18,519	*$55	11.2	$494	$0	$0	$150	$1,354
Age								
Under 25 years......	5,208	*36	8.7	*406	*0	*0	*66	*901
25-44 years.........	7,630	*78	11.7	*672	*0	*18	*140	*1,354
45-64 years.........	5,680	*43	12.9	*333	*0	*0	*180	*1,446
Sex								
Male................	10,082	*39	9.7	*405	0	0	50	1,868
Female..............	8,437	*75	13.0	*573	0	0	213	799
Race and ethnicity[1]								
White...............	15,786	*42	10.8	*386	0	0	145	799
Hispanic............	680	*216	*15.3	*1,413	*0	*0	*1,800	*6,500
Non-Hispanic........	15,106	*34	10.6	*319	0	0	111	616
Black...............	2,128	*135	15.6	*861	*0	*0	*35	*1,354
Other...............	*605	*136	*6.6	*2,067	*0	*3,217	*3,217	*3,217
Family dynamics								
Unchanging, full year......	15,487	*45	11.7	*381	0	0	100	901
Change in composition or existed less than full year......	3,032	*110	8.7	*1,273	*0	*89	*432	*1,950
Poverty status in 1980								
Below 150 percent..........	5,181	*132	16.0	*826	*0	*0	*223	*1,800
Below poverty level........	3,031	*109	18.2	*600	*0	*0	*183	*1,446
Poverty level to 149 percent......	2,149	*164	12.9	*1,275	*0	*0	*1,354	*1,985
150-199 percent...........	1,855	*72	9.7	*738	*0	*35	*330	*799
200-299 percent...........	4,250	*32	7.7	*410	*0	*12	*145	*2,196
300-499 percent...........	4,643	*13	10.9	*118	*0	*0	*50	*328
500 percent or more.......	2,590	*6	9.0	*66	*0	*0	*18	*400
Family income in 1980[2]								
Less than $10,000.........	8,222	*113	14.9	*760	0	0	223	1,868
$10,000-$19,999...........	7,113	*11	7.8	*143	*0	*0	*73	*333
$20,000-$34,999...........	2,529	*6	10.4	*61	*0	*0	*25	*400
$35,000 or more...........	*656	*0	*4.9	*0	*0	*0	*0	*0

Education[3]

None or elementary school	1,770	*7	14.6	*51	*0	*0	*0	*0
Some high school	2,546	*216	15.4	*1,396	*0	*15	*432	*1,985
High school graduate	5,759	*44	12.5	*353	*0	*0	*111	*1,354
Some college	4,037	*21	9.1	*226	*0	*40	*223	*901
College graduate or more	4,329	*29	7.8	*376	*0	*0	*27	*1,950

Employment status[4]

Worked full year	9,963	*10	7.3	*141	*0	*0	*25	*328
Worked part year	6,265	*116	14.0	*826	0	25	223	1,800
Never worked	2,264	*87	20.6	*421	*0	*0	*180	*1,446

Perceived health status[5]

Excellent	8,913	*37	7.4	*498	*0	*0	*73	*1,800
Good	6,852	*69	9.7	*711	*0	*0	*213	*616
Fair	1,866	*43	24.3	*177	*0	*0	*97	*432
Poor	803	*177	34.5	*513	*0	*0	*333	*1,868

Limitation in usual activity

None	16,928	*36	9.8	*366	0	0	145	616
Some limitation	*209	*142	*10.5	*1,354	*1,354	*1,354	*1,354	*1,354
Cannot perform usual activity	1,383	*282	28.7	*984	*0	*0	*140	*1,868

Bed days[2]

0	8,291	*0	*1.2	*30	*0	*0	*25	*150
1-5	5,721	*2	6.9	*24	*0	*0	*10	*89
6-10	2,013	*85	21.4	*396	*0	*0	*197	*400
11-20	1,222	*291	34.4	*845	*0	*0	*213	*901
More than 20	1,273	*383	57.6	*665	*0	*0	*394	*1,950

Family health care coverage

All members covered full year	12,974	*26	12.0	*218	*0	*0	40	447
Private insurance only	10,511	*17	8.9	*190	*0	*0	89	333
Medicaid only	*317	*0	*25.1	*0	*0	*0	*0	*0
Medicare only	*108	*187	*12.9	*1,446	*1,446	*1,446	*1,446	*1,446
Medicare and other public programs	—	—	—	—	—	—	—	—
Medicare and private insurance	—	—	—	—	—	—	—	—
Other public and private mixes	1,361	*77	19.6	*394	*15	*15	*40	*799
Other mixes of public programs	*186	*0	*8.5	*0	*0	*0	*0	*0
Source unknown	*491	*75	*50.3	*148	*0	*0	*0	*180
All members covered, some part year	3,223	*52	10.9	*475	*0	*0	*432	*1,985
Some members not covered	—	—	—	—	—	—	—	—
All members not covered	2,322	*224	*7.0	*3,202	*150	*330	*1,416	*9,220

[1]There were too few Hispanic of races other than white families for separate tabulation.
[2]Annual rate.
[3]Includes only families with heads 17 years of age and over.
[4]Excludes families with all members under 14 years of age.
[5]Excludes families with all members with health status unknown.

NOTE: 1-person families are families with average size less than 1.5. For 1-person families with more than 1 distinct individual, characteristics are those of head or of family as in Table 2.

Table 8

Out-of-pocket expenditures for inpatient hospital care for 1-person families under 65 years of age with health care coverage all year, by selected characteristics: United States, 1980

[Rate per family year. Civilian noninstitutionalized population with civilian family head]

| Characteristic | All families | | Families with discharges | | | | | |
| | Number in thousands | Mean expenditures | Percent | Mean expenditures | Expenditures at selected percentiles | | | |
					25th	50th	75th	90th
Total...............	12,974	*$26	12.0	*$218	$0	$0	$40	$447
Age								
Under 25 years............	3,166	*8	10.0	*76	*0	*0	*0	*179
25-44 years............	5,206	*34	12.3	*278	*0	*10	*97	*400
45-64 years............	4,601	*30	13.2	*228	*0	*0	*36	*650
Sex								
Male............	6,807	*25	11.1	*226	*0	*0	*35	*333
Female............	6,167	*28	13.1	*210	*0	*0	*89	*650
Race and ethnicity[1]								
White............	11,183	*22	11.5	*188	0	0	50	400
Hispanic............	*400	*0	*13.1	*0	*0	*0	*0	*0
Non-Hispanic............	10,782	*22	11.4	*196	0	0	66	400
Black............	1,428	*12	16.8	*68	*0	*0	*0	*197
Other............	*363	*226	*10.9	*2,067	*0	*3,217	*3,217	*3,217
Family dynamics								
Unchanging, full year......	11,017	*27	12.8	*208	0	0	35	400
Change in composition or existed less than full year......	1,957	*24	7.9	*301	*0	*66	*180	*1,950
Poverty status in 1980								
Below 150 percent............	2,775	*54	18.8	*284	*0	*0	*0	*650
Below poverty level............	1,638	*70	23.6	*295	*0	*0	*0	*650
Poverty level to 149 percent............	1,137	*30	*12.0	*252	*0	*0	*25	*1,868
150-199 percent............	1,072	*15	*11.1	*131	*0	*15	*36	*799
200-299 percent............	2,997	*36	9.6	*374	*0	*12	*145	*901
300-499 percent............	3,918	*15	11.8	*128	*0	*0	*73	*333
500 percent or more............	2,212	*4	7.7	*54	*0	*0	*18	*400
Family income in 1980[2]								
Less than $10,000............	4,620	*54	17.7	*307	*0	*0	*36	*799
$10,000-$19,999............	5,656	*14	9.8	*143	*0	*0	*73	*333
$20,000-$34,999............	2,114	*4	8.2	*53	*0	*0	*18	*100
$35,000 or more............	*584	*0	*2.6	*0	*0	*0	*0	*0

54

Education[3]

Characteristic							
None or elementary school	1,328	*10	19.5	*51	*0	*0	*0	*0
Some high school	1,538	*81	14.5	*560	*0	*12	*179	*1,868
High school graduate	4,047	*9	12.1	*73	*0	*0	*36	*145
Some college	2,830	*14	10.7	*131	*0	*35	*197	*333
College graduate or more	3,201	*40	9.0	*440	*0	*0	*97	*1,950

Employment status[4]

Worked full year	7,649	*10	8.3	*115	*0	*0	*25	*328
Worked part year	3,554	*28	13.7	*207	*0	*0	*40	*197
Never worked	1,769	*94	24.9	*377	*0	*0	*180	*1,446

Perceived health status[5]

Excellent	6,353	*9	6.8	*138	*0	*0	*18	*328
Good	4,537	*28	10.8	*260	*0	*0	*100	*447
Fair	1,425	*8	25.3	*30	*0	*0	*27	*145
Poor	*572	*249	*45.6	*545	*0	*0	*650	*1,868

Limitation in usual activity

None	11,652	*16	10.3	*159	0	0	40	333
Some limitation	*127	*0	*0.0	–	–	–	–	–
Cannot perform usual activity	1,195	*125	30.7	*407	*0	*0	*140	*1,446

Bed days[2]

0	5,669	0	*1.0	*0	*0	*0	*0	*0
1-5	4,146	*2	6.9	*34	*0	*0	*18	*100
6-10	1,247	*18	24.5	*73	*0	*0	*140	*333
11-20	984	*117	36.1	*326	*0	*0	*40	*901
More than 20	928	*208	60.6	*342	*0	*0	*97	*1,446

Family health care coverage

Private insurance only	10,511	*17	8.9	*190	0	0	89	333
Medicaid only	*317	*0	*25.1	*0	*0	*0	*0	*0
Medicare only	*108	*187	*12.9	*1,446	*1,446	*1,446	*1,446	*1,446
Medicare and other public programs	–	–	–	–	–	–	–	–
Medicare and private insurance	–	–	–	–	–	–	–	–
Other public and private mixes	1,361	*77	19.6	*394	*0	*15	*40	*799
Other mixes of public programs	*186	*0	*8.5	*0	*0	*0	*0	*0
Source unknown	*491	*75	*50.3	*148	*0	*0	*0	*180

[1]There were too few Hispanic families of races other than white for separate tabulation.
[2]Annual rate.
[3]Includes only families with heads 17 years of age and over.
[4]Excludes families with all members under 14 years of age.
[5]Excludes families with all members with health status unknown.

NOTE: 1-person families are families with average size less than 1.5. For 1-person families with more than 1 distinct individual, characteristics are those of head or of family as in Table 2.

Table 9

Out-of-pocket expenditures for inpatient hospital care for 1-person families under 65 years of age without health care coverage all year, by selected characteristics: United States, 1980

[Rate per family year. Civilian noninstitutionalized population with civilian family head]

Characteristic	All families			Families with discharges				
						Expenditures at selected percentiles		
	Number in thousands	Mean expenditures	Percent	Mean expenditures	25th	50th	75th	90th
Total....................	5,545	*$124	9.3	*$1,336	*$0	*$111	*$616	*$2,196
Age								
Under 25 years..........	2,042	*79	*6.8	*1,162	*0	*223	*1,416	*6,500
25-44 years.............	2,424	*173	*10.2	*1,689	*0	*111	*330	*1,354
45-64 years.............	1,079	*98	*11.8	*835	*0	*240	*1,800	*1,985
Sex								
Male....................	3,275	*69	6.8	*1,013	*0	*25	*1,800	*3,326
Female..................	2,270	*203	12.8	*1,584	*0	*183	*616	*2,196
Race and ethnicity[1]								
White...................	4,603	*90	9.1	*989	*0	*150	*432	*3,326
Hispanic................	*280	*525	*18.5	*2,840	*150	*1,800	*6,500	*6,500
Non-Hispanic............	4,323	*62	8.5	*729	*0	*25	*394	*2,196
Black...................	*700	*386	*13.3	*2,909	*0	*0	*1,354	*1,985
Other...................	*242	*0	*0.0	-	-	-	-	-
Family dynamics								
Unchanging, full year...	4,470	*89	9.1	*982	*0	*111	*616	*1,985
Change in composition or existed less than full year..............	1,075	*268	*10.0	*2,668	*0	*223	*1,416	*3,326
Poverty status in 1980								
Below 150 percent.......	2,405	*222	12.7	*1,757	*0	*183	*1,354	*1,985
Below poverty level.....	1,394	*156	*11.8	*1,317	*0	*183	*616	*9,220
Poverty level to 149 percent....	1,012	*314	*13.8	*2,276	*0	*223	*1,416	*1,985
150-199 percent.........	784	*150	*7.8	*1,919	*240	*330	*6,500	*6,500
200-299 percent.........	1,253	*22	*3.3	*662	*0	*111	*2,196	*2,196
300-499 percent.........	*725	*1	*6.1	*15	*0	*25	*25	*25
500 percent or more.....	*379	*17	*16.6	*100	*0	*0	*0	*432
Family income in 1980[2]								
Less than $10,000.......	3,602	*189	11.3	*1,672	*0	*223	*1,416	*3,326
$10,000-$19,999.........	1,457	0	0.0	-	-	-	-	-
$20,000-$34,999.........	*415	*17	*21.8	*77	*0	*0	*25	*432
$35,000 or more.........	*71	*0	*23.6	*0	*0	*0	*0	*0

Education[3]								
None or elementary school.........	*443	*0	*0.0	-	-	-	-	-
Some high school..................	1,008	*421	16.9	*2,488	*0	*150	*1,416	*9,220
High school graduate..............	1,713	*127	13.4	*952	*0	*111	*1,354	*3,326
Some college......................	1,208	*36	*5.3	*675	*223	*240	*1,800	*1,800
College graduate or more..........	1,127	0	*4.4	*0	*0	*0	*0	*0
Employment status[4]								
Worked full year..................	2,314	*13	*4.2	*309	*0	*0	*0	*1,985
Worked part year..................	2,711	*231	14.4	*1,599	*0	*223	*1,354	*2,196
Never worked......................	*495	*61	*5.1	*1,196	*0	*0	*3,326	*3,326
Perceived health status[5]								
Excellent.........................	2,559	*105	8.8	*1,191	*0	*25	*1,800	*2,196
Good..............................	2,314	*150	*7.7	*1,942	*0	*150	*394	*6,500
Fair..............................	*441	*158	*21.0	*752	*0	*240	*1,354	*1,354
Poor..............................	*231	*0	*7.0	*0	*0	*0	*0	*0
Limitation in usual activity								
None..............................	5,276	*79	8.8	*899	*0	*111	*432	*1,985
Some limitation...................	*82	*363	*26.8	*1,354	*1,354	*1,354	*1,354	*1,354
Cannot perform usual activity.....	*188	*1,279	*15.5	*8,231	*0	*0	*3,326	*53,732
Bed days[2]								
0.................................	2,622	*1	*1.6	*70	*25	*25	*150	*150
1-5...............................	1,575	0	*7.0	*0	*0	*0	*0	*0
6-10..............................	766	*194	*16.5	*1,176	*0	*183	*1,354	*6,500
11-20.............................	*237	*1,010	*27.3	*3,693	*0	*432	*616	*1,416
More than 20......................	*345	*855	*49.4	*1,731	*0	*394	*1,985	*9,220
Family health care coverage								
All members covered, some part year.....	3,223	*52	10.9	*475	*0	*0	*432	*1,985
Some members not covered..........	-	-	-	-	-	-	-	-
All members not covered...........	2,322	*224	*7.0	*3,202	*150	*330	*1,416	*9,220

[1] There were too few Hispanic families of races other than white for separate tabulation.
[2] Annual rate.
[3] Includes only families with heads 17 years of age and over.
[4] Excludes families with all members under 14 years of age.
[5] Excludes families with all members with health status unknown.

NOTE: 1-person families are families with average size less than 1.5. For 1-person families with more than 1 distinct individual, characteristics are those of head or of family as in Table 2.

Table 10

Out-of-pocket expenditures for inpatient hospital care for 1-person families 65 years of age and over, by selected characteristics: United States, 1980

[Rate per family year. Civilian noninstitutionalized population with civilian family head]

Characteristic	All families		Families with discharges					
	Number in thousands	Mean expenditures	Percent	Mean expenditures	Expenditures at selected percentiles			
					25th	50th	75th	90th
Total........................	7,714	$91	23.5	$388	$0	$0	$180	$871
Sex								
Male........................	1,784	*58	30.5	*189	*0	*0	*180	*355
Female......................	5,930	101	21.4	473	0	0	183	1,265
Race and ethnicity[1]								
White.......................	7,025	100	24.2	412	0	0	188	873
Hispanic....................	*138	*0	*46.9	*0	*0	*0	*0	*0
Non-Hispanic................	6,887	102	23.7	428	0	0	207	1,129
Black.......................	582	*8	*16.0	*47	*0	*12	*102	*143
Other.......................	*106	*0	*21.9	*0	*0	*0	*0	*0
Family dynamics								
Unchanging, full year.......	7,083	46	20.9	219	0	0	180	822
Change in composition or existed less than full year......	630	*601	52.7	*1,141	*0	*12	*207	*4,061
Poverty status in 1980								
Below 150 percent poverty level......	4,199	*66	23.7	*279	0	0	180	696
Below poverty level.........	2,220	*30	17.0	*179	0	*0	*102	*391
Poverty level to 149 percent......	1,979	*106	31.3	*339	0	0	188	767
150-199 percent.............	1,118	*54	19.0	*283	*0	*0	*159	*800
200-299 percent.............	1,313	*246	21.9	*1,124	*0	*180	*871	*1,484
300-499 percent.............	783	*45	29.4	*152	*0	*0	*83	*873
500 percent or more.........	*300	*27	30.1	*90	*0	*1	*172	*207
Family income in 1980[2]								
Less than $10,000...........	6,246	69	22.5	306	0	0	183	871
$10,000-$19,999.............	1,167	227	27.3	831	*0	*0	*180	*1,129
$20,000-$34,999.............	*136	*15	*20.9	*72	*0	*0	*172	*172
$35,000 or more.............	*165	37	*37.6	*98	*0	*1	*102	*207

Education

None or elementary school	3,012	*85	25.3	*336	0	0	180	871
Some high school	1,451	*31	21.0	*146	*0	*0	*24	*696
High school graduate	1,653	*200	17.9	*1,114	*6	*180	*800	*1,789
Some college	804	*68	26.1	*259	*0	*36	*352	*1,129
College graduate or more	793	*23	30.5	*77	*0	*0	*0	*83

Employment status

Worked full year	*411	*9	*15.3	*61	*6	*0	*27	*265
Worked part year	863	*286	19.7	*1,454	*0	*0	*211	*1,789
Never worked	6,439	70	24.6	286	0	0	180	871

Perceived health status[3]

Excellent	2,313	38	17.7	*213	*0	*0	*32	*1,129
Good	2,790	*123	21.0	*586	*0	*0	*225	*873
Fair	1,825	*76	26.8	*282	*0	*0	*207	*871
Poor	765	*177	43.5	*408	*0	*0	*180	*800

Limitation in usual activity

None	5,049	*36	16.1	226	0	*0	175	1,129
Some limitation	*523	*97	*33.8	*286	*0	*0	*295	*1,322
Cannot perform usual activity	2,142	*219	38.6	568	0	1	183	871

Bed days[2]

0	4,338	*3	*1.3	*199	*0	*175	*211	*580
1-5	867	*23	25.7	*88	*0	*6	*180	*265
6-10	658	124	49.1	*253	*0	*0	*159	*1,322
11-20	702	*232	56.9	*407	*0	*24	*352	*1,660
More than 20	1,149	*373	70.9	*526	0	0	180	800

Family health care coverage

All members covered full year	7,517	*81	23.6	*343	0	0	180	822
Private insurance only	*13	*207	100.0	*207	*207	*207	*207	*207
Medicaid only	–	–	–	–	–	–	–	–
Medicare only	1,154	*107	16.1	*662	*0	*180	*871	*2,668
Medicare and other public programs	993	*35	25.7	*137	*0	*0	*0	*180
Medicare and private insurance	4,819	*92	25.6	*358	0	0	180	767
Other public and private mixes	–	–	–	–	–	–	–	–
Other mixes of public programs	–	–	–	–	–	–	–	–
Source unknown	*538	*8	*15.6	*54	*0	*0	*102	*183
All members covered, some part year	–	–	–	–	–	–	–	–
Some members not covered	*24	*3,222	*100.0	*3,222	*0	*0	*7,144	*7,144
All members not covered	*172	*108	*11.1	*973	*353	*1,322	*1,322	*1,322

[1]There were too few Hispanic families of races other than white for separate tabulation.
[2]Annual rate.
[3]Excludes families with all members with health status unknown.

NOTE: 1-person families are families with average size less than 1.5. For 1-person families with more than 1 distinct individual, characteristics are those of head or of family as in Table 5.

59

Table 11

Out-of-pocket expenditures for inpatient physician care for multiple-person families, by selected characteristics: United States, 1980

[Rate per family year. Civilian noninstitutionalized population with civilian family head]

Characteristic	All families			Families with care				
	Number in thousands	Mean expenditures	Percent	Mean expenditures	Expenditures at selected percentiles			
					25th	50th	75th	90th
Total......................	58,135	$40	23.8	$167	$0	$43	$192	$452
Family size[1]								
2 persons.................	22,916	42	21.6	193	0	52	202	561
3 persons.................	12,567	38	24.0	159	0	62	210	441
4 persons.................	12,269	35	23.8	147	0	27	150	370
5 or more persons.........	10,383	43	28.3	153	0	30	174	385
Age of head								
Under 25 years............	4,308	26	23.6	108	0	16	110	334
25-44 years...............	25,173	34	22.4	150	0	30	178	394
45-64 years...............	20,129	40	22.4	179	0	41	192	433
65 years and over.........	8,525	65	31.4	206	0	71	239	601
Sex of head								
Male......................	44,874	41	24.7	166	0	50	194	442
Female....................	13,262	36	20.6	174	0	0	180	480
Race and ethnicity[2] of head								
White.....................	51,015	41	24.6	168	0	45	190	440
Hispanic	3,403	*44	19.9	*223	0	38	225	437
Non-Hispanic..............	47,613	41	24.9	164	0	45	185	440
Black.....................	6,090	27	17.7	153	0	25	198	526
Other.....................	1,030	*48	20.7	*232	*0	*74	*304	*388
Family structure								
Head and spouse present whole time......	42,556	39	24.7	157	0	50	190	432
Child under 17 years.....	22,442	40	26.0	153	0	43	183	378
No child under 17 years.....	20,114	38	23.3	163	0	60	202	475
Head only, no spouse at any time......	13,977	38	19.8	190	0	0	180	581
Child under 17 years.....	8,643	28	19.3	145	0	0	96	526
No child under 17 years.....	5,334	*53	20.6	*259	0	40	248	747
Other.....................	1,602	85	34.9	*244	*0	*45	*260	*744
Family dynamics								
Unchanging, full year.....	46,990	33	21.3	156	0	36	164	396
Change in composition or existed less than full year..............	11,145	68	34.2	197	0	60	240	645

Family poverty status in 1980							
Below 150 percent poverty level	10,938	29	22.2	130	0	0	120	385
Below poverty level	6,047	12	19.3	63	0	0	38	256
Poverty level to 149 percent	4,892	49	25.8	191	0	45	202	516
150-199 percent	6,355	56	24.1	233	0	75	273	688
200-299 percent	12,860	42	26.2	160	0	64	178	378
300-499 percent	17,047	44	23.7	184	0	57	200	529
500 percent or more	10,935	33	22.5	148	0	34	200	394
Family income in 1980[3]							
Less than $10,000	10,629	28	20.9	135	0	1	130	426
$10,000-$19,999	16,728	54	25.2	213	0	74	220	558
$20,000-$34,999	19,706	38	23.3	161	0	50	176	410
$35,000 or more	11,073	34	25.3	134	0	24	189	393
Education of head[4]							
None or elementary school	10,491	49	26.9	182	0	60	248	558
Some high school	9,267	41	23.2	174	0	38	194	584
High school graduate	20,605	38	24.0	157	0	20	161	427
Some college	8,651	30	21.2	143	0	60	180	333
College graduate or more	9,099	43	22.9	187	0	62	225	410
Family employment status[5]							
2 or more persons worked full year	14,607	29	21.0	138	0	33	160	348
Only 1 person worked full year	24,549	38	22.6	166	0	52	196	475
Some part-year work	11,303	42	26.2	161	0	29	201	461
No person worked	7,676	64	29.4	219	0	45	185	558
Worst perceived health status of any family member[6]							
Excellent	16,200	18	16.9	109	0	30	159	300
Good	24,467	35	22.5	155	0	52	193	396
Fair	11,131	54	28.1	191	0	28	177	529
Poor	6,318	90	39.0	231	0	55	256	715
Most severe limitation in usual activity of any family member							
None	43,941	29	19.8	147	0	42	190	393
Some limitation	3,679	*45	29.8	149	0	0	130	365
Cannot perform usual activity	10,515	83	38.4	216	0	50	219	687
Family's bed days[3]							
0	11,173	*3	*1.0	*281	*0	*125	*225	*1,652
1-5	14,527	17	13.1	126	0	50	162	391
6-10	8,834	24	24.2	97	0	18	118	260
11-20	9,982	38	32.1	118	0	20	120	385
More than 20	13,619	107	47.5	225	0	60	250	649

Table 11—continued

Out-of-pocket expenditures for inpatient physician care for multiple-person families, by selected characteristics: United States, 1980

[Rate per family year. Civilian noninstitutionalized population with civilian family head]

Characteristic	All families		Families with care					
	Number in thousands	Mean expenditures	Percent	Mean expenditures	Expenditures at selected percentiles			
					25th	50th	75th	90th
Family health care coverage								
All members covered full year..........	42,453	$38	24.5	$153	$0	$35	$175	$393
Private insurance only................	25,759	32	23.0	137	0	43	165	353
Medicaid only........................	1,621	*2	16.5	*10	*0	*0	*0	*0
Medicare only.......................	*574	*30	*19.3	*157	*71	*130	*239	*385
Medicare and other public programs....	*471	*19	*24.9	*75	*0	*0	*45	*70
Medicare and private insurance........	7,475	62	33.4	184	0	55	202	538
Other public and private mixes........	5,853	34	21.9	158	0	24	160	459
Other mixes of public programs........	*135	*5	*16.8	*27	*23	*30	*30	*30
Source unknown......................	*564	*164	*36.3	*453	*0	*0	*68	*3,256
All members covered, some part year.....	8,669	38	23.9	159	0	35	192	520
Some members not covered	4,963	65	24.0	272	0	116	305	755
All members not covered	2,051	*33	7.6	*436	*174	*432	*649	*678

[1]Average size during period of family's existence rounded to nearest integer; exactly half an integer rounded upward.
[2]There were too few Hispanic families of races other than white for separate tabulation.
[3]Annual rate.
[4]Includes only families with heads 17 years of age and over.
[5]Excludes families with all members under 14 years of age.
[6]Excludes families with all members with health status unknown.

NOTE: Multiple-person families are families with average size 1.5 or greater.

Table 12

Out-of-pocket expenditures for inpatient physician care for multiple-person families with all members under 65 years of age, by selected characteristics: United States, 1980

[Rate per family year. Civilian noninstitutionalized population with civilian family head]

Characteristic	All families		Families with care					
	Number in thousands	Mean expenditures	Percent	Mean expenditures	Expenditures at selected percentiles			
					25th	50th	75th	90th
Total...............	47,327	$435	21.8	$159	$0	$36	$180	$426
Family size[1]								
2 persons..............	14,958	33	17.1	192	0	58	202	572
3 persons..............	11,228	32	22.3	142	0	54	200	394
4 persons..............	11,546	34	23.1	149	0	21	139	370
5 or more persons......	9,595	41	26.9	151	0	32	165	385
Age of head								
Under 25 years.........	4,283	26	23.7	108	0	16	110	334
25–44 years............	24,783	33	22.2	147	0	28	175	394
45–64 years............	18,261	39	20.7	189	0	52	200	440
Sex of head								
Male...................	36,477	35	22.8	153	0	41	178	410
Female.................	10,850	33	18.2	183	0	0	200	526
Race and ethnicity[2] of head								
White..................	41,444	36	22.4	160	0	38	180	427
Hispanic...............	3,040	*48	19.9	*242	*0	*76	*243	*517
Non-Hispanic...........	38,405	35	22.6	155	0	38	169	410
Black..................	5,064	22	17.3	126	0	20	130	385
Other..................	819	*46	18.0	*256	*0	*0	*250	*832
Family structure								
Head and spouse present whole time......	34,963	36	23.1	154	0	45	183	410
Child under 17 years......	21,668	38	25.6	150	0	40	174	378
No child under 17 years...	13,295	31	19.1	162	0	67	225	436
Head only, no spouse at any time...	11,169	*32	17.3	187	0	0	161	526
Child under 17 years......	8,258	27	18.0	150	0	0	96	581
No child under 17 years...	2,911	*47	15.1	*310	*0	*60	*248	*273
Other..................	1,194	*27	23.8	*113	*0	*0	*191	*260
Family dynamics								
Unchanging, full year.......	37,714	30	19.2	157	0	29	153	386
Change in composition or existed less than full year.......	9,613	52	31.7	163	0	56	217	475

Table 12—continued

Out-of-pocket expenditures for inpatient physician care for multiple-person families with all members under 65 years of age, by selected characteristics: United States, 1980

[Rate per family year. Civilian noninstitutionalized population with civilian family head]

| | All families | | | Families with care | | | | | |
| | | | | | Expenditures at selected percentiles | | | | |
Characteristic	Number in thousands	Mean expenditures	Percent	Mean expenditures	25th	50th	75th	90th
Family poverty status in 1980								
Below 150 percent poverty level	8,770	$23	20.4	$114	$0	$0	$85	$371
Below poverty level	5,083	*10	18.8	55	0	0	0	209
Poverty level to 149 percent	3,687	*41	22.6	181	0	45	190	459
150-199 percent	4,825	54	22.4	238	0	60	269	715
200-299 percent	10,075	33	22.8	145	0	50	160	260
300-499 percent	14,307	39	22.3	174	0	52	200	515
500 percent or more	9,350	31	20.8	147	0	36	210	394
Family income in 1980[3]								
Less than $10,000	7,496	16	18.3	89	0	0	74	370
$10,000-$19,999	12,555	50	21.4	233	0	66	225	678
$20,000-$34,999	17,279	32	22.3	145	0	41	150	368
$35,000 or more	9,997	33	23.9	138	0	36	200	393
Education of head[4]								
None or elementary school	5,822	41	21.9	185	0	36	248	561
Some high school	7,546	35	21.1	167	0	37	189	610
High school graduate	18,299	32	22.7	142	0	16	130	371
Some college	7,556	25	20.0	125	0	60	166	315
College graduate or more	8,084	43	21.7	199	0	64	225	440
Family employment status[5]								
2 or more persons worked full year	13,629	26	19.9	131	0	33	135	322
Only 1 person worked full year	21,782	37	22.2	165	0	54	193	441
Some part-year work	9,021	38	24.4	156	0	20	200	459
No person worked	2,896	*47	19.5	*243	*0	*0	*38	*526
Worst perceived health status of any family member[6]								
Excellent	14,771	17	16.7	102	0	30	159	288
Good	20,837	31	21.6	143	0	40	191	380
Fair	8,021	56	26.0	216	0	41	250	612
Poor	3,678	*79	34.0	233	0	33	180	715

Most severe limitation in usual activity of any family member

	1	2	3	4	5	6	7	8
None.........	39,751	28	19.7	144	0	38	183	393
Some limitation......	2,814	*44	30.3	*144	0	0	105	273
Cannot perform usual activity......	4,762	82	34.2	238	0	45	208	715
Family's bed days[3]								
0.........	7,825	*2	*1.2	*134	*0	*125	*225	*510
1-5.........	12,427	16	11.3	139	0	40	190	500
6-10.........	7,470	21	20.3	102	0	25	132	260
11-20.........	8,884	34	29.9	114	0	10	110	385
More than 20.........	10,722	90	43.3	209	0	50	225	520
Family health care coverage								
All members covered full year.........	33,575	32	22.3	145	0	26	150	365
Private insurance only.........	25,502	31	22.6	139	0	45	175	365
Medicaid only.........	1,606	0	15.7	*0	*0	*0	*0	*0
Medicare only.........	-	-	-	-	-	-	-	-
Medicare and other public programs.........	*12	*0	*0.0	-	-	-	-	-
Medicare and private insurance.........	*95	*32	26.3	*121	*10	*225	*225	*225
Other public and private mixes.........	5,762	34	22.0	157	0	20	150	459
Other mixes of public programs.........	*135	*5	*16.8	*27	*23	*30	*30	*30
Source unknown.........	*463	*187	*35.9	*520	*0	*0	*68	*3,256
All members covered, some part year.........	7,968	35	23.2	152	0	30	160	500
Some members not covered.........	3,804	54	21.3	251	0	113	305	721
All members not covered.........	1,980	*31	7.4	*423	*174	*426	*600	*678

[1] Average size during period of family's existence rounded to nearest integer; exactly half an integer rounded upward.
[2] There were too few Hispanic families of races other than white for separate tabulation.
[3] Annual rate.
[4] Includes only families with heads 17 years of age and over.
[5] Excludes families with all members under 14 years of age.
[6] Excludes families with all members with health status unknown.

NOTE: Multiple-person families are families with average size 1.5 or greater.

Table 13

Out-of-pocket expenditures for inpatient physician care for multiple-person families with all members under 65 years of age and all members with health care coverage all year, by selected characteristics: United States, 1980

[Rate per family year. Civilian noninstitutionalized population with civilian family head]

Characteristic	All families			Families with care				
	Number in thousands	Mean expenditures	Percent	Mean expenditures	Expenditures at selected percentiles			
					25th	50th	75th	90th
Total.................	33,575	$32	22.3	$145	$0	$26	$150	$365
Family size[1]								
2 persons.................	10,994	36	18.4	196	0	56	193	561
3 persons.................	8,010	26	21.9	119	0	50	180	320
4 persons.................	8,464	34	24.9	138	0	10	124	327
5 or more persons.........	6,107	32	26.5	120	0	17	129	240
Age of head								
Under 25 years...........	2,585	20	22.4	89	0	13	95	328
25-44 years..............	18,256	29	23.1	127	0	20	150	308
45-64 years..............	12,733	40	21.2	186	0	41	185	433
Sex of head								
Male......................	27,351	34	23.5	145	0	33	159	373
Female....................	6,224	*25	17.3	*146	0	0	90	300
Race and ethnicity[2] of head								
White.....................	29,902	34	23.1	145	0	28	153	366
Hispanic.................	1,711	*54	25.0	*217	*0	*76	*200	*433
Non-Hispanic.............	28,191	32	23.0	140	0	26	141	365
Black....................	3,139	*17	15.5	*111	*0	*17	*105	*249
Other....................	533	*62	*18.6	*332	*0	*0	*250	*1,721
Family structure								
Head and spouse present whole time......	26,517	34	23.6	144	0	33	160	368
Child under 17 years.....	16,251	36	26.0	140	0	30	159	320
No child under 17 years..	10,266	30	19.7	152	0	51	175	412
Head only, no spouse at any time......	6,394	*26	16.3	*161	*0	0	90	273
Child under 17 years.....	5,051	9	15.4	*57	*0	*0	*62	*200
No child under 17 years..	1,343	*92	19.6	*472	*26	*60	*250	*1,790
Other....................	663	*35	31.7	*110	*0	*0	*150	*260
Family dynamics								
Unchanging, full year.....	28,266	29	19.9	147	0	22	130	353
Change in composition or existed less than full year.....	5,308	49	35.4	139	0	54	200	412

	Col 1	Col 2	Col 3	Col 4	Col 5	Col 6	Col 7	Col 8
Family poverty status in 1980								
Below 150 percent poverty level	4,640	*24	22.6	*106	0	0	74	231
Below poverty level	2,919	*9	18.3	*49	*0	*0	*0	*150
Poverty level to 149 percent	1,721	*49	29.9	*165	*0	*25	*166	*275
150-199 percent	2,657	37	23.3	159	0	26	216	442
200-299 percent	7,074	*33	24.7	*132	0	50	125	227
300-499 percent	11,427	37	21.8	170	0	30	159	480
500 percent or more	7,776	29	20.5	142	0	20	201	397
Family income in 1980[3]								
Less than $10,000	4,023	*15	19.6	75	0	0	71	232
$10,000-$19,999	7,715	51	23.1	220	0	60	206	517
$20,000-$34,999	13,970	30	22.7	132	0	30	125	310
$35,000 or more	7,867	28	22.3	125	0	20	189	373
Education of head[4]								
None or elementary school	3,188	40	24.7	163	0	25	225	561
Some high school	4,620	20	21.1	95	0	20	122	273
High school graduate	13,366	32	22.6	142	0	6	112	310
Some college	5,757	25	20.7	120	0	41	165	315
College graduate or more	6,625	45	23.0	195	0	63	210	397
Family employment status[5]								
2 or more persons worked full year	10,347	25	19.5	126	0	20	109	348
Only 1 person worked full year	16,128	32	23.5	138	0	50	160	349
Some part-year work	4,933	39	26.6	146	0	1	168	442
No person worked	2,167	*56	17.8	*313	*0	*0	*75	*832
Worst perceived health status of any family member[6]								
Excellent	11,162	15	17.3	86	0	5	125	240
Good	15,029	30	22.3	136	0	45	180	320
Fair	5,209	52	27.3	192	0	26	150	486
Poor	2,155	*90	36.5	*248	0	24	150	461
Most severe limitation in usual activity of any family member								
None	28,461	24	20.3	120	0	29	143	310
Some limitation	2,067	*56	31.3	*180	*0	*0	*150	*459
Cannot perform usual activity	3,047	*91	35.2	*259	0	26	153	786
Family's bed days[3]								
0	5,766	*1	*1.2	*88	*0	*125	*143	*225
1-5	8,806	9	10.6	89	0	26	115	196
6-10	5,513	22	22.0	98	0	25	112	260
11-20	6,162	30	30.7	97	0	7	110	268
More than 20	7,328	95	46.3	206	0	39	220	486

Table 13—continued

Out-of-pocket expenditures for inpatient physician care for multiple-person families with all members under 65 years of age and all members with health care coverage all year, by selected characteristics: United States, 1980

[Rate per family year. Civilian noninstitutionalized population with civilian family head]

Characteristic	All families		Families with care		Expenditures at selected percentiles			
	Number in thousands	Mean expenditures	Percent	Mean expenditures	25th	50th	75th	90th
Family health care coverage								
Private insurance only................	25,502	$31	22.6	$139	$0	$45	$175	$365
Medicaid only........................	1,606	0	15.7	*0	*0	*0	*0	*0
Medicare only........................	-	-	-	-	-	-	-	-
Medicare and other public programs......	*12	*0	*0.0	-	-	-	-	-
Medicare and private insurance..........	*95	*32	*26.3	*121	*10	*225	*225	*225
Other public and private mixes..........	5,762	34	22.0	157	0	20	150	459
Other mixes of public programs..........	*135	*5	*16.8	*27	*23	*30	*30	*30
Source unknown........................	*463	*187	*35.9	*520	*0	*0	*68	*3,256

[1]Average size during period of family's existence rounded to nearest integer; exactly half an integer rounded upward.
[2]There were too few Hispanic families of races other than white for separate tabulation.
[3]Annual rate.
[4]Includes only families with heads 17 years of age and over.
[5]Excludes families with all members under 14 years of age.
[6]Excludes families with all members with health status unknown.

NOTE: Multiple-person families are families with average size 1.5 or greater.

Table 14

Out-of-pocket expenditures for inpatient physician care for multiple-person families with all members under 65 years of age and some or all members without health care coverage all year, by selected characteristics: United States, 1980

[Rate per family year. Civilian noninstitutionalized population with civilian family head]

Characteristic	All families			Families with care				
	Number in thousands	Mean expenditures	Percent	Mean expenditures	Expenditures at selected percentiles			
					25th	50th	75th	90th
Total...............	13,752	$40	20.4	$195	$0	$57	$245	$600
Family size[1]								
2 persons............	3,964	24	13.6	*180	*0	*102	*250	*600
3 persons............	3,218	*45	23.0	197	0	56	243	526
4 persons............	3,082	*35	18.2	*193	*0	*55	*225	*621
5 or more persons....	3,488	56	27.6	202	0	52	245	613
Age of head								
Under 25 years.......	1,698	35	25.6	*135	*0	*34	*208	*456
25-44 years..........	6,527	42	19.8	213	0	68	250	660
45-64 years..........	5,528	38	19.4	197	0	59	269	600
Sex of head								
Male.................	9,126	37	20.9	180	0	62	245	520
Female...............	4,627	*44	19.4	227	0	38	243	1,028
Race and ethnicity[2] of head								
White................	11,542	42	20.5	205	0	62	243	621
Hispanic.............	1,328	*40	13.3	*302	*0	*85	*396	*645
Non-Hispanic.........	10,214	42	21.4	197	0	62	240	621
Black................	1,924	*29	20.3	*144	*0	*30	*281	*526
Other................	*286	*17	*16.7	*99	*0	*40	*100	*304
Family structure								
Head and spouse present whole time......	8,446	41	21.7	187	0	75	250	520
Child under 17 years.......	5,417	44	24.4	182	0	65	245	510
No child under 17 years....	3,029	34	17.1	*200	*0	*120	*300	*520
Head only, no spouse at any time......	4,775	*40	18.6	216	0	22	240	1,028
Child under 17 years......	3,207	*56	22.2	*252	*0	*20	*385	*1,028
No child under 17 years...	1,568	*8	11.4	*72	*0	*36	*161	*210
Other................	*532	*17	*13.9	*121	*0	*0	*208	*428
Family dynamics								
Unchanging, full year.......	9,448	33	17.3	189	0	57	225	526
Change in composition or existed less than full year........	4,304	55	27.1	202	0	60	281	625

69

Table 14--continued

Out-of-pocket expenditures for inpatient physician care for multiple-person families with all members under 65 years of age and some or all members without health care coverage all year, by selected characteristics: United States, 1980

[Rate per family year. Civilian noninstitutionalized population with civilian family head]

Characteristic	All families		Families with care						
	Number in thousands	Mean expenditures	Percent	Mean expenditures	Expenditures at selected percentiles				
					25th	50th	75th	90th	
Family poverty status in 1980									
Below 150 percent poverty level........	4,130	$22	17.9	$125	$0	$17	$111	$428	
Below poverty level.............	2,164	*12	19.4	*63	*0	*0	*38	*370	
Poverty level to 149 percent....	1,966	*33	16.1	*207	*27	*85	*385	*590	
150-199 percent.................	2,168	*74	21.4	*345	*16	*113	*432	*1,085	
200-299 percent.................	3,000	*34	18.1	*188	*0	*68	*240	*625	
300-499 percent.................	2,880	46	24.6	188	0	71	300	600	
500 percent or more.............	1,574	*37	22.1	*168	*0	*56	*238	*300	
Family income in 1980[3]									
Less than $10,000...............	3,473	*18	16.8	*108	*0	*0	*90	*428	
$10,000-$19,999.................	4,840	48	18.6	257	0	80	269	1,028	
$20,000-$34,999.................	3,310	43	20.6	207	0	105	300	520	
$35,000 or more.................	2,130	51	29.7	*172	*0	*52	*238	*621	
Education of head[4]									
None or elementary school.......	2,634	*41	18.6	*221	*0	*59	*385	*432	
Some high school................	2,926	*60	21.1	*282	*0	*50	*520	*1,028	
High school graduate............	4,934	33	23.1	143	0	40	208	380	
Some college....................	1,800	*25	17.7	*143	*0	*100	*240	*300	
College graduate or more........	1,459	*37	16.2	*227	*36	*97	*238	*600	
Family employment status[5]									
2 or more persons worked full year......	3,282	31	21.1	147	0	71	238	322	
Only 1 person worked full year..........	5,654	49	18.5	263	0	85	360	1,028	
Some part-year work.....................	4,087	37	21.7	172	0	40	225	520	
No person worked........................	*729	*22	*24.4	*90	*0	*0	*38	*526	
Worst perceived health status of any family member[6]									
Excellent.......................	3,609	23	14.7	*159	*0	*73	*240	*510	
Good............................	5,808	32	19.6	163	0	35	225	526	
Fair............................	2,812	63	23.7	268	0	85	304	1,070	
Poor............................	1,524	*63	30.5	*207	*0	*38	*269	*825	

70

Most severe limitation in usual activity
  of any family member

None........................	11,290	38	18.1	209	0	66	258	613
Some limitation.............	747	*9	27.3	*33	*0	*0	*38	*105
Cannot perform usual activity..........	1,715	*65	32.4	*200	*0	*62	*225	*687

Family's bed days³

0............................	2,059	*3	*1.1	*282	*30	*510	*510	*510
1-5..........................	3,620	31	12.9	*239	*22	*208	*396	*613
6-10.........................	1,957	*18	15.4	*118	*0	*57	*145	*269
11-20........................	2,722	44	28.1	157	0	22	200	526
More than 20.................	3,394	80	36.7	218	0	60	240	721

Family health care coverage

All members covered, some part year.....	7,968	35	23.2	152	0	30	160	500
Some members not covered........	3,804	54	21.3	251	0	113	305	721
All members not covered.........	1,980	*31	7.4	*423	*174	*426	*600	*678

[1]Average size during period of family's existence rounded to nearest integer; exactly half an integer rounded upward.
[2]There were too few Hispanic families of races other than white for separate tabulation.
[3]Annual rate.
[4]Includes only families with heads 17 years of age and over.
[5]Excludes families with all members under 14 years of age.
[6]Excludes families with all members with health status unknown.

NOTE: Multiple-person families are families with average size 1.5 or greater.

Table 15

Out-of-pocket expenditures for inpatient physician care for multiple-person families with members 65 years of age and over, by selected characteristics: United States, 1980

[Rate per family year. Civilian noninstitutionalized population with civilian family head]

Characteristic	All families		Families with care					
	Number in thousands	Mean expenditures	Percent	Mean expenditures	Expenditures at selected percentiles			
					25th	50th	75th	90th
Total............................	10,809	$63	32.7	$193	$0	$60	$219	$558
Family size[1]								
2 persons........................	7,958	58	30.1	194	0	50	200	538
3 persons........................	1,339	93	39.0	*238	*6	*132	*342	*601
4 persons........................	724	*46	35.5	*129	*0	*70	*210	*305
5 or more persons................	788	*76	45.6	*167	*0	*27	*191	*744
Family age								
All members 65 years and over....	4,141	78	30.5	254	0	71	350	739
Some members under 65............	6,668	54	34.1	159	0	52	191	475
Sex of head								
Male.............................	8,397	68	33.0	205	0	70	245	584
Female...........................	2,412	*48	31.5	*151	*0	*27	*172	*378
Race and ethnicity[2] of head								
White............................	9,571	64	34.1	189	0	57	202	530
Hispanic.........................	*363	*13	*19.8	*66	*0	*0	*70	*369
Non-Hispanic.....................	9,208	66	34.7	191	0	57	203	538
Black............................	1,027	*54	19.8	*270	*25	*180	*649	*744
Other............................	*211	*56	*31.6	*178	*74	*93	*388	*388
Family structure								
Head and spouse present whole time......	7,593	54	31.9	170	0	64	202	516
Child under 17 years.............	774	77	35.9	*215	*0	*98	*300	*755
No child under 17 years..........	6,819	52	31.5	164	0	57	193	516
Head only, no spouse at any time.......	2,808	*59	29.7	198	0	35	192	649
Child under 17 years.............	*384	*46	*45.5	*101	*0	*70	*180	*256
No child under 17 years..........	2,424	*61	27.2	*224	*0	*35	*342	*885
Other............................	*408	*256	*67.6	*379	*0	*110	*507	*1,119
Family dynamics								
Unchanging, full year............	9,276	46	29.8	154	0	53	193	403
Change in composition or existed less than full year..........	1,533	167	50.1	333	2	98	507	1,119

Family poverty status in 1980

Below 150 percent poverty level	2,169	*52	29.8	*174	*0	*45	*185	*516
Below poverty level	964	*22	22.2	*98	*0	*27	*142	*305
Poverty level to 149 percent	1,205	*76	35.8	*211	*0	*52	*202	*649
150-199 percent	1,530	65	29.4	*220	*0	*90	*300	*584
200-299 percent	2,785	73	38.5	191	0	80	270	538
300-499 percent	2,740	69	31.1	221	0	60	230	744
500 percent or more	1,585	*50	32.4	*153	*0	*25	*81	*309

Family income in 1980[3]

Less than $10,000	3,133	57	27.1	210	0	53	256	655
$10,000-$19,999	4,173	66	36.8	178	0	78	210	465
$20,000-$34,999	2,427	75	30.3	248	0	70	300	798
$35,000 or more	1,076	*44	38.5	*115	*0	*0	*75	*365

Education of head[4]

None or elementary school	4,669	59	33.1	179	0	70	250	558
Some high school	1,721	63	32.6	*195	*0	*45	*194	*584
High school graduate	2,306	80	34.1	233	0	71	192	764
Some college	1,095	*67	29.2	*230	*0	*81	*219	*755
College graduate or more	1,015	39	31.9	*121	*0	*57	*230	*378

Family employment status[5]

2 or more persons worked full year	979	*68	36.7	*185	*0	*31	*230	*465
Only 1 person worked full year	2,767	45	25.9	175	0	41	198	649
Some part-year work	2,282	58	33.4	174	0	70	256	530
No person worked	4,781	75	35.4	211	0	70	202	558

Worst perceived health status of any family member[6]

Excellent	1,429	*33	19.0	*172	*0	*35	*93	*739
Good	3,630	59	28.0	211	0	81	239	507
Fair	3,110	46	33.3	139	0	6	121	465
Poor	2,640	105	45.9	229	0	90	278	688

Most severe limitation in usual activity of any family member

None	4,190	38	20.9	179	0	70	200	397
Some limitation	865	*47	28.5	*166	*0	*71	*239	*389
Cannot perform usual activity	5,754	84	41.9	201	0	57	221	649

Family's bed days[3]

0	3,349	*6	*0.7	*853	*71	*71	*1,652	*1,652
1-5	2,100	22	24.1	*92	*0	*70	*121	*239
6-10	1,364	39	46.0	*85	*0	*14	*105	*193
11-20	1,098	66	49.4	*133	*0	*53	*182	*403
More than 20	2,897	169	63.4	267	0	92	365	798

Table 15--continued

Out-of-pocket expenditures for inpatient physician care for multiple-person families with members 65 years of age and over, by selected characteristics: United States, 1980

[Rate per family year. Civilian noninstitutionalized population with civilian family head]

Characteristic	All families		Families with care					
	Number in thousands	Mean expenditures	Percent	Mean expenditures	Expenditures at selected percentiles			
					25th	50th	75th	90th
Family health care coverage								
All members covered full year.........	8,879	$57	32.8	$174	$0	$53	$198	$529
Private insurance only...............	*258	*43	*58.8	*73	*0	*33	*83	*98
Medicaid only.......................	*15	*180	*100.0	*180	*180	*180	*180	*180
Medicare only.......................	*574	*30	*19.3	*157	*71	*130	*239	*385
Medicare and other public programs...	*459	*19	*25.6	*75	*0	*0	*45	*70
Medicare and private insurance.......	7,380	62	33.5	185	0	55	202	538
Other public and private mixes.......	*91	*35	*12.8	*275	*275	*275	*275	*275
Other mixes of public programs.......	-	-	-	-	-	-	-	-
Source unknown......................	*102	*63	*38.0	*165	*0	*53	*378	*378
All members covered, some part year..	701	*70	32.4	*216	*0	*110	*369	*649
Some members not covered............	1,159	*104	33.1	*315	*0	*172	*300	*1,004
All members not covered.............	*71	*87	*13.4	*649	*649	*649	*649	*649

[1] Average size during period of family's existence rounded to nearest integer; exactly half an integer rounded upward.
[2] There were too few Hispanic families of races other than white for separate tabulation.
[3] Annual rate.
[4] Includes only families with heads 17 years of age and over.
[5] Excludes families with all members under 14 years of age.
[6] Excludes families with all members with health status unknown.

NOTE: Multiple-person families are families with average size 1.5 or greater.

Table 16

Out-of-pocket expenditures for inpatient physician care for 1-person families, by selected characteristics: United States, 1980

[Rate per family year. Civilian noninstitutionalized population with civilian family head]

| Characteristic | All families | | Families with care | | | | | |
| | Number in thousands | Mean expenditures | Percent | Mean expenditures | Expenditures at selected percentiles | | | |
					25th	50th	75th	90th
Total.........................	26,233	$21	10.6	$201	$0	$28	$201	$660
Sex								
Male..........................	11,866	18	7.8	228	0	9	200	773
Female........................	14,367	24	12.9	188	0	43	203	660
Race and ethnicity[1]								
White.........................	22,811	20	10.7	182	0	33	199	627
Hispanic......................	818	*1	*7.4	*10	*0	*0	*33	*33
Non-Hispanic..................	21,993	20	10.9	186	0	45	200	627
Black.........................	2,711	*27	10.0	*271	*0	*0	*231	*773
Other.........................	*712	*55	*7.2	*764	*0	*0	*1,538	*1,538
Family dynamics								
Unchanging, full year.........	22,570	20	10.3	190	0	25	160	671
Change in composition or existed less than full year.....	3,662	32	12.2	*261	*0	*190	*331	*522
Poverty status in 1980								
Below 150 percent poverty level..........	9,379	24	12.7	187	0	16	190	606
Below poverty level...........	5,252	*13	11.6	*116	*0	*0	*108	*225
Poverty level to 149 percent..	4,128	37	14.1	*261	*0	*80	*296	*660
150-199 percent...............	2,974	*20	9.6	*210	*0	*80	*225	*690
200-299 percent...............	5,563	*28	8.8	*317	*0	*65	*398	*1,450
300-499 percent...............	5,426	*17	10.1	*171	*0	*15	*200	*644
500 percent or more...........	2,891	*9	8.9	*105	*0	*25	*215	*298
Family income in 1980[2]								
Less than $10,000.............	14,468	30	12.4	238	0	54	212	690
$10,000-$19,999...............	8,280	*11	8.2	*134	*0	*17	*133	*377
$20,000-$34,999...............	2,664	*12	8.4	*140	*0	*20	*231	*331
$35,000 or more...............	820	*11	*9.4	*120	*0	*25	*262	*298
Education[3]								
None or elementary school.....	4,782	33	15.2	216	0	18	200	671
Some high school..............	3,996	*30	11.8	*253	*0	*25	*298	*746
High school graduate..........	7,413	18	10.1	*179	*0	*33	*199	*522
Some college..................	4,842	13	8.6	*148	*0	*28	*220	*636
College graduate or more......	5,122	*17	8.0	*211	*0	*43	*201	*627

75

Table 16—continued

Out-of-pocket expenditures for inpatient physician care for 1-person families, by selected characteristics: United States, 1980

[Rate per family year. Civilian noninstitutionalized population with civilian family head]

| | All families | | Families with care | | | | | |
| | Number in thousands | Mean expenditures | Percent | Mean expenditures | Expenditures at selected percentiles | | | |
Characteristic					25th	50th	75th	90th
Employment status[4]								
Worked full year.........	10,374	*$4	5.0	*$74	*$0	*$0	*$62	*$200
Worked part year.........	7,129	31	11.3	272	0	80	231	682
Never worked.............	8,703	35	16.6	208	0	54	240	675
Perceived health status[5]								
Excellent................	11,226	*12	7.1	*172	0	17	109	606
Good.....................	9,642	22	8.6	254	0	43	231	746
Fair.....................	3,691	37	20.4	180	0	28	262	660
Poor.....................	1,568	*48	24.9	*190	*0	*75	*240	*690
Limitation in usual activity								
None.....................	21,977	14	8.1	169	0	25	146	474
Some limitation..........	731	*47	22.1	*213	*6	*54	*636	*660
Cannot perform usual activity.....	3,525	64	23.6	270	0	109	307	875
Bed days[2]								
0........................	12,629	*2	*0.6	*277	*0	*18	*117	*1,501
1-5......................	6,587	*3	6.4	*44	*0	*0	*55	*187
6-10.....................	2,671	*21	19.3	*107	*0	*45	*133	*259
11-20....................	1,924	*63	32.9	*192	*0	*25	*212	*377
More than 20.............	2,422	142	46.6	304	0	109	398	773
Family health care coverage								
All members covered full year.......	20,491	22	11.9	185	0	25	199	644
Private insurance only...	10,523	*11	7.0	*153	*0	*17	*187	*377
Medicaid only............	*317	*0	*6.9	*0	*0	*0	*0	*0
Medicare only............	1,262	*39	13.5	*289	*0	*80	*390	*1,266
Medicare and other public programs....	993	*13	16.8	*76	*0	*0	*0	*149
Medicare and private insurance........	4,819	50	20.4	246	0	66	240	738
Other public and private mixes.......	1,361	*24	*12.9	*184	*0	*48	*298	*918
Other mixes of public programs.......	*186	*0	*8.5	*0	*0	*0	*0	*0
Source unknown...........	1,030	*3	16.4	*20	*0	*0	*43	*68

All members covered, some part year.....	3,223	*11	*6.3	*167	*0	*53	*203	*660
Some members not covered...............	*24	*142	*54.9	*259	*259	*259	*259	*259
All members not covered................	2,495	*28	*4.8	*581	*80	*196	*682	*1,625

[1]There were too few Hispanic families of races other than white for separate tabulation.
[2]Annual rate.
[3]Includes only families with heads 17 years of age and over.
[4]Excludes families with all members under 14 years of age.
[5]Excludes families with all members with health status unknown.

NOTE: 1-person families are families with average size less than 1.5. For 1-person families with more than 1 distinct individual, characteristics are those of head or of family as in Table 1.

Table 17

Out-of-pocket expenditures for inpatient physician care for 1-person families under 65 years of age, by selected characteristics: United States, 1980

[Rate per family year. Civilian noninstitutionalized population with civilian family head]

Characteristic	All families		Families with care					
	Number in thousands	Mean expenditures	Percent	Mean expenditures	Expenditures at selected percentiles			
					25th	50th	75th	90th
Total............................	18,519	$13	7.5	$175	$0	$25	$190	$606
Age								
Under 25 years..................	5,208	*5	6.6	*73	*0	*0	*48	*190
25–44 years.....................	7,630	*16	7.4	*220	*0	*26	*133	*660
45–64 years.....................	5,680	*17	8.6	*193	*0	*75	*225	*682
Sex								
Male............................	10,082	*9	4.9	*172	*0	*0	*109	*606
Female..........................	8,437	19	10.6	176	0	26	196	660
Race and ethnicity[1]								
White...........................	15,786	8	7.3	113	0	17	124	331
Hispanic........................	680	*1	*5.1	*17	*0	*33	*33	*33
Non-Hispanic....................	15,106	9	7.4	116	0	17	133	331
Black...........................	2,128	*35	9.4	*370	*0	*196	*660	*918
Other...........................	*605	*65	*6.6	*988	*0	*1,538	*1,538	*1,538
Family dynamics								
Unchanging, full year...........	15,487	*11	7.5	*149	0	0	124	398
Change in composition or existed less than full year...........	3,032	*23	7.7	*303	*0	*190	*377	*606
Poverty status in 1980								
Below 150 percent...............	5,181	*21	9.1	*228	*0	*25	*190	*660
Below poverty level.............	3,031	*20	10.7	*187	*0	*0	*109	*918
Poverty level to 149 percent....	2,149	*22	*6.9	*318	*0	*124	*522	*660
150–199 percent.................	1,855	*10	*7.1	*135	*0	*75	*203	*682
200–299 percent.................	4,250	*16	6.5	*249	*0	*55	*190	*671
300–499 percent.................	4,643	*7	7.4	*99	*0	*15	*133	*220
500 percent or more.............	2,590	*6	6.5	*89	*0	*0	*187	*231
Family income in 1980[2]								
Less than $10,000...............	8,222	*23	9.4	*240	*0	*48	*203	*682
$10,000–$19,999.................	7,113	*4	5.8	*72	*0	*17	*133	*200
$20,000–$34,999.................	2,529	*11	7.8	*146	*0	*0	*231	*331
$35,000 or more.................	*656	*0	*2.3	*0	*0	*0	*0	*0

Education[3]

None or elementary school	1,770	*18	*245	*7.5	*48	*671	*918
Some high school	2,546	*25	*268	9.4	*53	*298	*606
High school graduate	5,759	*9	*95	9.5	*0	*124	*398
Some college	4,037	*12	*185	6.4	*133	*231	*682
College graduate or more	4,329	*11	*221	5.0	*28	*109	*1,538

Employment status[4]

Worked full year	9,963	*4	*83	4.6	*5	*109	*200
Worked part year	6,265	*27	*259	10.6	*80	*231	*671
Never worked	2,264	*15	*124	12.0	*0	*80	*522

Perceived health status[5]

Excellent	8,913	*6	*128	5.0	*0	*109	*220
Good	6,852	*14	*218	6.5	*33	*199	*377
Fair	1,866	*26	*143	18.0	*25	*225	*660
Poor	803	*51	*252	20.2	*75	*298	*918

Limitation in usual activity

None	16,928	*11	160	6.7	0	190	398
Some limitation	*209	*69	*660	*10.5	*660	*660	*660
Cannot perform usual activity	1,383	*35	*199	17.4	*0	*109	*918

Bed days[2]

0	8,291	0	*0	*0.3	*0	*0	*0
1–5	5,721	*2	*44	4.5	*0	*55	*199
6–10	2,013	*19	*118	16.3	*53	*133	*474
11–20	1,222	*58	*238	24.1	*0	*75	*606
More than 20	1,273	*97	*254	38.0	*108	*298	*773

Family health care coverage

All members covered full year	12,974	*11	*132	8.3	0	124	377
Private insurance only	10,511	*10	*151	6.9	*17	*187	*398
Medicaid only	*317	*0	*0	*6.9	*0	*0	*0
Medicare only	*108	*0	*0	*12.9	*0	*0	*0
Medicare and other public programs	–	–	–	–	–	–	–
Medicare and private insurance	–	–	–	–	–	–	–
Other public and private mixes	1,361	*24	*184	*12.9	*48	*298	*918
Other mixes of public programs	*186	*0	*0	*8.5	*0	*0	*0
Source unknown	*491	*3	*12	*26.0	*53	*0	*109
All members covered, some part year	3,223	*11	*167	*6.3	*0	*203	*660
Some members not covered	–	–	–	–	–	–	–
All members not covered	2,322	*29	*593	*4.9	*196	*682	*1,625

[1] There were too few Hispanic of races other than white families for separate tabulation.
[2] Annual rate.
[3] Includes only families with heads 17 years of age and over.
[4] Excludes families with all members under 14 years of age.
[5] Excludes families with all members with health status unknown.

NOTE: 1-person families are families with average size less than 1.5. For 1-person families with more than 1 distinct individual, characteristics are those of head or of family as in Table 2.

Table 18

Out-of-pocket expenditures for inpatient physician care for 1-person families under 65 years of age with health care coverage all year, by selected characteristics: United States, 1980

[Rate per family year. Civilian noninstitutionalized population with civilian family head]

Characteristic	All families		Families with care					
	Number in thousands	Mean expenditures	Percent	Mean expenditures	Expenditures at selected percentiles			
					25th	50th	75th	90th
Total...............	12,974	*$11	8.3	*$132	$0	$0	$124	$377
Age								
Under 25 years........	3,166	*5	8.0	*56	*0	*0	*33	*124
25-44 years........	5,206	*11	7.6	*146	*0	*25	*109	*231
45-64 years........	4,601	*15	9.3	*165	*0	*5	*220	*671
Sex								
Male..............	6,807	*10	6.2	*168	*0	*0	*109	*773
Female............	6,167	*12	10.6	*110	*0	*15	*141	*298
Race and ethnicity[1]								
White.............	11,183	6	7.9	73	0	0	109	220
Hispanic..........	*400	*2	*4.6	*33	*33	*33	*33	*33
Non-Hispanic......	10,782	6	8.0	74	0	0	109	220
Black.............	1,428	*27	10.7	*251	*0	*0	*231	*918
Other.............	*363	*108	*10.9	*988	*0	*1,538	*1,538	*1,538
Family dynamics								
Unchanging, full year.....	11,017	*10	8.5	*119	0	0	82	231
Change in composition or existed less than full year......	1,957	*16	*7.0	*224	*0	*109	*377	*773
Poverty status in 1980								
Below 150 percent......	2,775	*10	10.4	*99	*0	*0	*48	*298
Below poverty level......	1,638	*16	13.3	*118	*0	*0	*48	*298
Poverty level to 149 percent......	1,137	*2	*6.1	*39	*0	*0	*124	*124
150-199 percent......	1,072	*4	*6.7	*52	*0	*0	*75	*225
200-299 percent......	2,997	*22	8.3	*267	*0	*55	*398	*1,538
300-499 percent......	3,918	*9	8.1	*108	*0	*25	*133	*220
500 percent or more......	2,212	*5	6.9	*66	*0	*0	*187	*231
Family income in 1980[2]								
Less than $10,000......	4,620	*19	10.7	*180	*0	*0	*109	*671
$10,000-$19,999......	5,656	*5	7.3	*72	*0	*17	*133	*200
$20,000-$34,999......	2,114	*11	*7.4	*153	*0	*0	*231	*773
$35,000 or more......	*584	*0	*2.6	*0	*0	*0	*0	*0

Education[3]								
None or elementary school	1,328	*25	10.0	*245	*0	*48	*671	*918
Some high school	1,538	*5	*9.8	*55	*0	*25	*62	*298
High school graduate	4,047	*6	9.1	*63	*0	*0	*33	*225
Some college	2,830	*12	7.9	*152	*0	*109	*220	*377
College graduate or more	3,201	*14	6.3	*222	*0	*0	*82	*1,538
Employment status[4]								
Worked full year	7,649	*5	5.8	*86	*0	*15	*109	*200
Worked part year	3,554	*21	10.4	*204	*0	*0	*220	*671
Never worked	1,769	*16	14.8	*111	*0	*0	*80	*298
Perceived health status[5]								
Excellent	6,353	*3	5.0	*55	*0	*0	*62	*187
Good	4,537	*16	7.5	*208	*0	*25	*200	*671
Fair	1,425	*10	18.1	*54	*0	*5	*55	*225
Poor	*572	*71	*28.3	*252	*0	*75	*298	*918
Limitation in usual activity								
None	11,652	*10	7.3	*137	*0	*15	*133	*377
Some limitation	*127	*0	*0.0	-	-	-	-	-
Cannot perform usual activity	1,195	*22	19.1	*116	*0	*0	*55	*298
Bed days[2]								
0	5,669	0	0.0	-	-	-	-	-
1-5	4,146	*2	5.1	*40	*0	*0	*55	*187
6-10	1,247	*14	17.5	*81	*0	*0	*133	*225
11-20	984	*44	27.3	*163	*0	*0	*25	*141
More than 20	928	*78	41.0	*192	*0	*48	*298	*773
Family health care coverage								
Private insurance only	10,511	*10	6.9	*151	*0	*17	*187	*398
Medicaid only	*317	*0	*6.9	*0	*0	*0	*0	*0
Medicare only	*108	*0	*12.9	*0	*0	*0	*0	*0
Medicare and other public programs	-	-	-	-	-	-	-	-
Medicare and private insurance	-	-	-	-	-	-	-	-
Other public and private mixes	1,361	*24	*12.9	*184	*0	*48	*298	*918
Other mixes of public programs	*186	*0	*8.5	*0	*0	*0	*0	*0
Source unknown	*491	*3	*26.0	*12	*0	*0	*0	*109

[1] There were too few Hispanic families of races other than white for separate tabulation.
[2] Annual rate.
[3] Includes only families with heads 17 years of age and over.
[4] Excludes families with all members under 14 years of age.
[5] Excludes families with all members with health status unknown.

NOTE: 1-person families are families with average size less than 1.5. For 1-person families with more than 1 distinct individual, characteristics are those of head or of family as in Table 2.

81

Table 19

Out-of-pocket expenditures for inpatient physician care for 1-person families under 65 years of age without health care coverage all year, by selected characteristics: United States, 1980

[Rate per family year. Civilian noninstitutionalized population with civilian family head]

Characteristic	All families			Families with care				
	Number in thousands	Mean expenditures	Percent	Mean expenditures	Expenditures at selected percentiles			
					25th	50th	75th	90th
Total...............	5,545	*$18	5.7	*$319	*$0	*$108	*$331	*$682
Age								
Under 25 years........	2,042	*5	*4.3	*120	*0	*0	*190	*190
25-44 years..........	2,424	*28	*7.0	*395	*0	*80	*660	*1,625
45-64 years..........	1,079	*22	*5.4	*400	*196	*331	*522	*682
Sex								
Male..................	3,275	*5	*2.3	*193	*0	*0	*331	*606
Female................	2,270	*38	10.6	*359	*26	*190	*203	*682
Race and ethnicity[1]								
White.................	4,603	*14	5.9	*243	*0	*80	*203	*682
Hispanic..............	*280	*0	*6.0	*0	*0	*0	*0	*0
Non-Hispanic..........	4,323	*15	5.8	*259	*0	*80	*331	*682
Black.................	*700	*50	6.6	*761	*196	*660	*660	*660
Other.................	*242	*0	*0.0	-	-	-	-	-
Family dynamics								
Unchanging, full year......	4,470	*14	*4.9	*277	*0	*53	*196	*682
Change in composition or existed less than full year.......	1,075	*37	*8.9	*417	*190	*203	*331	*606
Poverty status in 1980								
Below 150 percent........	2,405	*33	*7.7	*429	*0	*190	*606	*1,625
Below poverty level......	1,394	*25	*7.6	*328	*0	*108	*196	*1,625
Poverty level to 149 percent.....	1,012	*44	*7.7	*567	*190	*522	*660	*660
150-199 percent.......	784	*18	*7.8	*231	*0	*80	*203	*682
200-299 percent.......	1,253	*2	*2.3	*91	*26	*26	*190	*190
300-499 percent.......	*725	*0	*3.7	*0	*0	*0	*0	*0
500 percent or more......	*379	*13	*3.9	*332	*331	*331	*331	*331
Family income in 1980[2]								
Less than $10,000........	3,602	*27	7.6	*350	*26	*190	*522	*682
$10,000-$19,999......	1,457	0	0.0	-	-	-	-	-
$20,000-$34,999......	*415	*12	*10.0	*117	*0	*0	*331	*331
$35,000 or more.......	*71	*0	*0.0	-	-	-	-	-

Education[3]

	Col 1	Col 2	Col 3	Col 4	Col 5	Col 6	Col 7	Col 8
None or elementary school	*443	*0	*0.0	–	–	–	–	–
Some high school	1,008	*55	*8.8	*626	*0	*53	*606	*1,625
High school graduate	1,713	*17	*10.5	*160	*0	*80	*196	*660
Some college	1,208	*11	*2.7	*412	*190	*190	*682	*682
College graduate or more	1,127	*3	*1.3	*203	*203	*203	*203	*203

Employment status[4]

	Col 1	Col 2	Col 3	Col 4	Col 5	Col 6	Col 7	Col 8
Worked full year	2,314	0	*0.7	*0	*0	*0	*0	*0
Worked part year	2,711	*35	10.7	*330	*0	*108	*331	*682
Never worked	*495	*10	*1.8	*522	*522	*522	*522	*522

Perceived health status[5]

	Col 1	Col 2	Col 3	Col 4	Col 5	Col 6	Col 7	Col 8
Excellent	2,559	*16	*5.1	*306	*0	*53	*203	*1,625
Good	2,314	*12	*4.7	*250	*0	*108	*190	*196
Fair	*441	*77	*17.6	*438	*331	*522	*660	*682
Poor	*231	*0	*0.0	–	–	–	–	–

Limitation in usual activity

	Col 1	Col 2	Col 3	Col 4	Col 5	Col 6	Col 7	Col 8
None	5,276	*12	5.3	*231	*0	*80	*196	*682
Some limitation	*82	*177	*26.8	*660	*660	*660	*660	*660
Cannot perform usual activity	*188	*114	*6.9	*1,653	*522	*522	*4,283	*4,283

Bed days[2]

	Col 1	Col 2	Col 3	Col 4	Col 5	Col 6	Col 7	Col 8
0	2,622	0	*1.0	*0	*0	*0	*0	*0
1–5	1,575	*2	*3.1	*62	*0	*0	*203	*203
6–10	766	*28	*14.3	*192	*26	*80	*196	*660
11–20	*237	*112	*11.3	*994	*331	*331	*606	*4,283
More than 20	*345	*145	*30.1	*482	*108	*190	*682	*1,625

Family health care coverage

	Col 1	Col 2	Col 3	Col 4	Col 5	Col 6	Col 7	Col 8
All members covered, some part year	3,223	*11	*6.3	*167	*0	*53	*203	*660
Some members not covered	–	–	–	–	–	–	–	–
All members not covered	2,322	*29	*4.9	*593	*80	*196	*682	*1,625

[1]There were too few Hispanic families of races other than white for separate tabulation.
[2]Annual rate.
[3]Includes only families with heads 17 years of age and over.
[4]Excludes families with all members under 14 years of age.
[5]Excludes families with all members with health status unknown.

NOTE: 1-person families are families with average size less than 1.5. For 1-person families with more than 1 distinct individual, characteristics are those of head or of family as in Table 2.

Table 20

Out-of-pocket expenditures for inpatient physician care for 1-person families 65 years of age and over, by selected characteristics: United States, 1980

[Rate per family year. Civilian noninstitutionalized population with civilian family head]

Characteristic	All families			Families with care				
	Number in thousands	Mean expenditures	Percent	Mean expenditures	Expenditures at selected percentiles			
					25th	50th	75th	90th
Total...............	7,714	$41	17.9	$228	$0	$54	$240	$690
Sex								
Male....................	1,784	*70	23.8	*293	*0	*66	*296	*1,100
Female..................	5,930	32	16.1	199	0	54	225	644
Race and ethnicity[1]								
White...................	7,025	45	18.5	243	0	68	259	720
Hispanic.............	*138	*0	*18.4	*0	*0	*0	*0	*0
Non-Hispanic.........	6,887	46	18.5	248	0	73	262	720
Black...................	582	0	12.5	*0	*0	*0	*0	*0
Other...................	*106	*0	*11.0	*0	*0	*0	*0	*0
Family dynamics								
Unchanging, full year........	7,083	38	16.5	231	0	54	212	720
Change in composition or existed less than full year...........	630	*73	33.8	*215	*0	*138	*298	*390
Poverty status in 1980								
Below 150 percent poverty level........	4,199	*27	17.1	*160	0	16	158	514
Below poverty level.........	2,220	*4	12.7	*33	*0	*0	*25	*149
Poverty level to 149 percent...........	1,979	*53	22.0	*242	*0	*80	*253	*675
150-199 percent.........	1,118	*38	13.8	*274	*0	*140	*690	*746
200-299 percent.........	1,313	*66	16.3	*406	*28	*76	*636	*1,450
300-499 percent.........	783	*76	26.2	*290	*0	*43	*627	*1,100
500 percent or more.........	*300	*40	*30.1	*134	*20	*191	*262	*298
Family income in 1980[2]								
Less than $10,000.........	6,246	39	16.4	236	0	66	225	720
$10,000-$19,999.........	1,167	*53	22.8	*231	*0	*28	*259	*644
$20,000-$34,999.........	*136	*21	*20.9	*100	*20	*20	*215	*215
$35,000 or more.........	*165	*56	*37.6	*149	*25	*191	*262	*298

Education

	Total	Percent[2]					
None or elementary school	3,012	19.8	210	0	6	160	644
Some high school	1,451	16.0	*237	*0	*0	*307	*875
High school graduate	1,653	12.1	*409	*146	*225	*675	*1,389
Some college	804	19.8	*90	*0	*3	*71	*240
College graduate or more	793	24.4	*201	*0	*54	*325	*627

Employment status

Worked full year	*411	*15.3	*11	*0	*0	*0	*54
Worked part year	863	16.5	*329	*0	*94	*307	*1,450
Never worked	6,439	18.2	228	0	66	259	690

Perceived health status[3]

Excellent	2,313	15.2	*229	*0	*45	*94	*675
Good	2,790	13.7	*296	*0	*54	*307	*1,389
Fair	1,825	22.9	*210	*0	*80	*296	*644
Poor	765	30.0	*147	*0	*93	*191	*542

Limitation in usual activity

None	5,049	12.9	*183	0	25	123	644
Some limitation	*523	*26.8	*143	*0	*20	*140	*636
Cannot perform usual activity	2,142	27.5	299	0	191	377	875

Bed days[2]

0	4,338	*1.0	*442	*71	*117	*1,501	*1,501
1–5	867	19.0	*44	*0	*9	*54	*76
6–10	658	28.5	*87	*0	*45	*73	*259
11–20	702	48.1	*151	*0	*80	*215	*377
More than 20	1,149	56.2	342	0	138	542	1,100

Family health care coverage

All members covered full year	7,517	18.1	227	0	54	225	690
Private insurance only	*13	*100.0	*298	*298	*298	*298	*298
Medicaid only	1,154	13.5	*314	*0	*93	*390	*1,266
Medicare only	993	16.8	*76	*0	*0	*0	*149
Medicare and other public programs	4,819	20.4	246	0	66	240	738
Medicare and private insurance	–	–	–	–	–	–	–
Other public and private mixes	–	–	–	–	–	–	–
Other mixes of public programs	*538	*7.6	*45	*25	*43	*43	*68
Source unknown	–	–	–	–	–	–	–
All members covered, some part year	*24	*54.9	*259	*259	*259	*259	*259
Some members not covered	*172	*4.0	*375	*375	*375	*375	*375
All members not covered	–	–	–	–	–	–	–

---

[1] There were too few Hispanic families of races other than white for separate tabulation.
[2] Annual rate.
[3] Excludes families with all members with health status unknown.

NOTE: 1-person families are families with average size less than 1.5. For 1-person families characteristics are those of head or of family as in Table 5.

85

Table 21

Out-of-pocket expenditures for ambulatory physician visits for multiple-person families, by selected characteristics: United States, 1980

[Rate per family year. Civilian noninstitutionalized population with civilian family head]

Characteristic	All families		Families with visits					
	Number in thousands	Mean expenditures	Percent	Mean expenditures	Expenditures at selected percentiles			
					25th	50th	75th	90th
Total.........................	58,135	$126	93.1	$136	$30	$88	$180	$303
Family size[1]								
2 persons......................	22,916	108	89.3	121	28	77	160	279
3 persons......................	12,567	125	94.9	132	30	87	171	284
4 persons......................	12,269	150	96.4	155	45	105	215	345
5 or more persons..............	10,383	142	95.6	148	24	97	201	352
Age of head								
Under 25 years.................	4,308	91	91.9	99	3	55	119	231
25-44 years....................	25,173	131	94.7	139	31	90	182	297
45-64 years....................	20,129	130	92.6	141	31	90	192	331
65 years and over..............	8,525	121	90.3	134	38	92	182	289
Sex of head								
Male...........................	44,874	139	93.8	149	41	101	194	324
Female.........................	13,262	83	90.9	91	0	46	120	223
Race and ethnicity[2] of head								
White..........................	51,015	132	93.8	141	35	94	186	314
Hispanic.......................	3,403	116	93.5	124	14	74	167	335
Non-Hispanic...................	47,613	133	93.8	142	37	96	187	309
Black..........................	6,090	82	88.5	93	3	42	120	248
Other..........................	1,030	98	85.8	114	24	56	128	203
Family structure								
Head and spouse present whole time......	42,556	141	94.4	150	43	102	196	331
Child under 17 years...........	22,442	157	96.4	163	50	111	217	355
No child under 17 years........	20,114	124	92.1	134	38	90	176	297
Head only, no spouse at any time......	13,977	79	89.2	88	3	46	117	214
Child under 17 years...........	8,643	75	92.8	81	0	38	105	207
No child under 17 years........	5,334	84	83.3	100	22	58	127	248
Other..........................	1,602	142	94.1	151	25	99	201	324
Family dynamics								
Unchanging, full year..........	46,990	126	93.2	135	31	88	180	300
Change in composition or existed less than full year.................	11,145	127	92.6	137	25	87	179	316

Family poverty status in 1980

Below 150 percent poverty level	10,938	80	90.3	88	0	38	120	220
Below poverty level	6,047	62	90.6	69	0	13	88	209
Poverty level to 149 percent	4,892	101	90.0	112	16	73	144	234
150-199 percent	6,355	128	92.1	139	35	93	189	331
200-299 percent	12,860	131	93.3	140	40	89	191	309
300-499 percent	17,047	139	94.5	147	43	103	192	305
500 percent or more	10,935	148	94.1	157	42	102	195	362

Family income in 1980[3]

Less than $10,000	10,629	79	89.9	87	0	39	122	220
$10,000-$19,999	16,728	119	91.2	131	34	83	173	294
$20,000-$34,999	19,706	135	94.7	142	40	97	185	297
$35,000 or more	11,073	168	96.2	175	52	123	237	377

Education of head[4]

None or elementary school	10,491	109	90.9	120	27	79	162	283
Some high school	9,267	99	92.8	107	15	66	142	253
High school graduate	20,605	123	92.9	133	30	87	179	296
Some college	8,651	136	93.8	144	40	105	195	335
College graduate or more	9,099	172	95.9	180	50	109	227	377

Family employment status[5]

2 or more persons worked full year	14,607	135	93.9	144	45	100	191	303
Only 1 person worked full year	24,549	138	93.6	147	38	96	190	319
Some part-year work	11,303	107	91.7	117	18	69	161	285
No person worked	7,676	101	91.9	109	0	62	164	268

Worst perceived health status of any family member[6]

Excellent	16,200	110	91.3	120	28	79	158	275
Good	24,467	131	93.7	140	34	90	184	307
Fair	11,131	130	93.0	140	29	92	184	338
Poor	6,318	141	95.8	147	22	98	208	350

Most severe limitation in usual activity of any family member

None	43,941	124	92.4	134	31	87	177	297
Some limitation	3,679	132	96.6	137	21	81	174	346
Cannot perform usual activity	10,515	135	94.8	142	27	97	193	350

Family's bed days[3]

0	11,173	86	85.0	101	25	66	139	234
1-5	14,527	106	91.8	116	30	76	144	258
6-10	8,834	131	96.0	136	28	89	174	297
11-20	9,982	144	95.9	151	40	105	213	329
More than 20	13,619	165	97.2	170	36	114	227	386

Table 21—continued

Out-of-pocket expenditures for ambulatory physician visits for multiple-person families, by selected characteristics: United States, 1980

[Rate per family year. Civilian noninstitutionalized population with civilian family head]

Characteristic	All families		Families with visits					
	Number in thousands	Mean expenditures	Percent	Mean expenditures	Expenditures at selected percentiles			
					25th	50th	75th	90th
Family health care coverage								
All members covered full year.............	42,453	$130	94.4	$138	$33	$92	$182	$303
Private insurance only.................	25,759	145	95.2	152	47	103	195	315
Medicaid only.....................	1,621	*11	93.5	*12	0	0	0	25
Medicare only....................	*574	*99	*87.6	*113	*45	*80	*149	*230
Medicare and other public programs....	*471	*34	*95.3	*36	*0	*0	*50	*97
Medicare and private insurance........	7,475	142	92.4	153	46	116	199	342
Other public and private mixes.......	5,853	105	94.6	111	12	62	139	283
Other mixes of public programs........	*135	*102	*91.4	*112	*0	*93	*157	*391
Source unknown..................	*564	*43	*93.1	*47	*0	*0	*40	*206
All members covered, some part year.....	8,669	118	90.6	131	28	79	176	300
Some members not covered.............	4,963	120	90.6	133	23	76	192	346
All members not covered	2,051	94	82.4	114	28	64	134	262

[1]Average size during period of family's existence rounded to nearest integer; exactly half an integer rounded upward.
[2]There were too few Hispanic families of races other than white for separate tabulation.
[3]Annual rate.
[4]Includes only families with heads 17 years of age and over.
[5]Excludes families with all members under 14 years of age.
[6]Excludes families with all members with health status unknown.

NOTE: Multiple-person families are families with average size 1.5 or greater.

Table 22

Out-of-pocket expenditures for ambulatory physician visits for multiple-person families with all members under 65 years of age, by selected characteristics: United States, 1980

[Rate per family year. Civilian noninstitutionalized population with civilian family head]

Characteristic	All families		Families with visits		Expenditures at selected percentiles			
	Number in thousands	Mean expenditures	Percent	Mean expenditures	25th	50th	75th	90th
Total..................	47,327	$126	93.6	$135	$30	$87	$176	$299
Family size[1]								
2 persons..............	14,958	102	88.7	115	23	71	142	265
3 persons..............	11,228	122	95.3	127	30	86	164	268
4 persons..............	11,546	148	96.6	153	45	103	210	339
5 or more persons.....	9,595	142	95.3	149	25	97	205	350
Age of head								
Under 25 years........	4,283	91	91.9	99	3	56	119	231
25-44 years...........	24,783	131	94.6	138	31	89	180	297
45-64 years...........	18,261	128	92.5	138	31	88	185	316
Sex of head								
Male..................	36,477	140	94.3	149	41	99	194	323
Female................	10,850	78	91.1	85	0	45	115	215
Race and ethnicity[2] of head								
White.................	41,444	132	94.2	140	34	93	184	309
Hispanic..............	3,040	119	93.4	128	15	80	175	335
Non-Hispanic..........	38,405	133	94.3	141	35	94	184	306
Black.................	5,064	77	89.4	86	0	39	102	231
Other.................	819	112	85.1	132	25	65	138	214
Family structure								
Head and spouse present whole time......	34,963	142	94.8	150	42	100	196	325
Child under 17 years...	21,668	156	96.5	162	50	110	216	346
No child under 17 years......	13,295	118	92.0	128	34	83	159	286
Head only, no spouse at any time......	11,169	74	89.7	83	0	45	113	208
Child under 17 years...	8,258	73	92.4	79	0	37	105	207
No child under 17 years......	2,911	77	81.8	95	20	58	119	230
Other.................	1,194	142	93.9	152	20	82	201	353
Family dynamics								
Unchanging, full year......	37,714	126	93.8	134	30	87	176	297
Change in composition or existed less than full year......	9,613	126	92.5	137	25	87	178	315

Table 22—continued

Out-of-pocket expenditures for ambulatory physician visits for multiple-person families with all members under 65 years of age, by selected characteristics: United States, 1980

[Rate per family year. Civilian noninstitutionalized population with civilian family head]

Characteristic	All families		Families with visits		Expenditures at selected percentiles			
	Number in thousands	Mean expenditures	Percent	Mean expenditures	25th	50th	75th	90th
Family poverty status in 1980								
Below 150 percent poverty level......	8,770	$77	91.0	$85	$0	$30	$112	$219
Below poverty level...............	5,083	63	91.6	69	0	6	87	213
Poverty level to 149 percent......	3,687	97	90.2	107	15	62	130	219
150-199 percent...................	4,825	132	91.7	144	36	94	197	346
200-299 percent...................	10,075	126	93.6	135	36	87	183	296
300-499 percent...................	14,307	139	95.3	146	44	102	192	299
500 percent or more...............	9,350	147	94.2	156	42	99	190	354
Family income in 1980[3]								
Less than $10,000.................	7,496	68	89.9	76	0	20	96	206
$10,000-$19,999...................	12,555	116	91.4	127	35	81	164	285
$20,000-$34,999...................	17,279	133	95.3	140	39	96	184	291
$35,000 or more...................	9,997	168	95.9	176	54	122	236	380
Education of head[4]								
None or elementary school........	5,822	103	91.6	113	20	73	152	270
Some high school.................	7,546	98	93.7	105	15	62	134	244
High school graduate.............	18,299	120	92.7	129	30	86	173	289
Some college.....................	7,556	133	94.3	141	40	105	196	315
College graduate or more.........	8,084	175	96.0	182	55	106	230	380
Family employment status[5]								
2 or more persons worked full year.....	13,629	135	94.0	143	44	98	190	304
Only 1 person worked full year........	21,782	138	93.8	147	39	96	190	316
Some part-year work..............	9,021	105	92.6	113	15	64	147	267
No person worked.................	2,896	57	92.5	62	0	0	87	204
Worst perceived health status of any family member[6]								
Excellent........................	14,771	111	92.0	121	28	80	160	275
Good.............................	20,837	130	93.8	138	32	90	182	304
Fair.............................	8,021	130	94.0	139	27	88	180	338
Poor.............................	3,678	149	97.2	153	18	96	208	350

Most severe limitation in usual activity of any family member							
None........................	39,751	125	92.9	134	30	87	177	296
Some limitation.............	2,814	130	97.1	133	14	75	159	347
Cannot perform usual activity.......	4,762	133	97.2	137	22	86	180	331
Family's bed days³							
0...........................	7,825	84	85.6	98	22	64	138	231
1-5.........................	12,427	103	91.6	112	26	76	140	257
6-10........................	7,470	131	96.2	136	26	85	168	299
11-20.......................	8,884	145	95.6	151	40	105	215	329
More than 20................	10,722	164	98.0	167	37	110	221	377
Family health care coverage							
All members covered full year.......	33,575	129	95.0	135	30	89	175	297
Private insurance only......	25,502	144	95.2	151	47	103	195	309
Medicaid only...............	1,606	*11	93.4	*11	0	0	0	23
Medicare only...............	–	*0	–	–	–	–	–	*0
Medicare and other public programs....	*12	*0	*100.0	*0	*0	*0	*0	*230
Medicare and private insurance.......	*95	*65	*74.0	*87	*46	*80	*83	*284
Other public and private mixes.......	5,762	104	94.7	110	12	60	135	*391
Other mixes of public programs.......	*135	*102	*91.4	*112	*0	*93	*157	*117
Source unknown..............	*463	*34	*95.3	*35	*0	*0	*35	300
All members covered, some part year....	7,968	120	90.8	132	28	82	179	381
Some members not covered....	3,804	130	91.9	141	25	83	208	265
All members not covered.....	1,980	97	83.8	115	27	64	136	

[1] Average size during period of family's existence rounded to nearest integer; exactly half an integer rounded upward.
[2] There were too few Hispanic families of races other than white for separate tabulation.
[3] Annual rate.
[4] Includes only families with heads 17 years of age and over.
[5] Excludes families with all members under 14 years of age.
[6] Excludes families with all members with health status unknown.

NOTE: Multiple-person families are families with average size 1.5 or greater.

Table 23

Out-of-pocket expenditures for ambulatory physician visits for multiple-person families with all members under 65 years of age and all members with health care coverage all year, by selected characteristics: United States, 1980

[Rate per family year. Civilian noninstitutionalized population with civilian family head]

Characteristic	All families		Families with visits					
	Number in thousands	Mean expenditures	Percent	Mean expenditures	Expenditures at selected percentiles			
					25th	50th	75th	90th
Total...................	33,575	$129	95.0	$135	$30	$89	$175	$297
Family size[1]								
2 persons..................	10,994	110	92.3	119	25	75	146	275
3 persons..................	8,010	125	95.6	130	30	88	167	263
4 persons..................	8,464	146	96.5	152	45	104	213	338
5 or more persons..........	6,107	143	96.8	147	25	97	196	352
Age of head								
Under 25 years.............	2,585	82	93.0	88	1	56	115	217
25-44 years................	18,256	131	95.8	137	31	92	180	293
45-64 years................	12,733	134	94.2	142	34	91	182	325
Sex of head								
Male.......................	27,351	141	95.2	148	42	100	192	316
Female.....................	6,224	74	94.0	78	0	35	102	201
Race and ethnicity[2] of head								
White......................	29,902	136	95.6	142	35	96	185	306
Hispanic...................	1,711	118	95.8	123	9	74	163	340
Non-Hispanic...............	28,191	137	95.6	143	38	97	185	303
Black......................	3,139	63	90.6	70	0	30	90	171
Other......................	533	*117	85.6	*137	*30	*64	*138	*204
Family structure								
Head and spouse present whole time......	26,517	142	95.6	149	44	101	194	317
Child under 17 years.......	16,251	156	96.7	161	53	110	215	345
No child under 17 years....	10,266	120	93.9	128	36	85	158	281
Head only, no spouse at any time........	6,394	71	92.3	77	0	35	102	184
Child under 17 years.......	5,051	65	93.5	69	0	23	91	172
No child under 17 years....	1,343	97	87.8	111	29	65	136	281
Other......................	663	140	94.8	*148	*0	*50	*159	*302
Family dynamics								
Unchanging, full year......	28,266	130	95.4	136	32	90	177	295
Change in composition or existed less than full year....	5,308	120	92.8	129	20	81	169	308

Family poverty status in 1980								
Below 150 percent poverty level	4,640	65	92.9	70	0	10	87	180
Below poverty level	2,919	49	93.3	53	0	0	35	170
Poverty level to 149 percent	1,721	93	92.0	101	0	58	114	207
150-199 percent	2,657	132	94.2	140	42	97	175	331
200-299 percent	7,074	125	94.8	132	36	87	183	285
300-499 percent	11,427	141	96.4	146	43	104	192	293
500 percent or more	7,776	150	94.7	159	44	100	189	367
Family income in 1980[3]								
Less than $10,000	4,023	56	92.0	61	0	0	74	164
$10,000-$19,999	7,715	116	93.7	123	35	84	159	268
$20,000-$34,999	13,970	133	95.6	139	36	97	184	289
$35,000 or more	7,867	170	96.7	176	55	118	230	385
Education of head[4]								
None or elementary school	3,188	102	94.0	108	15	72	140	265
Some high school	4,620	87	94.6	92	12	59	123	222
High school graduate	13,366	119	94.3	127	32	86	169	281
Some college	5,757	133	95.0	140	35	105	198	304
College graduate or more	6,625	185	97.0	191	57	109	243	398
Family employment status[5]								
2 or more persons worked full year	10,347	141	95.9	147	44	100	192	312
Only 1 person worked full year	16,128	137	94.6	145	40	98	184	304
Some part-year work	4,933	105	94.7	111	14	66	140	256
No person worked	2,167	60	94.2	64	0	0	87	214
Worst perceived health status of any family member[6]								
Excellent	11,162	116	94.9	123	28	81	159	275
Good	15,029	134	94.5	142	35	96	189	299
Fair	5,209	125	96.0	130	27	88	167	291
Poor	2,155	151	96.6	156	15	93	205	369
Most severe limitation in usual activity of any family member								
None	28,461	127	94.6	135	32	90	175	290
Some limitation	2,067	149	97.7	152	15	89	213	409
Cannot perform usual activity	3,047	126	97.0	130	19	83	167	331
Family's bed days[3]								
0	5,766	90	89.0	101	23	67	142	234
1-5	8,806	105	92.9	113	27	77	137	257
6-10	5,513	128	97.7	131	26	88	168	279
11-20	6,162	150	96.8	155	42	111	216	329
More than 20	7,328	170	98.5	172	35	110	230	385

Table 23--continued

Out-of-pocket expenditures for ambulatory physician visits for multiple-person families with all members under 65 years of age and all members with health care coverage all year, by selected characteristics: United States, 1980

[Rate per family year. Civilian noninstitutionalized population with civilian family head]

Characteristic	All families		Families with visits		Expenditures at selected percentiles			
	Number in thousands	Mean expenditures	Percent	Mean expenditures	25th	50th	75th	90th
Family health care coverage								
Private insurance only................	25,502	$144	95.2	$151	$47	$103	$195	$309
Medicaid only........................	1,606	*11	93.4	*11	0	0	0	23
Medicare only........................	–	–	–	–	–	–	–	–
Medicare and other public programs.....	*12	*0	*100.0	*0	*0	*0	*0	*0
Medicare and private insurance.........	*95	*65	*74.0	*87	*46	*80	*83	*230
Other public and private mixes.........	5,762	104	94.7	110	12	60	135	284
Other mixes of public programs.........	*135	*102	*91.4	*112	*0	*93	*157	*391
Source unknown.......................	*463	*34	*95.3	*35	*0	*0	*35	*117

[1]Average size during period of family's existence rounded to nearest integer; exactly half an integer rounded upward.
[2]There were too few Hispanic families of races other than white for separate tabulation.
[3]Annual rate.
[4]Includes only families with heads 17 years of age and over.
[5]Excludes families with all members under 14 years of age.
[6]Excludes families with all members with health status unknown.

NOTE: Multiple-person families are families with average size 1.5 or greater.

Table 24

Out-of-pocket expenditures for ambulatory physician visits for multiple-person families with all members under 65 years of age and some or all members without health care coverage all year, by selected characteristics: United States, 1980

[Rate per family year. Civilian noninstitutionalized population with civilian family head]

Characteristic	All families		Families with visits					
	Number in thousands	Mean expenditures	Percent	Mean expenditures	Expenditures at selected percentiles			
					25th	50th	75th	90th
Total............................	13,752	$119	90.1	$133	$27	$82	$179	$307
Family size[1]								
2 persons........................	3,964	80	78.7	101	19	55	125	236
3 persons........................	3,218	114	94.7	120	30	83	157	285
4 persons........................	3,082	151	97.0	156	45	102	208	358
5 or more persons................	3,488	142	92.6	153	26	95	216	350
Age of head								
Under 25 years...................	1,698	105	90.1	116	10	56	140	315
25–44 years......................	6,527	128	91.4	140	31	82	181	304
45–64 years......................	5,528	113	88.5	128	26	85	191	307
Sex of head								
Male.............................	9,126	138	91.5	151	35	90	200	345
Female...........................	4,627	83	87.3	95	10	58	127	247
Race and ethnicity[2] of head								
White............................	11,542	123	90.7	136	30	85	181	314
Hispanic.......................	1,328	120	90.2	133	25	95	208	310
Non-Hispanic...................	10,214	123	90.7	136	30	84	179	316
Black............................	1,924	100	87.3	114	5	56	136	283
Other............................	*286	*102	*84.2	*122	*20	*87	*176	*231
Family structure								
Head and spouse present whole time......	8,446	141	92.1	153	35	93	203	348
Child under 17 years...........	5,417	158	95.8	165	42	112	220	363
No child under 17 years........	3,029	111	85.7	130	27	73	170	299
Head only, no spouse at any time........	4,775	78	86.1	91	14	56	121	230
Child under 17 years...........	3,207	87	90.7	95	4	60	140	247
No child under 17 years........	1,568	61	76.8	79	16	46	111	213
Other............................	*532	*146	*92.8	*157	*35	*117	*210	*429
Family dynamics								
Unchanging, full year............	9,448	112	89.1	126	27	73	173	300
Change in composition or existed less than full year..........	4,304	135	92.1	146	29	97	190	316

Table 24—continued

Out-of-pocket expenditures for ambulatory physician visits for multiple-person families with all members under 65 years of age and some or all members without health care coverage all year, by selected characteristics: United States, 1980

[Rate per family year. Civilian noninstitutionalized population with civilian family head]

| Characteristic | All families | | | Families with visits | | | | | |
| | Number in thousands | Mean expenditures | Percent | Mean expenditures | Expenditures at selected percentiles | | | | |
					25th	50th	75th	90th	
Family poverty status in 1980									
Below 150 percent poverty level	4,130	$91	88.9	$102	$6	$56	$133	$250	
Below poverty level	2,164	82	89.2	92	0	44	120	256	
Poverty level to 149 percent	1,966	100	88.6	113	18	63	147	222	
150–199 percent	2,168	133	88.6	150	28	83	209	355	
200–299 percent	3,000	130	90.9	143	36	88	191	316	
300–499 percent	2,880	132	91.1	144	45	92	191	314	
500 percent or more	1,574	133	91.6	145	27	93	195	315	
Family income in 1980[3]									
Less than $10,000	3,473	83	87.6	95	0	42	122	222	
$10,000–$19,999	4,840	117	87.7	134	30	76	181	316	
$20,000–$34,999	3,310	133	94.2	142	45	89	181	308	
$35,000 or more	2,130	162	93.3	173	50	141	251	369	
Education of head[4]									
None or elementary school	2,634	106	88.7	119	25	74	166	292	
Some high school	2,926	115	92.2	125	20	72	177	276	
High school graduate	4,934	121	88.5	137	25	85	189	316	
Some college	1,800	133	92.1	144	50	90	181	339	
College graduate or more	1,459	129	91.2	141	45	99	190	295	
Family employment status[5]									
2 or more persons worked full year	3,282	115	88.1	131	42	88	185	286	
Only 1 person worked full year	5,654	142	91.6	155	36	90	208	348	
Some part-year work	4,087	104	90.0	116	15	62	152	285	
No person worked	*729	*47	*87.5	*54	*0	*0	*86	*174	
Worst perceived health status of any family member[6]									
Excellent	3,609	94	83.2	113	30	70	161	268	
Good	5,808	118	92.2	128	26	82	173	315	
Fair	2,812	141	90.2	156	27	89	213	380	
Poor	1,524	145	98.0	148	21	99	210	271	

Most severe limitation in usual activity of any family member							
None	11,290	118	88.6	133	28	83	180	308
Some limitation	747	77	95.6	80	6	46	117	180
Cannot perform usual activity	1,715	145	97.3	149	30	90	210	338
Family's bed days[3]							
0	2,059	67	75.9	88	22	55	120	226
1-5	3,620	98	88.5	111	25	65	143	273
6-10	1,957	137	92.1	148	25	74	167	421
11-20	2,722	134	92.9	144	30	92	213	316
More than 20	3,394	152	96.9	157	50	117	219	355
Family health care coverage							
All members covered, some part year	7,968	120	90.8	132	28	82	179	300
Some members not covered	3,804	130	91.9	141	25	83	208	381
All members not covered	1,980	97	83.8	115	27	64	136	265

[1]Average size during period of family's existence rounded to nearest integer; exactly half an integer rounded upward.
[2]There were too few Hispanic families of races other than white for separate tabulation.
[3]Annual rate.
[4]Includes only families with heads 17 years of age and over.
[5]Excludes families with all members under 14 years of age.
[6]Excludes families with all members with health status unknown.

NOTE: Multiple-person families are families with average size 1.5 or greater.

Table 25

Out-of-pocket expenditures for ambulatory physician visits for multiple-person families with members 65 years of age and over, by selected characteristics: United States, 1980

[Rate per family year. Civilian noninstitutionalized population with civilian family head]

Characteristic	All families		Families with visits		Expenditures at selected percentiles			
	Number in thousands	Mean expenditures	Percent	Mean expenditures	25th	50th	75th	90th
Total..................	10,809	$129	91.2	$141	$37	$101	$190	$319
Family size[1]								
2 persons..................	7,958	119	90.3	132	38	100	182	289
3 persons..................	1,339	153	90.8	169	39	90	247	422
4 persons..................	724	182	93.3	195	43	140	253	434
5 or more persons..........	788	131	98.6	133	18	96	188	354
Family age								
All members 65 years and over..........	4,141	129	91.2	141	45	107	187	289
Some members under 65......	6,668	129	91.1	141	30	90	193	360
Sex of head								
Male.......................	8,397	136	91.5	148	43	108	196	342
Female.....................	2,412	105	89.9	117	24	59	146	253
Race and ethnicity[2] of head								
White......................	9,571	133	92.0	145	40	104	193	320
Hispanic...................	*363	*89	*94.3	*94	*0	*40	*85	*362
Non-Hispanic...............	9,208	135	91.9	147	43	106	194	320
Black......................	1,027	107	84.2	127	15	60	188	300
Other......................	*211	*41	*88.7	*46	*0	*33	*101	*127
Family structure								
Head and spouse present whole time......	7,593	140	92.5	151	46	110	200	354
Child under 17 years......	774	185	94.9	195	43	153	280	478
No child under 17 years...	6,819	135	92.2	146	46	108	193	319
Head only, no spouse at any time........	2,808	96	87.1	110	21	57	135	253
Child under 17 years......	*384	*127	*100.0	*127	*0	*50	*129	*415
No child under 17 years...	2,424	91	85.1	107	24	58	135	253
Other......................	*408	*141	*94.7	*149	*35	*125	*190	*317
Family dynamics								
Unchanging, full year......	9,276	129	90.8	142	39	102	190	318
Change in composition or existed less than full year....	1,533	129	93.4	138	25	90	190	319

Family poverty status in 1980							
Below 150 percent poverty level	2,169	89	87.6	102	15	70	155	232
Below poverty level	964	58	85.5	68	0	39	104	193
Poverty level to 149 percent	1,205	114	89.2	128	39	116	183	285
150–199 percent	1,530	113	93.2	121	30	73	175	262
200–299 percent	2,785	146	92.2	159	44	106	206	384
300–499 percent	2,740	137	90.4	151	40	110	200	342
500 percent or more	1,585	152	93.6	163	42	111	229	373
Family income in 1980[3]							
Less than $10,000	3,133	103	89.7	115	30	81	164	256
$10,000–$19,999	4,173	129	90.7	142	32	90	188	342
$20,000–$34,999	2,427	145	90.4	160	45	104	199	370
$35,000 or more	1,076	166	99.0	168	42	129	237	373
Education of head[4]							
None or elementary school	4,669	116	89.9	129	40	87	175	283
Some high school	1,721	103	89.0	115	17	81	184	290
High school graduate	2,306	152	93.9	162	44	122	233	368
Some college	1,095	153	90.1	170	42	110	190	385
College graduate or more	1,015	150	95.3	158	40	116	217	374
Family employment status[5]							
2 or more persons worked full year	979	143	93.3	153	65	125	196	288
Only 1 person worked full year	2,767	135	92.1	147	33	92	190	373
Some part-year work	2,282	118	88.3	134	30	78	185	319
No person worked	4,781	127	91.6	139	38	103	187	303
Worst perceived health status of any family member[6]							
Excellent	1,429	94	83.7	113	28	70	153	289
Good	3,630	141	92.6	152	42	107	191	319
Fair	3,110	129	90.6	142	40	104	186	326
Poor	2,640	130	93.9	139	28	98	201	354
Most severe limitation in usual activity of any family member							
None	4,190	117	88.2	132	37	80	175	307
Some limitation	865	141	94.7	149	45	104	194	309
Cannot perform usual activity	5,754	136	92.8	146	32	105	199	357
Family's bed days[3]							
0	3,349	89	83.7	106	33	72	152	234
1–5	2,100	126	93.1	135	42	83	164	316
6–10	1,364	133	94.8	140	46	122	189	289
11–20	1,098	142	97.9	145	40	116	190	362
More than 20	2,897	169	94.1	180	32	128	253	461

99

Table 25--continued

Out-of-pocket expenditures for ambulatory physician visits for multiple-person families with members 65 years of age and over, by selected characteristics: United States, 1980

[Rate per family year. Civilian noninstitutionalized population with civilian family head]

Characteristic	All families			Families with visits				
	Number in thousands	Mean expenditures	Percent	Mean expenditures	Expenditures at selected percentiles			
					25th	50th	75th	90th
Family health care coverage								
All members covered full year...........	8,879	$137	92.3	$148	$43	$110	$194	$320
Private insurance only.................	*258	*274	*95.1	*288	*70	*183	*317	*802
Medicaid only.........................	*15	*60	*100.0	*60	*60	*60	*60	*60
Medicare only........................	*574	*99	*87.6	*113	*45	*80	*149	*230
Medicare and other public programs....	*459	*35	*95.2	*36	*0	*0	*50	*97
Medicare and private insurance........	7,380	143	92.6	154	47	116	200	342
Other public and private mixes........	*91	*126	*88.7	*142	*62	*146	*266	*283
Other mixes of public programs........	-	-	-	-	-	-	-	-
Source unknown.......................	*102	*88	*82.9	*106	*19	*21	*206	*445
All members covered, some part year.....	701	98	89.1	*110	*22	*50	*111	*257
Some members not covered...............	1,159	89	86.3	104	15	60	130	297
All members not covered.................	*71	*28	*42.9	*66	*37	*44	*127	*127

[1]Average size during period of family's existence rounded to nearest integer; exactly half an integer rounded upward.
[2]There were too few Hispanic families of races other than white for separate tabulation.
[3]Annual rate.
[4]Includes only families with heads 17 years of age and over.
[5]Excludes families with all members under 14 years of age.
[6]Excludes families with all members with health status unknown.

NOTE: Multiple-person families are families with average size 1.5 or greater.

100

Characteristic								
Education[3]								
None or elementary school	1,328	65.4	42	65	10	49	82	185
Some high school	1,538	66.1	36	55	12	40	70	145
High school graduate	4,047	74.0	45	61	7	30	78	158
Some college	2,830	73.6	44	60	0	34	87	163
College graduate or more	3,201	73.3	67	91	5	47	102	210
Employment status[4]								
Worked full year	7,649	73.7	47	64	11	39	86	150
Worked part year	3,554	69.0	57	82	0	43	103	199
Never worked	1,769	69.8	41	59	0	20	69	196
Perceived health status[5]								
Excellent	6,353	67.9	39	57	0	26	69	150
Good	4,537	75.0	60	80	14	48	102	190
Fair	1,425	79.1	46	58	0	51	74	143
Poor	*572	*75.7	*77	*101	*0	*44	*128	*285
Limitation in usual activity								
None	11,652	71.9	48	66	4	37	88	170
Some limitation	*127	*87.4	*83	*95	*33	*74	*158	*159
Cannot perform usual activity	1,195	70.8	57	81	0	20	129	185
Bed days[2]								
0	5,669	62.4	40	65	0	32	90	161
1–5	4,146	72.9	46	63	5	35	80	154
6–10	1,247	89.3	69	78	9	60	104	221
11–20	984	82.4	65	*79	*12	*43	*82	*190
More than 20	928	91.1	67	73	7	40	100	220
Family health care coverage								
Private insurance only	10,511	71.1	50	70	10	40	90	173
Medicaid only	*317	*53.7	*4	*8	*0	*0	*0	*20
Medicare only	*108	*53.8	*64	*118	*45	*60	*103	*320
Medicare and other public programs	-	-	-	-	-	-	-	-
Medicare and private insurance	-	-	-	-	-	-	-	-
Other public and private mixes	1,361	80.7	64	80	0	56	100	185
Other mixes of public programs	*186	*49.3	*16	*32	*0	*8	*32	*139
Source unknown	*491	*88.4	*26	*29	*0	*0	*16	*50

[2]Annual rate.
[3]Includes only families with heads 17 years of age and over.
[4]Excludes families with all members under 14 years of age.
[5]Excludes families with all members with health status unknown.

NOTE: 1-person families are families with average size less than 1.5. For 1-person families with more than 1 distinct individual, characteristics are those of head or of family as in Table 2.

Table 29

Out-of-pocket expenditures for ambulatory physician visits for 1-person families under 65 years of age without health care coverage all year, by selected characteristics: United States, 1980

[Rate per family year. Civilian noninstitutionalized population with civilian family head]

Characteristic	All families		Families with visits					
	Number in thousands	Mean expenditures	Percent	Mean expenditures	Expenditures at selected percentiles			
					25th	50th	75th	90th
Total.................	5,545	$43	61.4	$70	$4	$30	$72	$185
Age								
Under 25 years..............	2,042	48	65.0	75	0	28	74	229
25-44 years.................	2,424	42	63.9	66	3	29	68	156
45-64 years.................	1,079	33	49.1	*67	*12	*41	*81	*161
Sex								
Male........................	3,275	19	50.3	38	0	15	36	80
Female......................	2,270	77	77.5	99	26	47	117	229
Race and ethnicity[1]								
White.......................	4,603	41	63.5	64	0	30	72	161
Hispanic....................	*280	*13	*47.6	*27	*0	*25	*60	*70
Non-Hispanic................	4,323	43	64.5	66	0	30	75	161
Black.......................	*700	*66	*54.4	*121	*14	*46	*104	*326
Other.......................	*242	*17	*42.7	*40	*26	*40	*45	*65
Family dynamics								
Unchanging, full year.......	4,470	39	62.9	63	4	27	68	156
Change in composition or existed less than full year.......	1,075	57	55.5	102	15	40	123	253
Poverty status in 1980								
Below 150 percent...........	2,405	41	58.7	69	7	30	74	188
Below poverty level.........	1,394	29	55.9	51	0	25	68	139
Poverty level to 149 percent..........	1,012	57	62.6	*91	*10	*33	*106	*253
150-199 percent.............	784	30	57.2	*52	*8	*28	*65	*139
200-299 percent.............	1,253	*47	62.1	*75	*0	*18	*66	*123
300-499 percent.............	*725	*60	*71.0	*84	*15	*31	*110	*232
500 percent or more.........	*379	*39	*66.8	*59	*0	*40	*81	*208
Family income in 1980[2]								
Less than $10,000...........	3,602	44	61.0	72	7	30	68	188
$10,000-$19,999.............	1,457	43	61.5	70	4	30	78	156
$20,000-$34,999.............	*415	*36	*62.1	*57	*0	*20	*81	*208
$35,000 or more.............	*71	*13	*81.0	*16	*0	*0	*45	*45

108

Education[3]

None or elementary school	*443	*20	*39.2	*50	*0	*30	*60	*221
Some high school	1,008	*35	50.4	*68	*18	*27	*68	*121
High school graduate	1,713	39	64.5	61	0	37	74	188
Some college	1,208	*46	70.7	*64	0	20	45	124
College graduate or more	1,127	62	64.6	*96	*12	*34	*110	*340

Employment status[4]

Worked full year	2,314	56	65.3	86	0	33	78	224
Worked part year	2,711	36	63.5	57	6	29	72	161
Never worked	*495	*17	*31.7	*52	*15	*22	*56	*188

Perceived health status[5]

Excellent	2,559	32	61.7	52	0	20	55	139
Good	2,314	54	57.9	93	16	40	97	214
Fair	*441	*55	*79.1	*69	*0	*45	*81	*197
Poor	*231	*28	*59.8	*46	*0	*15	*30	*224

Limitation in usual activity

None	5,276	41	61.2	67	6	30	72	180
Some limitation	*82	*226	*61.8	*365	*0	*326	*875	*875
Cannot perform usual activity	*188	*15	*67.9	*22	*0	*0	*22	*56

Bed days[2]

0	2,622	27	44.7	59	0	25	60	161
1-5	1,575	52	76.6	68	0	29	74	180
6-10	766	72	78.8	*91	*15	*39	*65	*229
11-20	*237	*69	*74.2	*93	*35	*76	*98	*224
More than 20	*345	*41	*72.4	*57	*0	*30	*56	*161

Family health care coverage

All members covered, some part year	3,223	43	68.2	63	0	23	62	151
Some members not covered	-	-	-	-	-	-	-	-
All members not covered	2,322	42	52.1	81	20	45	97	221

[1]There were too few Hispanic families of races other than white for separate tabulation.
[2]Annual rate.
[3]Includes only families with heads 17 years of age and over.
[4]Excludes families with all members under 14 years of age.
[5]Excludes families with all members with health status unknown.

NOTE: 1-person families are families with average size less than 1.5. For 1-person families with more than 1 distinct individual, characteristics are those of head or of family as in Table 2.

Table 30

Out-of-pocket expenditures for ambulatory physician visits for 1-person families 65 years of age and over, by selected characteristics: United States, 1980

[Rate per family year. Civilian noninstitutionalized population with civilian family head]

Characteristic	All families		Families with visits					
	Number in thousands	Mean expenditures	Percent	Mean expenditures	Expenditures at selected percentiles			
					25th	50th	75th	90th
Total..................	7,714	$74	79.3	$94	$15	$54	$109	$203
Sex								
Male.................	1,784	61	74.0	82	0	31	96	228
Female...............	5,930	78	80.8	97	18	55	110	197
Race and ethnicity[1]								
White................	7,025	78	80.5	97	16	55	114	204
Hispanic.............	*138	*20	*81.9	*25	*0	*0	*14	*65
Non-Hispanic.........	6,887	79	80.4	98	17	56	115	206
Black................	582	33	68.8	*48	*0	*25	*74	*118
Other................	*106	*69	*57.2	*121	*0	*0	*101	*452
Family dynamics								
Unchanging, full year.......	7,083	71	79.4	90	15	51	108	203
Change in composition or existed less than full year...........	630	*110	77.9	*141	0	60	125	196
Poverty status in 1980								
Below 150 percent poverty level......	4,199	73	79.4	92	7	40	101	182
Below poverty level.............	2,220	76	79.6	95	5	30	82	156
Poverty level to 149 percent...........	1,979	70	79.2	89	8	56	121	197
150-199 percent..........	1,118	73	81.3	90	15	48	115	237
200-299 percent..........	1,313	66	74.3	89	29	71	115	197
300-499 percent..........	783	84	84.1	100	31	83	138	232
500 percent or more......	*300	*104	*78.9	*132	*30	*56	*125	*543
Family income in 1980[2]								
Less than $10,000........	6,246	70	77.8	90	9	44	104	193
$10,000-$19,999..........	1,167	88	87.4	100	36	83	138	218
$20,000-$34,999..........	*136	*113	*63.2	*179	*42	*56	*274	*747
$35,000 or more..........	*165	*97	*91.9	*105	*25	*40	*125	*144

Education

None or elementary school	3,012	80.3	93	8	41	104	174
Some high school	1,451	69.1	81	2	55	106	193
High school graduate	1,653	82.5	98	16	54	102	197
Some college	804	73.0	*80	*21	*56	*103	*162
College graduate or more	793	93.5	115	36	71	182	257

Employment status

Worked full year	*411	*76.6	*78	*25	*57	*94	*156
Worked part year	863	75.3	85	14	57	104	221
Never worked	6,439	80.0	96	15	50	114	197

Perceived health status[3]

Excellent	2,313	72.4	97	20	58	120	208
Good	2,790	78.2	91	10	48	101	206
Fair	1,825	87.8	103	15	53	118	204
Poor	765	82.9	68	9	56	106	182

Limitation in usual activity

None	5,049	76.9	92	15	55	106	197
Some limitation	*523	*80.1	*98	*21	*42	*114	*226
Cannot perform usual activity	2,142	84.5	96	12	47	115	204

Bed days[2]

0	4,338	70.3	84	15	50	103	169
1-5	867	83.5	83	31	60	116	208
6-10	658	93.5	67	0	30	83	183
11-20	702	97.0	145	0	65	128	298
More than 20	1,149	90.7	112	15	56	110	245

Family health care coverage

All members covered full year	7,517	80.0	94	14	55	109	203
Private insurance only	*13	*100.0	*84	*84	*84	*84	*84
Medicaid only	—	—	—	—	—	—	—
Medicare only	1,154	66.9	*139	22	72	134	204
Medicare and other public programs	993	79.8	*61	0	0	28	81
Medicare and private insurance	4,819	83.7	95	20	60	118	216
Other public and private mixes	—	—	—	—	—	—	—
Other mixes of public programs	—	—	—	—	—	—	—
Source unknown	*538	*74.4	*68	*8	*41	*79	*130
All members covered, some part year	—	—	—	—	—	—	—
Some members not covered	*24	*100.0	*110	*30	*175	*175	*175
All members not covered	*172	*46.3	*54	*36	*40	*45	*115

[1] There were too few Hispanic families of races other than white for separate tabulation.
[2] Annual rate.
[3] Excludes families with all members with health status unknown.

NOTE: 1-person families are families with average size less than 1.5. For 1-person families with more than 1 distinct individual, characteristics are those of head or of family as in Table 5.

111

Table 31

Out-of-pocket expenditures for hospital emergency room and outpatient visits for multiple-person families, by selected characteristics: United States, 1980

[Rate per family year. Civilian noninstitutionalized population with civilian family head]

Characteristic	All families		Families with visits					
	Number in thousands	Mean expenditures	Percent	Mean expenditures	Expenditures at selected percentiles			
					25th	50th	75th	90th
Total...............	58,135	$32	60.0	$53	$0	$9	$59	$145
Family size[1]								
2 persons.................	22,916	25	48.6	52	0	5	51	141
3 persons.................	12,567	31	61.2	50	0	8	64	148
4 persons.................	12,269	35	64.8	53	0	9	55	143
5 or more persons.........	10,383	44	78.2	57	0	13	66	160
Age of head								
Under 25 years............	4,308	32	67.1	47	0	0	55	153
25–44 years...............	25,173	34	65.9	51	0	8	55	135
45–64 years...............	20,129	32	56.6	57	0	8	66	160
65 years and over.........	8,525	26	47.0	55	0	14	60	144
Sex of head								
Male......................	44,874	31	58.6	53	0	12	62	145
Female....................	13,262	34	65.0	53	0	0	44	147
Race and ethnicity[2] of head								
White.....................	51,015	32	59.6	53	0	10	59	145
Hispanic..................	3,403	42	61.9	68	0	21	90	180
Non-Hispanic..............	47,613	31	59.4	52	0	10	58	142
Black.....................	6,090	34	64.4	53	0	0	44	150
Other.....................	1,030	36	55.1	66	0	14	77	172
Family structure								
Head and spouse present whole time......	42,556	30	58.7	52	0	12	60	143
Child under 17 years.....	22,442	33	67.3	49	0	13	59	141
No child under 17 years.....	20,114	28	49.1	57	0	10	61	149
Head only, no spouse at any time......	13,977	33	62.8	53	0	0	47	147
Child under 17 years.....	8,643	38	71.5	53	0	6	44	147
No child under 17 years.....	5,334	26	48.7	53	0	6	54	144
Other.....................	1,602	57	71.5	80	0	11	101	259

Family dynamics

Unchanging, full year	46,990	27	58.0	46	0	7	52	128
Change in composition or existed less than full year	11,145	53	68.4	77	0	15	84	190

Family poverty status in 1980

Below 150 percent poverty level	10,938	31	65.7	47	0	0	48	147
Below poverty level	6,047	30	67.8	44	0	0	38	120
Poverty level to 149 percent	4,892	33	63.1	52	0	6	59	165
150-199 percent	6,355	53	60.0	88	0	16	88	194
200-299 percent	12,860	32	62.0	52	0	17	60	141
300-499 percent	17,047	26	58.4	45	0	6	48	128
500 percent or more	10,935	29	54.5	53	0	7	64	152

Family income in 1980[3]

Less than $10,000	10,629	31	60.9	51	0	0	47	154
$10,000-$19,999	16,728	37	58.7	63	0	15	73	169
$20,000-$34,999	19,706	29	60.1	49	0	11	54	135
$35,000 or more	11,073	30	61.0	49	0	8	59	142

Education of head[4]

None or elementary school	10,491	38	54.4	69	0	15	74	182
Some high school	9,267	42	65.2	65	0	2	65	150
High school graduate	20,605	28	60.9	46	0	7	58	128
Some college	8,651	28	62.9	44	0	9	45	124
College graduate or more	9,099	27	56.6	47	0	6	57	145

Family employment status[5]

2 or more persons worked full year	14,607	28	61.5	45	0	6	59	133
Only 1 person worked full year	24,549	37	58.7	62	0	15	65	165
Some part-year work	11,303	34	65.6	52	0	4	56	147
No person worked	7,676	21	53.1	40	0	0	35	133

Worst perceived health status of any family member[6]

Excellent	16,200	21	53.0	40	0	5	42	107
Good	24,467	28	59.6	47	0	8	53	136
Fair	11,131	44	66.3	66	0	13	72	165
Poor	6,318	54	68.8	79	0	13	100	264

Most severe limitation in usual activity of any family member

None	43,941	29	58.2	50	0	9	55	135
Some limitation	3,679	36	66.6	55	0	6	47	119
Cannot perform usual activity	10,515	42	65.5	64	0	11	84	182

Table 31--continued

Out-of-pocket expenditures for hospital emergency room and outpatient visits for multiple-person families, by selected characteristics: United States, 1980

[Rate per family year. Civilian noninstitutionalized population with civilian family head]

| | All families | | | Families with visits | | | | |
| | | | | | | Expenditures at selected percentiles | | |
Characteristic	Number in thousands	Mean expenditures	Percent	Mean expenditures	25th	50th	75th	90th
Family's bed days³								
0.........	11,173	17	37.7	45	0	7	53	136
1-5........	14,527	22	52.5	42	0	7	49	125
6-10.......	8,834	33	62.6	52	0	7	57	135
11-20......	9,982	31	68.4	45	0	12	52	123
More than 20......	13,619	55	78.6	70	0	10	73	186
Family health care coverage								
All members covered full year.........	42,453	$24	59.7	$40	$0	$4	$44	$112
Private insurance only..............	25,759	24	58.8	41	0	8	46	120
Medicaid only......................	1,621	*5	69.7	*8	0	0	0	0
Medicare only.....................	*574	*16	*27.6	*58	*11	*26	*83	*142
Medicare and other public programs....	*471	*12	*61.9	*20	*0	*0	*11	*73
Medicare and private insurance........	7,475	26	50.4	51	0	14	60	138
Other public and private mixes........	5,853	27	73.1	38	0	0	41	103
Other mixes of public programs........	*135	*2	*64.0	*3	*0	*0	*2	*20
Source unknown.....................	*564	*17	*83.6	*21	*0	*0	*0	*70
All members covered, some part year.....	8,669	40	63.0	63	0	15	74	169
Some members not covered.............	4,963	79	61.3	129	0	41	169	343
All members not covered..............	2,051	51	51.9	99	30	51	118	248

¹Average size during period of family's existence rounded to nearest integer; exactly half an integer rounded upward.
²There were too few Hispanic families of races other than white for separate tabulation.
³Annual rate.
⁴Includes only families with heads 17 years of age and over.
⁵Excludes families with all members under 14 years of age.
⁶Excludes families with all members with health status unknown.

NOTE: Multiple-person families are families with average size 1.5 or greater.

Table 32

Out-of-pocket expenditures for hospital emergency room and outpatient visits for multiple-person families with all members under 65 years of age, by selected characteristics: United States, 1980

[Rate per family year. Civilian noninstitutionalized population with civilian family head]

| Characteristic | All families | | Families with visits | | | | | |
| | Number in thousands | Mean expenditures | Percent | Mean expenditures | Expenditures at selected percentiles | | | |
					25th	50th	75th	90th
Total........................	47,327	$33	62.3	$52	$0	$8	$56	$145
Family size[1]								
2 persons....................	14,958	26	50.0	51	0	1	44	121
3 persons....................	11,228	31	62.5	49	0	7	63	143
4 persons....................	11,546	34	64.8	52	0	8	53	140
5 or more persons...........	9,595	45	78.1	57	0	15	64	160
Age of head								
Under 25 years...............	4,283	31	67.1	46	0	0	51	153
25–44 years..................	24,783	34	65.8	51	0	8	55	134
45–64 years..................	18,261	32	56.2	56	0	10	64	155
Sex of head								
Male.........................	36,477	32	60.6	53	0	12	60	144
Female.......................	10,850	35	67.9	51	0	0	44	145
Race and ethnicity[2] of head								
White........................	41,444	32	61.7	53	0	9	57	143
Hispanic...................	3,040	47	64.1	73	0	25	92	181
Non-Hispanic...............	38,405	31	61.5	51	0	8	55	136
Black........................	5,064	32	67.5	48	0	0	44	145
Other........................	819	45	59.3	*76	*0	*24	*128	*180
Family structure								
Head and spouse present whole time......	34,963	31	60.7	51	0	12	59	142
Child under 17 years.......	21,668	32	67.1	48	0	12	59	137
No child under 17 years....	13,295	29	50.3	57	0	10	60	148
Head only, no spouse at any time.......	11,169	36	66.2	55	0	0	45	152
Child under 17 years.......	8,258	38	71.1	54	0	0	44	147
No child under 17 years....	2,911	31	52.3	60	0	0	52	185
Other........................	1,194	48	70.0	68	0	8	94	210
Family dynamics								
Unchanging, full year........	37,714	28	60.7	46	0	6	50	125
Change in composition or existed less than full year.........	9,613	50	68.2	73	0	15	80	180

115

Table 32--continued

Out-of-pocket expenditures for hospital emergency room and outpatient visits for multiple-person families with all members under 65 years of age, by selected characteristics: United States, 1980

[Rate per family year. Civilian noninstitutionalized population with civilian family head]

| | All families | | Families with visits | | | | | |
| | Number in thousands | Mean expenditures | Percent | Mean expenditures | Expenditures at selected percentiles | | | |
Characteristic					25th	50th	75th	90th
Family poverty status in 1980								
Below 150 percent poverty level	8,770	$31	69.5	$45	$0	$0	$47	$143
Below poverty level	5,083	28	71.7	39	0	0	30	101
Poverty level to 149 percent	3,687	37	66.4	55	0	13	68	172
150-199 percent	4,825	61	62.4	97	0	24	90	219
200-299 percent	10,075	35	65.6	53	0	15	62	149
300-499 percent	14,307	26	60.2	44	0	5	44	117
500 percent or more	9,350	27	55.0	49	0	7	64	143
Family income in 1980[3]								
Less than $10,000	7,496	32	66.2	49	0	0	46	143
$10,000-$19,999	12,555	41	62.6	65	0	15	73	170
$20,000-$34,999	17,279	29	61.1	47	0	11	52	132
$35,000 or more	9,997	30	60.9	49	0	8	59	142
Education of head[4]								
None or elementary school	5,822	43	60.9	70	0	14	60	208
Some high school	7,546	45	66.8	67	0	0	64	149
High school graduate	18,299	29	61.7	46	0	8	59	128
Some college	7,556	28	64.4	43	0	5	44	120
College graduate or more	8,084	28	58.3	47	0	6	57	141
Family employment status[5]								
2 or more persons worked full year	13,629	28	61.7	45	0	8	56	135
Only 1 person worked full year	21,782	37	59.6	61	0	15	61	167
Some part-year work	9,021	35	68.3	51	0	0	56	142
No person worked	2,896	20	66.0	30	0	0	2	60
Worst perceived health status of any family member[6]								
Excellent	14,771	19	54.7	36	0	4	41	101
Good	20,837	29	61.4	48	0	7	54	136
Fair	8,021	52	70.6	73	0	17	75	176
Poor	3,678	63	79.2	79	0	12	91	272

Most severe limitation in usual activity
of any family member

None................................	39,751	29	59.7	49	0	8	54	132
Some limitation.....................	2,814	35	72.8	48	0	1	47	119
Cannot perform usual activity.......	4,762	58	77.1	76	0	11	94	257

Family's bed days[3]

0...................................	7,825	19	42.0	45	0	4	41	143
1-5.................................	12,427	22	54.2	40	0	5	49	121
6-10................................	7,470	31	63.5	48	0	5	57	132
11-20...............................	8,884	30	69.0	43	0	14	51	116
More than 20........................	10,722	59	79.8	74	0	11	70	198

Family health care coverage

All members covered full year.......	33,575	23	62.0	38	0	0	41	106
Private insurance only..............	25,502	24	58.7	40	0	8	46	114
Medicaid only.......................	1,606	*5	69.4	*8	0	0	0	0
Medicare only.......................	*12	–	–	–	–	–	–	–
Medicare and other public programs..	*95	*0	*0.0	–	*0	*30	*133	*133
Medicare and private insurance......	5,762	*21	*49.5	*42	*0	0	42	105
Other public and private mixes......	*135	28	73.0	38	0	0	*2	*20
Other mixes of public programs......	*463	*2	*64.0	*3	*0	*0	*0	*16
Source unknown......................	.*463	*17	*89.9	*19	*0	*0	*0	169
All members covered, some part year.	7,968	40	64.1	63	0	18	70	335
Some members not covered............	3,804	88	65.1	135	0	44	169	248
All members not covered.............	1,980	53	53.2	100	30	51	118	

[1]Average size during period of family's existence rounded to nearest integer; exactly half an integer rounded upward.
[2]There were too few Hispanic families of races other than white for separate tabulation.
[3]Annual rate.
[4]Includes only families with heads 17 years of age and over.
[5]Excludes families with all members under 14 years of age.
[6]Excludes families with all members with health status unknown.

NOTE: Multiple-person families are families with average size 1.5 or greater.

Table 33

Out-of-pocket expenditures for hospital emergency room and outpatient visits for multiple-person families with all members under 65 years of age and all members with health care coverage all year, by selected characteristics: United States, 1980

[Rate per family year. Civilian noninstitutionalized population with civilian family head]

Characteristic	All families		Families with visits					
	Number in thousands	Mean expenditures	Percent	Mean expenditures	Expenditures at selected percentiles			
					25th	50th	75th	90th
Total.................	33,575	$23	62.0	$38	$0	$0	$41	$106
Family size[1]								
2 persons............	10,994	20	50.3	39	0	0	35	94
3 persons............	8,010	23	63.5	36	0	0	42	99
4 persons............	8,464	25	64.6	39	0	5	47	132
5 or more persons....	6,107	28	77.9	36	0	3	47	120
Age of head								
Under 25 years.......	2,585	22	70.9	31	0	0	40	95
25-44 years..........	18,256	24	65.8	36	0	3	42	99
45-64 years..........	12,733	23	54.8	42	0	4	41	128
Sex of head								
Male.................	27,351	25	60.7	41	0	6	47	115
Female...............	6,224	16	68.2	23	0	0	25	72
Race and ethnicity[2] of head								
White................	29,902	23	61.6	38	0	3	41	106
Hispanic.............	1,711	24	58.5	41	0	4	57	134
Non-Hispanic.........	28,191	23	61.8	38	0	3	40	105
Black................	3,139	19	67.1	29	0	0	40	95
Other................	533	*36	58.3	*72	*0	*15	*130	*172
Family structure								
Head and spouse present whole time.....	26,517	25	60.8	41	0	7	46	112
Child under 17 years..........	16,251	26	67.7	38	0	8	47	112
No child under 17 years.......	10,266	24	49.9	47	0	4	44	114
Head only, no spouse at any time........	6,394	16	65.6	24	0	0	27	78
Child under 17 years..........	5,051	16	69.1	23	0	0	21	78
No child under 17 years.......	1,343	14	52.6	27	0	0	35	67
Other................	663	*36	77.5	*46	*0	*0	*56	*138
Family dynamics								
Unchanging, full year....	28,266	22	61.2	35	0	0	40	99
Change in composition or existed less than full year....	5,308	32	66.7	49	0	2	63	154

Family poverty status in 1980							
Below 150 percent poverty level	4,640	21	72.6	29	0	0	27	99
Below poverty level	2,919	14	73.7	19	0	0	0	60
Poverty level to 149 percent	1,721	33	70.9	47	0	7	59	154
150-199 percent	2,657	27	65.3	42	0	4	48	112
200-299 percent	7,074	26	65.8	40	0	11	48	106
300-499 percent	11,427	20	59.5	34	0	2	37	89
500 percent or more	7,776	26	55.0	47	0	5	60	143
Family income in 1980[3]							
Less than $10,000	4,023	18	69.2	26	0	0	12	78
$10,000-$19,999	7,715	27	63.1	42	0	4	43	106
$20,000-$34,999	13,970	22	60.5	36	0	5	44	100
$35,000 or more	7,867	26	60.1	44	0	6	48	141
Education of head[4]							
None or elementary school	3,188	25	59.8	42	0	0	39	147
Some high school	4,620	23	65.0	35	0	0	40	89
High school graduate	13,366	20	61.3	33	0	0	41	100
Some college	5,757	24	64.5	37	0	2	40	90
College graduate or more	6,625	28	60.5	47	0	7	52	135
Family employment status[5]							
2 or more persons worked full year	10,347	21	61.5	34	0	4	43	112
Only 1 person worked full year	16,128	27	59.3	45	0	11	48	120
Some part-year work	4,933	22	71.6	31	0	0	32	95
No person worked	2,167	*13	63.3	*20	0	0	0	48
Worst perceived health status of any family member[6]							
Excellent	11,162	18	56.3	32	0	0	35	91
Good	15,029	22	62.0	36	0	3	44	102
Fair	5,209	29	67.8	42	0	4	53	132
Poor	2,155	44	78.2	56	0	0	58	158
Most severe limitation in usual activity of any family member							
None	28,461	21	59.9	35	0	3	41	100
Some limitation	2,067	35	71.3	49	0	0	33	132
Cannot perform usual activity	3,047	38	75.6	50	0	0	58	165
Family's bed days[3]							
0	5,766	13	42.8	30	0	0	31	85
1-5	8,806	16	52.9	31	0	3	38	101
6-10	5,513	21	62.8	34	0	0	41	100
11-20	6,162	26	71.3	37	0	5	43	100
More than 20	7,328	39	79.8	49	0	2	50	135

Table 33—continued

Out-of-pocket expenditures for hospital emergency room and outpatient visits for multiple-person families with all members under 65 years of age and all members with health care coverage all year, by selected characteristics: United States, 1980

[Rate per family year. Civilian noninstitutionalized population with civilian family head]

| | All families | | Families with visits | | | | | |
| | | | | | Expenditures at selected percentiles | | | |
Characteristic	Number in thousands	Mean expenditures	Percent	Mean expenditures	25th	50th	75th	90th
Family health care coverage								
Private insurance only..............	25,502	$24	58.7	$40	$0	$8	$46	$114
Medicaid only......................	1,606	*5	69.4	*8	0	0	0	0
Medicare only......................	-	-	-	-	-	-	-	-
Medicare and other public programs..	*12	*0	*0.0	-	-	-	-	-
Medicare and private insurance......	*95	*21	*49.5	*42	*0	*30	*133	*133
Other public and private mixes......	5,762	28	73.0	38	0	0	42	105
Other mixes of public programs......	*135	*2	*64.0	*3	*0	*0	*2	*20
Source unknown.....................	*463	*17	*89.9	*19	*0	*0	*0	*16

1Average size during period of family's existence rounded to nearest integer; exactly half an integer rounded upward.
2There were too few Hispanic families of races other than white for separate tabulation.
3Annual rate.
4Includes only families with heads 17 years of age and over.
5Excludes families with all members under 14 years of age.
6Excludes families with all members with health status unknown.

NOTE: Multiple-person families are families with average size 1.5 or greater.

120

Table 34

Out-of-pocket expenditures for hospital emergency room and outpatient visits for multiple-person families with all members under 65 years of age and some or all members without health care coverage all year, by selected characteristics: United States, 1980

[Rate per family year. Civilian noninstitutionalized population with civilian family head]

Characteristic	All families		Families with visits					
	Number in thousands	Mean expenditures	Percent	Mean expenditures	Expenditures at selected percentiles			
					25th	50th	75th	90th
Total..................	13,752	$55	62.8	$88	$0	$30	$96	$223
Family size[1]								
2 persons..................	3,964	41	49.1	84	0	25	75	243
3 persons..................	3,218	50	60.0	84	0	43	110	257
4 persons..................	3,082	*57	65.4	*87	0	22	78	165
5 or more persons..........	3,488	74	78.5	94	0	32	109	229
Age of head								
Under 25 years.............	1,698	45	61.4	73	0	30	85	195
25–44 years................	6,527	61	65.9	92	0	30	97	225
45–64 years................	5,528	52	59.5	88	0	30	97	249
Sex of head								
Male.......................	9,126	53	60.4	87	0	36	100	225
Female.....................	4,627	61	67.5	90	0	21	80	223
Race and ethnicity[2] of head								
White......................	11,542	56	61.9	90	0	32	97	223
Hispanic...................	1,328	75	71.3	106	0	45	153	240
Non-Hispanic...............	10,214	53	60.7	88	0	32	94	221
Black......................	1,924	53	68.2	78	0	10	88	212
Other......................	*286	*51	*61.0	*83	*0	*25	*76	*305
Family structure								
Head and spouse present whole time......	8,446	50	60.6	82	0	35	97	219
Child under 17 years.......	5,417	52	65.5	79	0	33	98	201
No child under 17 years....	3,029	46	51.7	89	0	38	94	223
Head only, no spouse at any time.......	4,775	64	67.0	96	0	25	88	227
Child under 17 years.......	3,207	73	74.3	99	0	25	88	223
No child under 17 years....	1,568	46	52.0	88	0	15	56	243
Other......................	*532	*62	*60.7	*103	*0	*23	*145	*369
Family dynamics								
Unchanging, full year......	9,448	48	59.5	80	0	32	94	223
Change in composition or existed less than full year...........	4,304	72	70.0	103	0	26	113	243

121

Table 34—continued

Out-of-pocket expenditures for hospital emergency room and outpatient visits for multiple-person families with all members under 65 years of age and some or all members without health care coverage all year, by selected characteristics: United States, 1980

[Rate per family year. Civilian noninstitutionalized population with civilian family head]

| | All families | | Families with visits | | | | | |
| | Number in thousands | Mean expenditures | Percent | Mean expenditures | Expenditures at selected percentiles | | | |
Characteristic					25th	50th	75th	90th
Family poverty status in 1980								
Below 150 percent poverty level......	4,130	$43	65.9	$65	$0	$18	$64	$221
Below poverty level......	2,164	46	69.0	67	0	15	62	180
Poverty level to 149 percent......	1,966	40	62.4	63	0	20	72	223
150-199 percent......	2,168	101	58.9	171	7	71	169	369
200-299 percent......	3,000	56	65.3	86	0	39	98	272
300-499 percent......	2,880	51	62.8	81	0	24	98	229
500 percent or more......	1,574	31	55.2	56	0	30	80	175
Family income in 1980[3]								
Less than $10,000......	3,473	49	62.7	78	0	20	68	259
$10,000-$19,999......	4,840	63	61.8	103	0	41	126	223
$20,000-$34,999......	3,310	58	63.6	92	0	35	109	257
$35,000 or more......	2,130	42	63.9	66	0	20	83	142
Education of head[4]								
None or elementary school......	2,634	63	62.3	102	0	35	148	346
Some high school......	2,926	80	69.5	115	0	29	100	272
High school graduate......	4,934	51	62.9	81	0	33	98	221
Some college......	1,800	42	64.1	65	0	26	75	189
College graduate or more......	1,459	24	48.2	49	0	6	74	167
Family employment status[5]								
2 or more persons worked full year......	3,282	49	62.2	79	0	31	95	197
Only 1 person worked full year......	5,654	64	60.5	106	0	36	113	272
Some part-year work......	4,087	50	64.3	78	0	29	97	185
No person worked......	*729	*40	*74.0	*54	*0	*0	*47	*330
Worst perceived health status of any family member[6]								
Excellent......	3,609	23	49.7	47	0	23	80	120
Good......	5,808	48	60.0	80	0	30	87	219
Fair......	2,812	94	75.7	124	0	37	119	293
Poor......	1,524	89	80.5	111	0	27	193	351

Most severe limitation in usual activity
of any family member

None.....................	11,290	59.2	51	85	0	30	94	201
Some limitation..............	747	77.2	35	*46	*0	*20	*48	*85
Cannot perform usual activity..........	1,715	79.8	95	119	0	38	172	361

Family's bed days[3]

0...........	2,059	39.9	36	90	0	38	113	212
1-5...........	3,620	57.3	35	61	0	24	80	165
6-10...........	1,957	65.7	57	87	0	25	80	297
11-20...........	2,722	63.8	38	60	0	35	85	173
More than 20...........	3,394	80.0	102	127	0	35	150	305

Family health care coverage

All members covered, some part year......	7,968	64.1	40	63	0	18	70	169
Some members not covered........	3,804	65.1	88	135	0	44	169	335
All members not covered........	1,980	53.2	53	100	30	51	118	248

[1] Average size during period of family's existence rounded to nearest integer; exactly half an integer rounded upward.
[2] There were too few Hispanic families of races other than white for separate tabulation.
[3] Annual rate.
[4] Includes only families with heads 17 years of age and over.
[5] Excludes families with all members under 14 years of age.
[6] Excludes families with all members with health status unknown.

NOTE: Multiple-person families are families with average size 1.5 or greater.

123

Table 35

Out-of-pocket expenditures for hospital emergency room and outpatient visits for multiple-person families with members 65 years of age and over, by selected characteristics: United States, 1980

[Rate per family year. Civilian noninstitutionalized population with civilian family head]

Characteristic	All families		Families with visits					
	Number in thousands	Mean expenditures	Percent	Mean expenditures	Expenditures at selected percentiles			
					25th	50th	75th	90th
Total..............................	10,809	$28	50.2	$56	$0	$12	$70	$150
Family size[1]								
2 persons.........................	7,958	25	46.0	55	0	14	60	144
3 persons.........................	1,339	*31	50.3	*62	0	13	74	165
4 persons.........................	724	*51	64.9	*78	*0	*13	*116	*230
5 or more persons.................	788	36	79.6	*45	*0	*6	*84	*165
Family age								
All members 65 years and over.....	4,141	17	45.1	38	0	8	47	117
Some members under 65.............	6,668	35	53.4	66	0	15	80	182
Sex of head								
Male..............................	8,397	27	49.8	55	0	13	73	150
Female............................	2,412	*32	51.9	*62	0	12	60	182
Race and ethnicity[2] of head								
White.............................	9,571	27	50.6	54	0	14	74	150
Hispanic..........................	*363	*6	*43.0	*14	*0	*0	*21	*55
Non-Hispanic......................	9,208	28	50.9	55	0	14	79	150
Black.............................	1,027	*43	49.0	*88	*0	*0	*44	*186
Other.............................	*211	*3	*38.7	*7	*0	*0	*0	*50
Family structure								
Head and spouse present whole time.....	7,593	28	49.2	57	0	13	73	150
Child under 17 years..............	774	48	71.9	66	0	31	102	145
No child under 17 years...........	6,819	26	46.6	55	0	11	61	150
Head only, no spouse at any time......	2,808	21	49.2	43	0	12	54	143
Child under 17 years..............	*384	*35	*80.4	*44	*0	*0	*21	*73
No child under 17 years...........	2,424	19	44.3	43	0	14	54	143
Other.............................	*408	*85	*76.0	*112	*0	*32	*179	*514
Family dynamics								
Unchanging, full year.............	9,276	21	47.0	45	0	11	60	136
Change in composition or existed less than full year..............	1,533	71	69.7	102	0	30	138	241

Family poverty status in 1980

Below 150 percent poverty level	2,169	*30	50.3	*59	0	2	73	182
Below poverty level	964	*41	47.0	*88	*0	*20	*102	*264
Poverty level to 149 percent	1,205	21	53.0	39	0	0	32	144
150-199 percent	1,530	*28	52.5	*54	0	20	34	192
200-299 percent	2,785	23	49.0	46	0	13	60	123
300-499 percent	2,740	26	49.3	53	0	9	85	143
500 percent or more	1,585	41	51.8	78	0		80	228

Family income in 1980[3]

Less than $10,000	3,133	27	48.3	56	0	0	59	182
$10,000-$19,999	4,173	25	47.1	54	0	18	75	145
$20,000-$34,999	2,427	35	53.2	67	0	14	77	165
$35,000 or more	1,076	28	61.2	46	0	6	59	135

Education of head[4]

None or elementary school	4,669	32	46.2	69	0	20	84	162
Some high school	1,721	31	58.1	53	0	7	70	150
High school graduate	2,306	24	54.6	43	0	5	54	143
Some college	1,095	25	52.3	*48	*0	*13	*68	*125
College graduate or more	1,015	*22	42.9	*51	*0	*6	*42	*169

Family employment status[5]

2 or more persons worked full year	979	30	59.8	*49	*0	*6	*81	*133
Only 1 person worked full year	2,767	37	51.7	72	0	15	85	145
Some part-year work	2,282	31	54.8	56	0	16	58	184
No person worked	4,781	22	45.2	49	0	8	61	150

Worst perceived health status of any family member[6]

Excellent	1,429	*39	35.1	*110	*0	*21	*70	*350
Good	3,630	19	49.0	39	0	12	50	136
Fair	3,110	23	55.2	41	0	9	60	127
Poor	2,640	42	54.3	78	0	14	115	215

Most severe limitation in usual activity of any family member

None	4,190	26	43.2	59	0	16	62	162
Some limitation	865	*41	46.1	*90	*0	*8	*70	*169
Cannot perform usual activity	5,754	28	56.0	51	0	8	73	150

Family's bed days[3]

0	3,349	12	27.5	43	0	15	70	136
1-5	2,100	23	42.0	54	0	20	47	156
6-10	1,364	44	57.3	77	0	18	60	177
11-20	1,098	*38	63.5	*59	0	7	55	228
More than 20	2,897	41	74.1	55	0	4	85	165

Table 35—continued

Out-of-pocket expenditures for hospital emergency room and outpatient visits for multiple-person families with members 65 years of age and over, by selected characteristics: United States, 1980

[Rate per family year. Civilian noninstitutionalized population with civilian family head]

Characteristic	All families		Families with visits		Expenditures at selected percentiles			
	Number in thousands	Mean expenditures	Percent	Mean expenditures	25th	50th	75th	90th
Family health care coverage								
All members covered full year	8,879	$25	50.7	$50	$0	$12	$60	$142
Private insurance only	*258	*67	*72.1	*93	*0	*12	*179	*215
Medicaid only	*15	*0	*100.0	*0	*0	*0	*0	*0
Medicare only	*574	*16	*27.6	*58	*11	*26	*83	*142
Medicare and other public programs	*459	*13	*63.5	*20	*0	*0	*11	*73
Medicare and private insurance	7,380	26	50.4	51	0	14	60	138
Other public and private mixes	*91	*7	*75.6	*9	*0	*0	*16	*42
Other mixes of public programs	-	-	-	-	-	-	-	-
Source unknown	*102	*17	*55.1	*31	*0	*0	*0	*150
All members covered, some part year	701	*34	50.9	*67	*0	*0	*82	*192
Some members not covered	1,159	*50	48.9	*102	*0	*21	*177	*343
All members not covered	*71	*0	*13.4	*0	*0	*0	*0	*0

1Average size during period of family's existence rounded to nearest integer; exactly half an integer rounded upward.
2There were too few Hispanic families of races other than white for separate tabulation.
3Annual rate.
4Includes only families with heads 17 years of age and over.
5Excludes families with all members under 14 years of age.
6Excludes families with all members with health status unknown.

NOTE: Multiple-person families are families with average size 1.5 or greater.

Table 36

Out-of-pocket expenditures for hospital emergency room and outpatient visits for 1-person families, by selected characteristics: United States, 1980

[Rate per family year. Civilian noninstitutionalized population with civilian family head]

Characteristic	All families		Families with visits					
	Number in thousands	Mean expenditures	Percent	Mean expenditures	Expenditures at selected percentiles			
					25th	50th	75th	90th
Total................	26,233	$11	34.2	$33	$0	$0	$38	$95
Sex								
Male.......................	11,866	8	32.9	25	0	0	29	80
Female.....................	14,367	14	35.3	39	0	7	47	97
Race and ethnicity[1]								
White......................	22,811	11	33.2	32	0	0	38	93
Hispanic...................	818	*11	40.7	*28	*0	*0	*37	*100
Non-Hispanic...............	21,993	11	32.9	33	0	0	39	93
Black......................	2,711	15	42.7	*34	0	0	38	95
Other......................	*712	*10	*34.9	*28	*0	*0	*48	*86
Family dynamics								
Unchanging, full year......	22,570	11	35.0	31	0	0	38	90
Change in composition or existed less than full year.....	3,662	13	29.2	46	0	0	40	119
Poverty status in 1980								
Below 150 percent poverty level....	9,379	12	35.1	34	0	0	40	93
Below poverty level........	5,252	11	34.4	31	0	0	35	93
Poverty level to 149 percent....	4,128	13	36.1	37	0	4	49	91
150-199 percent...........	2,974	8	34.0	23	0	0	32	83
200-299 percent...........	5,563	12	31.6	39	0	7	46	95
300-499 percent...........	5,426	12	38.3	31	0	0	37	84
500 percent or more........	2,891	9	28.6	31	0	0	38	97
Family income in 1980[2]								
Less than $10,000.........	14,468	11	34.5	33	0	0	38	95
$10,000-$19,999..........	8,280	12	35.7	33	0	5	37	89
$20,000-$34,999..........	2,664	11	32.2	33	0	0	45	97
$35,000 or more...........	820	*3	20.2	*16	*0	*0	*32	*37

Table 36—continued

Out-of-pocket expenditures for hospital emergency room and outpatient visits for 1-person families, by selected characteristics: United States, 1980

[Rate per family year. Civilian noninstitutionalized population with civilian family head]

Characteristic	All families			Families with visits					
	Number in thousands	Mean expenditures	Percent	Mean expenditures	Expenditures at selected percentiles				
					25th	50th	75th	90th	
Education[3]									
None or elementary school..........	4,782	10	35.9	28	0	0	32	80	
Some high school...................	3,996	13	31.3	40	0	0	40	141	
High school graduate...............	7,413	11	33.4	32	0	0	39	89	
Some college.......................	4,842	12	37.5	32	0	0	44	95	
College graduate or more...........	5,122	11	32.7	34	0	5	39	96	
Employment status[4]									
Worked full year...................	10,374	$10	30.4	$32	$0	$0	$42	$95	
Worked part year...................	7,129	12	34.7	36	0	0	44	96	
Never worked.......................	8,703	12	38.2	31	0	0	33	83	
Perceived health status[5]									
Excellent..........................	11,226	9	30.1	29	0	0	35	89	
Good...............................	9,642	10	31.6	32	0	5	48	95	
Fair...............................	3,691	20	45.0	44	0	6	48	126	
Poor...............................	1,568	*16	54.7	*30	0	0	4	77	
Limitation in usual activity									
None...............................	21,977	10	30.8	33	0	0	40	95	
Some limitation....................	731	*30	52.3	*57	*0	*30	*76	*118	
Cannot perform usual activity......	3,525	14	51.4	27	0	0	28	89	
Bed days[2]									
0..................................	12,629	8	23.1	34	0	6	43	95	
1-5................................	6,587	11	34.3	31	0	0	35	80	
6-10...............................	2,671	15	47.7	32	0	0	44	106	
11-20..............................	1,924	17	55.3	31	0	0	28	96	
More than 20.......................	2,422	20	60.1	33	0	0	30	80	
Family health care coverage									
All members covered full year......	20,491	10	35.6	28	0	0	32	82	
Private insurance only.............	10,523	10	31.6	33	0	0	39	97	
Medicaid only......................	*317	*0	*29.3	*0	*0	*0	*0	*0	
Medicare only......................	1,262	*12	28.9	*43	*0	*25	*50	*84	
Medicare and other public programs..	993	*4	42.5	*9	*0	*0	*0	*38	
Medicare and private insurance......	4,819	12	36.1	34	0	8	36	77	
Other public and private mixes.....	1,361	*10	48.3	*20	*0	*0	*5	*61	
Other mixes of public programs.....	*186	*0	*68.6	*0	*0	*0	*0	*0	
Source unknown.....................	1,030	*6	54.4	*11	*0	*0	*0	*45	

All members covered, some part year......	3,223	13	36.3	35	0	20	51	97
Some members not covered.................	*24	*13	*100.0	*13	*0	*0	*29	*29
All members not covered..................	2,495	18	19.5	*92	*22	*60	*106	*313

1There were too few Hispanic families of races other than white for separate tabulation.
2Annual rate.
3Includes only families with heads 17 years of age and over.
4Excludes families with all members under 14 years of age.
5Excludes families with all members with health status unknown.

NOTE: 1-person families are families with average size less than 1.5. For 1-person families with more than 1 distinct individual, characteristics are those of head or of family as in Table 1.

Table 37

Out-of-pocket expenditures for hospital emergency room and outpatient visits for 1-person families under 65 years of age, by selected characteristics: United States, 1980

[Rate per family year. Civilian noninstitutionalized population with civilian family head]

Characteristic	All families		Families with visits		Expenditures at selected percentiles			
	Number in thousands	Mean expenditures	Percent	Mean expenditures	25th	50th	75th	90th
Total..............	18,519	$11	33.6	$33	$0	$0	$44	$97
Age								
Under 25 years..........	5,208	14	35.3	39	0	8	55	96
25–44 years............	7,630	9	33.0	26	0	0	29	82
45–64 years............	5,680	12	32.7	36	0	0	48	121
Sex								
Male..................	10,082	8	32.1	24	0	0	29	80
Female................	8,437	15	35.3	43	0	8	52	126
Race and ethnicity[1]								
White.................	15,786	10	32.1	33	0	0	44	97
Hispanic............	680	*13	39.8	*33	*0	*16	*37	*100
Non-Hispanic........	15,106	10	31.8	33	0	0	44	97
Black.................	2,128	*16	43.7	*37	*0	0	41	105
Other.................	*605	*10	*35.4	*28	*0	*0	*48	*86
Family dynamics								
Unchanging, full year..........	15,487	11	35.3	31	0	0	40	96
Change in composition or existed less than full year..........	3,032	12	24.8	47	0	0	50	142
Poverty status in 1980								
Below 150 percent...........	5,181	13	34.3	38	0	0	48	136
Below poverty level...........	3,031	13	34.8	37	0	0	44	142
Poverty level to 149 percent...........	2,149	14	33.6	*41	*0	*0	*50	*136
150–199 percent...........	1,855	8	35.0	*22	*0	*0	*30	*102
200–299 percent...........	4,250	10	30.5	33	0	5	41	95
300–499 percent...........	4,643	13	38.5	34	0	3	45	86
500 percent or more...........	2,590	8	27.3	*28	*0	*0	*32	*97
Family income in 1980[2]								
Less than $10,000...........	8,222	12	34.6	35	0	0	45	106
$10,000–$19,999...........	7,113	12	34.7	33	0	6	39	89
$20,000–$34,999...........	2,529	9	31.6	*28	*0	*0	*45	*97
$35,000 or more...........	*656	*4	*15.9	*26	*0	*0	*37	*121

Characteristic	Number							
Education[3]								
None or elementary school	1,770	*10	33.6	*29	*0	*0	*22	*75
Some high school	2,546	14	30.8	45	0	0	50	148
High school graduate	5,759	11	34.4	32	0	0	41	95
Some college	4,037	12	38.8	31	0	0	45	95
College graduate or more	4,329	9	28.7	32	0	0	34	97
Employment status[4]								
Worked full year	9,963	10	30.5	32	0	6	44	95
Worked part year	6,265	12	34.8	36	0	0	48	102
Never worked	2,264	*13	43.2	*31	0	0	15	154
Perceived health status[5]								
Excellent	8,913	9	31.6	27	0	0	30	86
Good	6,852	11	30.0	37	0	6	58	97
Fair	1,866	23	46.0	51	0	0	75	154
Poor	803	*10	57.9	*18	*0	*0	*0	*45
Limitation in usual activity								
None	16,928	10	31.5	33	0	0	44	96
Some limitation	*209	*20	*48.5	*42	*0	*0	*50	*118
Cannot perform usual activity	1,383	*18	57.0	*31	*0	*0	*8	*163
Bed days[2]								
0	8,291	8	23.5	35	0	3	49	96
1–5	5,721	11	33.9	32	0	0	35	82
6–10	2,013	15	41.8	35	0	6	48	123
11–20	1,222	*16	56.9	*27	*0	*0	*15	*105
More than 20	1,273	*21	61.9	*34	*0	*0	*45	*136
Family health care coverage								
All members covered full year	12,974	10	35.7	28	0	0	29	89
Private insurance only	10,511	10	31.5	33	0	0	40	97
Medicaid only	*317	*0	*29.3	*0	*0	*0	*0	*0
Medicare only	*108	*23	*38.8	*60	*0	*0	*180	*180
Medicare and other public programs	–	–	–	–	–	–	–	–
Medicare and private insurance	–	–	–	–	–	–	–	–
Other public and private mixes	1,361	*10	48.3	*20	*0	*0	*5	*61
Other mixes of public programs	*186	*0	*68.6	*0	*0	*0	*0	*0
Source unknown	*491	*6	*79.6	*7	*0	*0	*0	*45
All members covered, some part year	3,223	13	36.3	35	0	20	51	97
Some members not covered	–	–	–	–	–	–	–	–
All members not covered	2,322	16	18.1	*87	*22	*60	*106	*255

[1]There were too few Hispanic of races other than white families for separate tabulation.
[2]Annual rate.
[3]Includes only families with heads 17 years of age and over.
[4]Excludes families with all members under 14 years of age.
[5]Excludes families with all members with health status unknown.

NOTE: 1-person families are families with average size less than 1.5. For 1-person families with more than 1 distinct individual, characteristics are those of head or of family as in Table 2.

Table 38

Out-of-pocket expenditures for hospital emergency room and outpatient visits for 1-person families under 65 years of age with health care coverage all year, by selected characteristics: United States, 1980

[Rate per family year. Civilian noninstitutionalized population with civilian family head]

Characteristic	All families		Families with visits					
	Number in thousands	Mean expenditures	Percent	Mean expenditures	Expenditures at selected percentiles			
					25th	50th	75th	90th
Total..............	12,974	$10	35.7	$28	$0	$0	$29	$89
Age								
Under 25 years.......	3,166	13	37.6	34	0	0	32	89
25-44 years.........	5,206	8	35.2	22	0	0	15	53
45-64 years.........	4,601	10	34.9	29	0	0	44	98
Sex								
Male................	6,807	6	34.0	18	0	0	9	48
Female..............	6,167	14	37.5	38	0	0	46	121
Race and ethnicity[1]								
White...............	11,183	10	34.2	29	0	0	32	95
Hispanic...........	*400	*13	*40.0	*31	*0	*30	*40	*100
Non-Hispanic.......	10,782	10	34.0	29	0	0	29	95
Black...............	1,428	*12	46.1	*25	*0	*0	*15	*55
Other...............	*363	*3	*39.8	*8	*0	*0	*0	*28
Family dynamics								
Unchanging, full year.....	11,017	10	37.2	26	0	0	28	89
Change in composition or existed less than full year........	1,957	*12	27.1	*43	0	0	39	96
Poverty status in 1980								
Below 150 percent..........	2,775	*7	35.6	21	0	0	0	71
Below poverty level......	1,638	*8	39.9	*21	*0	*0	*0	*71
Poverty level to 149 percent......	1,137	*6	29.4	*21	*0	*0	*44	*61
150-199 percent........	1,072	*6	37.1	*16	*0	*0	*9	*49
200-299 percent........	2,997	10	34.8	30	0	0	40	95
300-499 percent........	3,918	14	41.5	33	0	0	35	89
500 percent or more.....	2,212	*7	25.8	*28	*0	*0	*28	*121
Family income in 1980[2]								
Less than $10,000.........	4,620	7	36.6	20	0	0	8	57
$10,000-$19,999..........	5,656	13	38.9	33	0	0	36	95
$20,000-$34,999..........	*2,114	*9	31.3	*28	*0	*0	*44	*100
$35,000 or more..........	*584	*4	*12.6	*31	*0	*0	*37	*121

Education[3]

None or elementary school	1,328	*6	37.5	*16	*0	*0	*8	*60
Some high school	1,538	*8	33.1	*23	*0	*0	*10	*66
High school graduate	4,047	11	37.7	30	0	0	34	89
Some college	2,830	12	39.6	29	0	0	36	96
College graduate or more	3,201	*9	30.1	*31	0	0	25	98

Employment status[4]

Worked full year	7,649	10	31.5	32	0	0	39	96
Worked part year	3,554	9	36.9	23	0	0	8	71
Never worked	1,769	*12	51.2	*23	0	0	7	66

Perceived health status[5]

Excellent	6,353	7	31.2	24	0	0	22	82
Good	4,537	11	34.3	32	0	0	44	95
Fair	1,425	*19	48.3	*38	*0	*0	*45	*126
Poor	*572	*8	*66.3	*13	*0	*0	*0	*15

Limitation in usual activity

None	11,652	9	33.0	27	0	0	30	82
Some limitation	*127	*28	*52.2	*54	*0	*0	*50	*118
Cannot perform usual activity	1,195	*17	59.5	*28	*0	*0	*8	*123

Bed days[2]

0	5,669	8	25.7	29	0	0	37	96
1-5	4,146	11	34.2	32	0	0	32	71
6-10	1,247	14	47.5	*28	*0	*0	*38	*100
11-20	984	*11	58.7	*19	*0	*0	*8	*89
More than 20	928	*14	62.7	*23	*0	*0	*0	*53

Family health care coverage

Private insurance only	10,511	10	31.5	33	0	0	40	97
Medicaid only	*317	*0	*29.3	*0	*0	*0	*0	*0
Medicare only	*108	*23	*38.8	*60	*0	*0	*180	*180
Medicare and other public programs	—	—	—	—	—	—	—	—
Medicare and private insurance	—	—	—	—	—	—	—	—
Other public and private mixes	1,361	*10	48.3	*20	*0	*0	*5	*61
Other mixes of public programs	*186	*0	*68.6	*0	*0	*0	*0	*0
Source unknown	*491	*6	*79.6	*7	*0	*0	*45	*45

[1]There were too few Hispanic families of races other than white for separate tabulation.
[2]Annual rate.
[3]Includes only families with heads 17 years of age and over.
[4]Excludes families with all members under 14 years of age.
[5]Excludes families with all members with health status unknown.

NOTE: 1-person families are families with average size less than 1.5. For 1-person families with more than 1 distinct individual, characteristics are those of head or of family as in Table 2.

133

Table 39

Out-of-pocket expenditures for hospital emergency room and outpatient visits for 1-person families under 65 years of age without health care coverage all year, by selected characteristics: United States, 1980

[Rate per family year. Civilian noninstitutionalized population with civilian family head]

| Characteristic | All families | | Families with visits | | | | | |
	Number in thousands	Mean expenditures	Percent	Mean expenditures	25th	50th	75th	90th
Total..............	5,545	$14	28.6	$49	$0	$27	$65	$136
Age								
Under 25 years..........	2,042	16	31.8	*49	*0	*35	*84	*142
25–44 years..........	2,424	11	28.4	*37	*0	*26	*50	*95
45–64 years..........	1,079	*19	23.3	*79	*0	*22	*115	*187
Sex								
Male...............	3,275	11	28.1	39	0	20	60	115
Female.............	2,270	18	29.5	*63	*9	*48	*84	*142
Race and ethnicity[1]								
White..............	4,603	12	27.1	44	0	26	60	141
Hispanic...........	*280	*14	*39.4	*36	*0	*0	*29	*187
Non-Hispanic.......	4,323	12	26.3	45	0	26	60	141
Black..............	*700	*26	*38.9	*66	*0	*50	*85	*136
Other..............	*242	*20	*28.6	*70	*48	*48	*86	*115
Family dynamics								
Unchanging, full year.....	4,470	15	30.6	48	0	27	60	115
Change in composition or existed less than full year...........	1,075	*11	20.7	*55	*0	*16	*102	*142
Poverty status in 1980								
Below 150 percent.....	2,405	20	32.8	*60	*0	*29	*80	*173
Below poverty level......	1,394	*18	28.8	*62	*9	*40	*77	*173
Poverty level to 149 percent....	1,012	*22	38.4	*58	*0	*22	*80	*142
150–199 percent...	784	*10	32.0	*32	*0	*0	*36	*106
200–299 percent...	1,253	*9	20.2	*45	*12	*27	*86	*115
300–499 percent...	*725	*10	*22.1	*44	*12	*50	*60	*84
500 percent or more....	*379	*9	35.8	*25	*0	*0	*32	*97
Family income in 1980[2]								
Less than $10,000......	3,602	18	32.0	55	0	27	85	142
$10,000–$19,999......	1,457	*6	18.3	*33	*12	*29	*51	*60
$20,000–$34,999......	*415	*10	*33.2	*31	*0	*0	*65	*97
$35,000 or more......	*71	*6	*42.6	*14	*0	*0	*32	*32

Education[3]

None or elementary school	*443	*21	*22.0	*94	*0	*23	*58	*362
Some high school	1,008	24	27.4	*86	*4	*50	*141	*187
High school graduate	1,713	11	26.8	*41	*0	*16	*60	*142
Some college	1,208	14	37.2	*37	*0	*36	*60	*85
College graduate or more	1,127	*8	24.8	*34	*0	*27	*50	*97

Employment status[4]

Worked full year	2,314	9	27.3	*34	*0	*23	*51	*95
Worked part year	2,711	17	31.9	54	0	35	85	142
Never worked	*495	*19	*14.7	*127	*4	*22	*362	*362

Perceived health status[5]

Excellent	2,559	12	32.6	*36	*0	*26	*48	*95
Good	2,314	12	21.5	*54	*9	*52	*85	*141
Fair	*441	*39	*38.7	*101	*0	*80	*148	*362
Poor	*231	*16	*37.1	*42	*0	*4	*22	*187

Limitation in usual activity

None	5,276	14	28.0	49	0	27	77	115
Some limitation	*82	*8	*42.6	*19	*0	*0	*50	*50
Cannot perform usual activity	*188	*25	*41.3	*59	*0	*4	*154	*187

Bed days[2]

0	2,622	*10	18.8	*53	*0	*27	*84	*115
1-5	1,575	11	33.1	*32	*0	*12	*60	*97
6-10	766	*17	32.5	*51	*0	*40	*60	*142
11-20	*237	*34	49.7	*69	*35	*50	*51	*173
More than 20	*345	*39	59.8	*66	*0	*4	*106	*154

Family health care coverage

All members covered, some part year	3,223	13	36.3	35	0	20	51	97
Some members not covered	-	-	-	-	-	-	-	-
All members not covered	2,322	16	18.1	*87	*22	*60	*106	*255

[1] There were too few Hispanic families of races other than white for separate tabulation.
[2] Annual rate.
[3] Includes only families with heads 17 years of age and over.
[4] Excludes families with all members under 14 years of age.
[5] Excludes families with all members with health status unknown.

NOTE: 1-person families are families with average size less than 1.5. For 1-person families with more than 1 distinct individual, characteristics are those of head or of family as in Table 2.

Table 40

Out-of-pocket expenditures for hospital emergency room and outpatient visits for 1-person families 65 years of age and over, by selected characteristics: United States, 1980

[Rate per family year. Civilian noninstitutionalized population with civilian family head]

Characteristic	All families		Families with visits		Expenditures at selected percentiles			
	Number in thousands	Mean expenditures	Percent	Mean expenditures	25th	50th	75th	90th
Total..................	7,714	$11	35.7	$32	$0	$5	$35	$80
Sex								
Male..................	1,784	*11	37.5	*30	0	0	30	72
Female................	5,930	11	35.2	32	0	6	37	82
Race and ethnicity[1]								
White.................	7,025	12	35.5	32	0	5	35	77
Hispanic.............	*138	*2	*45.1	*4	*0	*0	*0	*20
Non-Hispanic.........	6,887	12	35.3	33	0	6	36	77
Black.................	582	*9	39.0	*23	*0	*8	*30	*80
Other.................	*106	*9	*32.4	*28	*0	*10	*84	*84
Family dynamics								
Unchanging, full year.....	7,083	10	34.4	30	0	6	37	80
Change in composition or existed less than full year......	630	*22	50.4	*43	*0	*0	*29	*80
Poverty status in 1980								
Below 150 percent poverty level........	4,199	10	36.2	28	0	0	34	80
Below poverty level.........	2,220	*8	33.8	24	0	0	33	52
Poverty level to 149 percent.....	1,979	*13	38.8	32	0	5	35	89
150-199 percent........	1,118	8	32.5	*25	*0	*22	*35	*72
200-299 percent........	1,313	*19	35.1	*55	*0	*12	*50	*82
300-499 percent........	783	*5	37.4	*13	*0	*0	*25	*48
500 percent or more.....	*300	*19	*40.0	*48	*0	*0	*42	*80
Family income in 1980[2]								
Less than $10,000.......	6,246	11	34.4	31	0	6	35	82
$10,000-$19,999........	1,167	*13	41.5	*31	*0	*0	*37	*65
$20,000-$34,999........	*136	*42	*43.4	*97	*38	*42	*80	*494
$35,000 or more........	*165	*0	*37.2	*0	*0	*0	*0	*0

Education

None or elementary school	3,012	10	37.2	0	28	6	34	82
Some high school	1,451	*11	32.2	*0	*33	*0	*28	*72
High school graduate	1,653	*9	29.9	*0	*30	*0	*35	*50
Some college	804	*11	30.5	*0	*34	*0	*35	*106
College graduate or more	793	*22	54.2	*0	*40	*23	*50	*77

Employment status

Worked full year	*411	*6	*28.3	*0	*22	*0	*15	*146
Worked part year	863	*13	34.4	*0	*38	*8	*37	*50
Never worked	6,439	11	36.4	0	31	6	35	82

Perceived health status[3]

Excellent	2,313	*9	24.3	*0	*36	*18	*42	*90
Good	2,790	7	35.8	0	20	5	30	57
Fair	1,825	16	43.9	0	37	9	36	89
Poor	765	*23	51.4	*0	*44	*0	*14	*80

Limitation in usual activity

None	5,049	9	28.8	0	31	0	35	57
Some limitation	*523	*34	*53.8	*0	*63	*38	*80	*106
Cannot perform usual activity	2,142	11	47.7	0	23	5	30	77

Bed days[2]

0	4,338	7	22.2	0	32	19	41	68
1-5	867	*10	37.4	*0	*26	*7	*37	*80
6-10	658	*18	65.6	*0	*27	*0	*33	*106
11-20	702	*21	52.4	*0	*39	*0	*50	*91
More than 20	1,149	*19	58.1	0	*32	0	29	53

Family health care coverage

All members covered full year	7,517	10	35.5	0	29	5	35	76
Private insurance only	*13	*0	*100.0	*0	*0	*0	*0	*0
Medicaid only	—	—	—	—	—	—	—	—
Medicare only	1,154	*11	28.0	*0	*41	*30	*42	*83
Medicare and other public programs	993	*4	42.5	*0	*9	*0	*0	*38
Medicare and private insurance	4,819	12	36.1	0	34	8	36	77
Other public and private mixes	—	—	—	—	—	—	—	—
Other mixes of public programs	—	—	—	—	—	—	—	—
Source unknown	*538	*6	*31.4	*0	*20	*0	*23	*66
All members covered, some part year	—	—	—	—	—	—	—	—
Some members not covered	*24	*13	*100.0	*0	*13	*0	*29	*29
All members not covered	*172	*47	*38.8	*18	*122	*82	*106	*360

[1]There were too few Hispanic families of races other than white for separate tabulation.
[2]Annual rate.
[3]Excludes families with all members with health status unknown.

NOTE: 1-person families are families with average size less than 1.5. For 1-person families with more than 1 distinct individual, characteristics are those of head or of family as in Table 5.

Table 41

Out-of-pocket expenditures for dental visits for multiple-person families, by selected characteristics: United States, 1980

[Rate per family year. Civilian noninstitutionalized population with civilian family head]

Characteristic	All families		Families with visits		Expenditures at selected percentiles			
	Number in thousands	Mean expenditures	Percent	Mean expenditures	25th	50th	75th	90th
Total.........	58,135	$159	71.3	$223	$25	$79	$241	$567
Family size								
2 persons......	22,916	110	60.7	181	21	60	190	429
3 persons......	12,567	132	73.1	180	20	70	193	513
4 persons......	12,269	203	80.1	254	35	109	301	622
5 or more persons......	10,383	249	82.1	303	27	108	322	779
Age of head								
Under 25 years......	4,308	57	55.4	103	0	35	110	276
25-44 years......	25,173	172	78.0	221	24	82	232	563
45-64 years......	20,129	188	73.0	257	28	92	310	632
65 years and over......	8,525	105	55.6	190	26	66	205	456
Sex of head								
Male......	44,874	181	73.0	248	33	94	280	622
Female......	13,262	86	65.7	130	0	36	134	315
Race and ethnicity[2] of head								
White......	51,015	171	72.7	235	28	87	253	580
Hispanic......	3,403	151	63.3	239	14	66	166	713
Non-Hispanic......	47,613	172	73.4	234	29	90	256	578
Black......	6,090	64	59.5	108	0	25	103	302
Other......	1,030	156	70.8	220	20	39	322	772
Family structure								
Head and spouse present whole time......	42,556	184	73.5	251	34	98	281	625
Child under 17 years......	22,442	227	80.6	282	40	111	316	724
No child under 17 years......	20,114	136	65.5	208	28	79	246	513
Head only, no spouse at any time......	13,977	86	64.5	134	0	38	136	345
Child under 17 years......	8,643	91	70.8	128	0	25	110	335
No child under 17 years......	5,334	79	54.3	145	20	53	165	387
Other......	1,602	132	72.6	182	15	53	200	533
Family dynamics								
Unchanging, full year......	46,990	163	71.5	228	26	81	244	581
Change in composition or existed less than full year......	11,145	144	70.3	205	18	66	225	512

Family poverty status in 1980

Below 150 percent poverty level	10,938	69	59.1	117	0	25	110	280
Below poverty level	6,047	56	60.6	92	0	10	75	239
Poverty level to 149 percent	4,892	86	57.3	149	15	40	148	341
150-199 percent	6,355	118	62.0	191	23	60	203	449
200-299 percent	12,860	148	69.9	211	26	88	225	550
300-499 percent	17,047	192	76.0	253	36	99	283	613
500 percent or more	10,935	235	83.1	283	39	117	335	700

Family income in 1980[3]

Less than $10,000	10,629	55	53.8	103	0	20	75	265
$10,000-$19,999	16,728	109	63.3	172	24	66	176	416
$20,000-$34,999	19,706	184	78.3	235	35	96	255	595
$35,000 or more	11,073	290	87.8	331	47	144	395	849

Education of head[4]

None or elementary school	10,491	80	52.0	154	15	43	146	452
Some high school	9,267	106	63.6	166	17	60	193	420
High school graduate	20,605	163	74.9	217	24	85	237	540
Some college	8,651	207	79.8	260	32	97	292	675
College graduate or more	9,099	251	85.1	295	40	114	324	727

Family employment status[5]

2 or more persons worked full year	14,607	231	80.2	288	38	109	322	767
Only 1 person worked full year	24,549	172	74.8	230	30	90	253	560
Some part-year work	11,303	88	62.8	141	8	50	154	395
No person worked	7,676	86	55.7	154	0	40	142	402

Worst perceived health status of any family member[6]

Excellent	16,200	191	75.5	253	33	97	275	635
Good	24,467	164	74.3	221	26	80	232	564
Fair	11,131	127	64.3	197	15	61	240	532
Poor	6,318	115	61.6	186	12	48	171	480

Most severe limitation in usual activity of any family member

None	43,941	168	73.2	230	26	82	242	580
Some limitation	3,679	168	71.0	236	18	82	286	681
Cannot perform usual activity	10,515	118	63.5	185	16	65	205	486

Family's bed days[3]

0	11,173	125	63.4	197	22	66	230	500
1-5	14,527	147	71.8	205	26	83	228	531
6-10	8,834	168	74.1	227	28	80	254	576
11-20	9,982	177	75.7	234	27	94	256	606
More than 20	13,619	181	72.2	251	20	76	250	629

Table 41—continued

Out-of-pocket expenditures for dental visits for multiple-person families, by selected characteristics: United States, 1980

[Rate per family year.   Civilian noninstitutionalized population with civilian family head]

Characteristic	All families		Families with visits		Expenditures at selected percentiles			
	Number in thousands	Mean expenditures	Percent	Mean expenditures	25th	50th	75th	90th
Family health care coverage								
All members covered full year..........	42,453	$177	74.8	$237	$25	$85	$253	$605
Private insurance only............	25,759	220	80.3	275	40	106	299	675
Medicaid only..............	1,621	*20	67.9	*30	0	0	0	65
Medicare only..............	*574	*53	*48.0	*111	*30	*75	*151	*250
Medicare and other public programs....	*471	*24	*38.7	*61	*0	*0	*25	*456
Medicare and private insurance........	7,475	131	60.7	216	30	74	250	578
Other public and private mixes........	5,853	128	76.5	167	3	60	177	440
Other mixes of public programs........	*135	*172	*81.1	*212	*64	*130	*210	*767
Source unknown................	*564	*32	*73.6	*44	*0	*0	*26	*160
All members covered, some part year.....	8,66C	129	65.2	199	21	66	222	514
Some members not covered.....	4,963	97	59.9	161	20	55	183	447
All members not covered	2,051	64	51.3	126	28	58	138	279

[1]Average size during period of family's existence rounded to nearest integer; exactly half an integer rounded upward.
[2]There were too few Hispanic families of races other than white for separate tabulation.
[3]Annual rate.
[4]Includes only families with heads 17 years of age and over.
[5]Excludes families with all members under 14 years of age.
[6]Excludes families with all members with health status unknown.

NOTE: Multiple-person families are families with average size 1.5 or greater.

Table 42

Out-of-pocket expenditures for dental visits for multiple-person families with all members under 65 years of age, by selected characteristics: United States, 1980

[Rate per family year. Civilian noninstitutionalized population with civilian family head]

Characteristic	All families		Families with visits					
	Number in thousands	Mean expenditures	Percent	Mean expenditures	Expenditures at selected percentiles			
					25th	50th	75th	90th
Total........................	47,327	$168	74.2	$226	$25	$81	$244	$574
Family size[1]								
2 persons.................	14,958	119	64.7	183	20	60	187	423
3 persons.................	11,228	128	74.2	173	19	70	187	490
4 persons.................	11,546	198	80.3	246	35	108	299	612
5 or more persons.........	9,595	253	81.6	310	27	114	328	809
Age of head								
Under 25 years............	4,283	56	55.1	102	0	34	104	276
25-44 years...............	24,783	171	77.9	220	24	82	231	560
45-64 years...............	18,261	189	73.6	257	28	99	317	617
Sex of head								
Male......................	36,477	190	76.0	250	34	99	283	622
Female....................	10,850	93	68.1	136	0	30	136	329
Race and ethnicity[2] of head								
White.....................	41,444	180	75.7	237	28	91	258	581
Hispanic................	3,040	149	64.6	231	14	66	160	630
Non-Hispanic............	38,405	182	76.6	237	29	93	260	581
Black.....................	5,064	70	62.4	113	0	25	116	302
Other.....................	819	168	70.9	236	10	39	347	810
Family structure								
Head and spouse present whole time.....	34,963	193	76.3	253	35	102	284	629
Child under 17 years......	21,668	225	80.4	280	40	112	316	710
No child under 17 years...	13,295	141	69.7	203	26	81	242	491
Head only, no spouse at any time......	11,169	93	67.4	138	0	36	134	345
Child under 17 years......	8,258	94	71.6	131	0	25	110	335
No child under 17 years...	2,911	91	55.6	164	20	57	179	495
Other.....................	1,194	121	75.2	161	14	60	209	449
Family dynamics								
Unchanging, full year.....	37,714	175	75.0	234	25	85	246	600
Change in composition or existed less than full year.....	9,613	137	71.1	193	18	67	228	509

Table 42—continued

Out-of-pocket expenditures for dental visits for multiple-person families with all members under 65 years of age, by selected characteristics: United States, 1980

[Rate per family year. Civilian noninstitutionalized population with civilian family head]

Characteristic	All families		Families with visits		Expenditures at selected percentiles			
	Number in thousands	Mean expenditures	Percent	Mean expenditures	25th	50th	75th	90th
Family poverty status in 1980								
Below 150 percent poverty level......	8,770	$80	64.4	$124	$0	$21	$122	$300
Below poverty level.............	5,083	61	63.7	96	0	0	79	242
Poverty level to 149 percent......	3,687	105	65.4	161	15	41	153	348
150-199 percent.................	4,825	130	66.6	195	23	61	196	449
200-299 percent.................	10,075	162	72.7	222	26	94	238	558
300-499 percent.................	14,307	198	77.9	255	37	100	283	619
500 percent or more.............	9,350	229	83.4	275	40	115	335	678
Family income in 1980[3]								
Less than $10,000...............	7,496	59	60.7	97	0	15	70	230
$10,000-$19,999.................	12,555	115	64.7	178	24	67	190	449
$20,000-$34,999.................	17,279	185	79.0	235	35	96	253	590
$35,000 or more.................	9,997	284	88.0	323	48	144	393	805
Education of head[4]								
None or elementary school.......	5,822	97	58.6	165	14	40	160	481
Some high school................	7,546	106	66.0	160	17	61	183	393
High school graduate............	18,299	165	75.2	219	24	86	240	545
Some college....................	7,556	203	80.1	253	30	93	265	616
College graduate or more........	8,084	251	85.5	293	40	115	326	729
Family employment status[5]								
2 or more persons worked full year......	13,629	229	79.6	287	38	109	324	750
Only 1 person worked full year.........	21,782	173	75.6	228	30	91	256	555
Some part-year work.............	9,021	89	66.1	135	3	47	150	371
No person worked................	2,896	86	63.4	135	0	4	86	283
Worst perceived health status of any family member[6]								
Excellent.......................	14,771	196	76.4	257	35	98	275	640
Good............................	20,837	169	75.6	224	25	81	234	560
Fair............................	8,021	134	69.0	195	13	58	240	519
Poor............................	3,678	118	69.3	171	4	48	176	480

Most severe limitation in usual activity of any family member

None..................................	39,751	171	74.8	229	26	83	244	576
Some limitation.......................	2,814	173	72.6	238	14	67	258	765
Cannot perform usual activity.........	4,762	135	70.6	191	6	65	225	519

Family's bed days[3]

0.....................................	7,825	140	67.5	207	22	75	250	535
1-5...................................	12,427	150	73.1	206	25	84	229	518
6-10..................................	7,470	172	77.1	223	29	80	247	576
11-20.................................	8,884	181	77.5	233	27	94	260	564
More than 20..........................	10,722	194	75.7	256	18	77	250	668

Family health care coverage

All members covered full year.........	33,575	190	79.0	240	25	89	257	608
Private insurance only................	25,502	218	80.4	271	40	105	297	668
Medicaid only.........................	1,606	*21	67.5	*30	0	0	0	65
Medicare only.........................	-	*0	-	-	-	-	-	-
Medicare and other public programs....	*12	*0	*0.0	-	-	-	-	-
Medicare and private insurance........	*95	*3	*25.7	*11	*4	*18	*18	*18
Other public and private mixes........	5,762	128	76.9	166	3	60	177	423
Other mixes of public programs........	*135	*172	*81.1	*212	*64	*130	*210	*767
Source unknown........................	*463	*35	*81.8	*43	*0	*0	*25	*160
All members covered, some part year...	7,968	129	65.3	198	20	66	233	514
Some members not covered..............	3,804	107	62.7	171	21	66	192	449
All members not covered...............	1,980	66	51.2	128	29	56	144	279

[1]Average size during period of family's existence rounded to nearest integer; exactly half an integer rounded upward.
[2]There were too few Hispanic families of races other than white for separate tabulation.
[3]Annual rate.
[4]Includes only families with heads 17 years of age and over.
[5]Excludes families with all members under 14 years of age.
[6]Excludes families with all members with health status unknown.

NOTE: Multiple-person families are families with average size 1.5 or greater.

Table 43

Out-of-pocket expenditures for dental visits for multiple-person families with all members under 65 years of age and all members with health care coverage all year, by selected characteristics: United States, 1980

[Rate per family year. Civilian noninstitutionalized population with civilian family head]

Characteristic	All families		Families with visits		Expenditures at selected percentiles			
	Number in thousands	Mean expenditures	Percent	Mean expenditures	25th	50th	75th	90th
Total..................	33,575	$190	79.0	$240	$25	$89	$257	$608
Family size[1]								
2 persons..............	10,994	139	69.6	200	20	65	211	484
3 persons..............	8,010	149	78.8	189	19	76	209	535
4 persons..............	8,464	220	84.6	260	40	116	313	661
5 or more persons......	6,107	292	88.4	330	33	128	326	897
Age of head								
Under 25 years........	2,585	54	61.5	88	0	30	94	246
25–44 years...........	18,256	198	82.2	241	25	91	241	635
45–64 years...........	12,733	205	77.9	263	31	106	328	617
Sex of head								
Male..................	27,351	206	80.1	258	35	102	292	647
Female................	6,224	116	74.4	156	0	28	148	329
Race and ethnicity[2] of head								
White.................	29,902	200	80.3	250	30	95	275	612
Hispanic..............	1,711	172	71.5	241	3	52	165	713
Non-Hispanic..........	28,191	202	80.8	250	30	98	277	608
Black.................	3,139	81	67.1	121	0	21	129	302
Other.................	533	228	78.7	*290	*20	*94	*528	*871
Family structure								
Head and spouse present whole time......	26,517	209	80.2	261	36	105	293	651
Child under 17 years...	16,251	245	84.8	289	43	116	324	732
No child under 17 years...	10,266	152	72.7	209	26	82	246	507
Head only, no spouse at any time......	6,394	116	74.3	156	0	30	136	358
Child under 17 years...	5,051	111	76.7	145	0	20	117	330
No child under 17 years...	1,343	132	65.3	202	28	64	240	581
Other.................	663	125	78.5	*159	*0	*65	*210	*342
Family dynamics								
Unchanging, full year...	28,266	197	79.6	248	26	92	260	630
Change in composition or existed less than full year...	5,308	148	76.0	194	19	70	210	504

Family poverty status in 1980

Below 150 percent poverty level	4,640	96	73.4	131	0	12	136	288
Below poverty level	2,919	63	72.1	87	0	0	65	230
Poverty level to 149 percent	1,721	153	75.5	203	8	52	180	376
150-199 percent	2,657	171	70.0	245	22	69	230	517
200-299 percent	7,074	182	78.5	232	28	95	242	591
300-499 percent	11,427	206	79.5	259	39	100	276	653
500 percent or more	7,776	234	85.1	275	38	111	355	686

Family income in 1980[3]

Less than $10,000	4,023	70	70.2	100	0	0	65	230
$10,000-$19,999	7,715	136	69.3	196	24	76	223	450
$20,000-$34,999	13,970	197	80.6	245	37	96	250	629
$35,000 or more	7,867	290	90.3	321	45	133	395	788

Education of head[4]

None or elementary school	3,188	113	63.1	179	12	46	187	535
Some high school	4,620	124	72.8	171	14	68	225	395
High school graduate	13,366	178	78.9	225	24	91	238	550
Some college	5,757	221	82.4	268	30	92	294	700
College graduate or more	6,625	269	88.4	304	44	116	346	750

Family employment status[5]

2 or more persons worked full year	10,347	245	82.7	297	40	114	337	752
Only 1 person worked full year	16,128	190	79.2	240	34	98	260	590
Some part-year work	4,933	112	76.0	147	0	42	157	429
No person worked	2,167	*97	66.7	*145	0	0	86	283

Worst perceived health status of any family member[6]

Excellent	11,162	224	80.7	277	37	106	315	689
Good	15,029	188	80.4	233	26	86	241	576
Fair	5,209	150	74.9	200	12	66	250	532
Poor	2,155	124	70.7	176	1	56	157	384

Most severe limitation in usual activity of any family member

None	28,461	194	79.7	243	28	91	260	612
Some limitation	2,067	199	77.9	256	14	88	286	765
Cannot perform usual activity	3,047	143	73.4	195	4	65	205	540

Family's bed days[3]

0	5,766	158	73.0	217	21	78	276	535
1-5	8,806	171	78.3	218	27	90	233	591
6-10	5,513	187	80.6	232	28	80	240	637
11-20	6,162	202	80.9	249	39	103	293	612
More than 20	7,328	228	81.7	279	18	82	268	713

Table 43--continued

Out-of-pocket expenditures for dental visits for multiple-person families with all members under 65 years of age and all members with health care coverage all year, by selected characteristics: United States, 1980

[Rate per family year. Civilian noninstitutionalized population with civilian family head]

| | All families | | Families with visits | | | | | |
| | | | | | Expenditures at selected percentiles | | | |
Characteristic	Number in thousands	Mean expenditures	Percent	Mean expenditures	25th	50th	75th	90th
Family health care coverage								
Private insurance only............	25,502	$218	80.4	$271	$40	105	$297	$668
Medicaid only....................	1,606	*21	67.5	*30	0	0	0	65
Medicare only...................	-	-	-	-	-	-	-	-
Medicare and other public programs.....	*12	*0	*0.0	-	-	-	-	-
Medicare and private insurance.........	*95	*3	*25.7	*11	*4	*18	*18	*18
Other public and private mixes........	5,762	128	76.9	166	3	60	177	423
Other mixes of public programs........	*135	*172	*81.1	*212	*64	*130	*210	*767
Source unknown..................	*463	*35	*81.8	*43	*0	*0	*25	*160

1Average size during period of family's existence rounded to nearest integer; exactly half an integer rounded upward.
2There were too few Hispanic families of races other than white for separate tabulation.
3Annual rate.
4Includes only families with heads 17 years of age and over.
5Excludes families with all members under 14 years of age.
6Excludes families with all members with health status unknown.

NOTE: Multiple-person families are families with average size 1.5 or greater.

Table 44

Out-of-pocket expenditures for dental visits for multiple-person families with all members under 65 years of age and some or all members without health care coverage all year, by selected characteristics: United States, 1980

[Rate per family year. Civilian noninstitutionalized population with civilian family head]

Characteristic	All families		Families with visits		Expenditures at selected percentiles			
	Number in thousands	Mean expenditures	Percent	Mean expenditures	25th	50th	75th	90th
Total............	13,752	$114	62.5	$182	$22	$63	$200	$483
Family size[1]								
2 persons............	3,964	63	51.3	122	20	50	148	335
3 persons............	3,218	78	62.8	124	20	56	155	290
4 persons............	3,082	137	68.6	199	26	75	259	506
5 or more persons....	3,488	186	69.7	266	21	91	355	687
Age of head								
Under 25 years........	1,698	*60	45.3	132	15	45	140	323
25–44 years...........	6,527	95	66.0	144	21	60	179	382
45–64 years...........	5,528	153	63.7	240	25	75	275	632
Sex of head								
Male................	9,126	141	64.0	220	30	85	259	533
Female..............	4,627	61	59.6	103	15	40	126	315
Race and ethnicity[2] of head								
White...............	11,542	126	64.0	196	26	74	227	506
Hispanic............	1,328	120	55.7	216	21	70	160	511
Non-Hispanic........	10,214	126	65.1	194	26	74	231	506
Black...............	1,924	53	54.6	97	3	30	84	300
Other...............	*286	*55	*56.5	*98	*0	*20	*40	*545
Family structure								
Head and spouse present whole time......	8,446	143	64.4	222	30	90	253	514
Child under 17 years.....	5,417	164	67.1	245	30	92	279	608
No child under 17 years......	3,029	104	59.6	175	28	80	231	415
Head only, no spouse at any time......	4,775	63	58.2	108	15	40	131	345
Child under 17 years.....	3,207	66	63.5	104	8	36	100	345
No child under 17 years......	1,568	56	47.3	118	20	55	171	212
Other...............	*532	*116	*71.1	*163	*15	*56	*168	*533
Family dynamics								
Unchanging, full year........	9,448	109	61.4	178	25	65	192	452
Change in composition or existed less than full year........	4,304	124	65.1	191	15	62	265	512

Table 44—continued

Out-of-pocket expenditures for dental visits for multiple-person families with all members under 65 years of age and some or all members without health care coverage all year, by selected characteristics: United States, 1980

[Rate per family year. Civilian noninstitutionalized population with civilian family head]

| | All families | | Families with visits | | | | | |
| Characteristic | Number in thousands | Mean expenditures | Percent | Mean expenditures | Expenditures at selected percentiles | | | |
					25th	50th	75th	90th
Family poverty status in 1980								
Below 150 percent poverty level	4,130	$61	54.3	$112	$8	$35	$116	$300
Below poverty level	2,164	59	52.3	113	0	24	119	300
Poverty level to 149 percent	1,966	63	56.6	111	18	40	115	323
150–199 percent	2,168	79	62.4	126	25	55	135	410
200–299 percent	3,000	114	59.1	193	25	75	215	511
300–499 percent	2,880	166	71.2	234	29	105	330	563
500 percent or more	1,574	206	74.9	275	50	146	286	636
Family income in 1980[3]								
Less than $10,000	3,473	45	49.7	91	4	28	82	235
$10,000–$19,999	4,840	82	57.4	143	23	56	150	449
$20,000–$34,999	3,310	136	72.5	187	26	85	259	506
$35,000 or more	2,130	265	79.5	333	56	168	386	889
Education of head[4]								
None or elementary school	2,634	77	53.1	145	15	35	131	449
Some high school	2,926	76	55.2	138	21	53	138	350
High school graduate	4,934	129	65.1	198	23	73	242	533
Some college	1,800	146	72.9	200	35	94	213	480
College graduate or more	1,459	168	72.5	231	27	76	250	545
Family employment status[5]								
2 or more persons worked full year	3,282	178	70.0	254	25	75	265	729
Only 1 person worked full year	5,654	122	65.5	187	27	70	249	506
Some part-year work	4,087	62	54.1	115	15	47	148	279
No person worked	*729	*54	*53.7	*101	*0	*21	*116	*387
Worst perceived health status of any family member[6]								
Excellent	3,609	110	63.0	175	28	73	188	410
Good	5,808	122	63.1	193	25	74	205	496
Fair	2,812	106	58.1	182	15	55	213	512
Poor	1,524	110	67.4	163	20	43	250	532

Most severe limitation in usual activity
of any family member

None.............................	11,290	114	62.3	183	25	63	192	460
Some limitation..................	747	99	58.1	*170	*15	*40	*227	*501
Cannot perform usual activity....	1,715	121	65.8	184	15	75	290	512

Family's bed days[3]

0................................	2,059	89	52.3	169	25	63	192	483
1-5..............................	3,620	101	60.3	167	20	61	200	422
6-10.............................	1,957	130	67.3	193	30	80	279	480
11-20............................	2,722	132	69.7	190	21	61	182	501
More than 20.....................	3,394	119	62.6	191	20	62	205	525

Family health care coverage

All members covered, some part year.....	7,968	129	65.3	198	20	66	233	514
Some members not covered.............	3,804	107	62.7	171	21	66	192	449
All members not covered..............	1,980	66	51.2	128	29	56	144	279

[1]Average size during period of family's existence rounded to nearest integer; exactly half an integer rounded upward.
[2]There were too few Hispanic families of races other than white for separate tabulation.
[3]Annual rate.
[4]Includes only families with heads 17 years of age and over.
[5]Excludes families with all members under 14 years of age.
[6]Excludes families with all members with health status unknown.

NOTE: Multiple-person families are families with average size 1.5 or greater.

Table 45

Out-of-pocket expenditures for dental visits for multiple-person families with members 65 years of age and over, by selected characteristics: United States, 1980

[Rate per family year. Civilian noninstitutionalized population with civilian family head]

Characteristic	All families		Families with visits					
	Number in thousands	Mean expenditures	Percent	Mean expenditures	Expenditures at selected percentiles			
					25th	50th	75th	90th
Total....................	10,809	$122	58.5	$209	$26	$67	$208	$557
Family size[1]								
2 persons................	7,958	94	53.2	176	27	60	193	431
3 persons................	1,339	157	63.7	247	25	102	390	694
4 persons................	724	*289	75.4	*383	*22	*128	*325	*1,117
5 or more persons........	788	196	87.5	224	33	83	159	700
Family age								
All members 65 years and over...	4,141	94	52.2	180	30	67	208	401
Some members under 65....	6,668	140	62.5	224	22	67	222	644
Sex of head								
Male.....................	8,397	142	59.5	238	30	75	272	625
Female...................	2,412	55	55.0	99	10	39	131	250
Race and ethnicity[2] of head								
White....................	9,571	132	59.7	221	29	74	240	578
Hispanic...............	*363	*168	*52.3	*322	*0	*40	*302	*1,237
Non-Hispanic...........	9,208	130	60.0	217	30	75	230	557
Black....................	1,027	*36	45.2	*79	*0	*33	*67	*398
Other....................	211	*111	*70.3	*157	*20	*30	*66	*772
Family structure								
Head and spouse present whole time.....	7,593	143	60.3	237	30	75	272	600
Child under 17 years....	774	289	85.6	337	48	108	390	1,144
No child under 17 years..	6,819	127	57.4	221	30	71	250	578
Head only, no spouse at any time.....	2,808	59	52.9	112	11	45	139	315
Child under 17 years....	*384	*29	*53.9	*55	*0	*0	*90	*131
No child under 17 years..	2,424	64	52.8	122	20	50	150	387
Other....................	*408	*166	*64.8	*256	*19	*40	*171	*1,184
Family dynamics								
Unchanging, full year....	9,276	111	57.4	194	28	70	215	520
Change in composition or existed less than full year....	1,533	187	65.4	286	20	65	197	772

Family poverty status in 1980								
Below 150 percent poverty level	2,169	27	37.7	71	10	38	67	151
Below poverty level	964	*28	44.1	*64	*10	*37	*70	*99
Poverty level to 149 percent	1,205	26	32.5	*79	*20	*40	*67	*155
150-199 percent	1,530	82	47.7	172	20	47	272	486
200-299 percent	2,785	97	59.7	162	26	70	134	351
300-499 percent	2,740	161	66.5	242	30	82	280	597
500 percent or more	1,585	268	81.6	329	35	139	310	805
Family income in 1980[3]								
Less than $10,000	3,133	48	37.2	128	20	40	90	401
$10,000-$19,999	4,173	90	59.1	153	25	60	139	304
$20,000-$34,999	2,427	175	72.9	240	36	108	280	686
$35,000 or more	1,076	344	85.8	401	34	139	475	1,193
Education of head[4]								
None or elementary school	4,669	60	43.8	136	21	49	125	401
Some high school	1,721	107	53.4	201	25	59	222	557
High school graduate	2,306	149	72.8	205	20	70	208	430
Some college	1,095	238	77.8	306	40	131	374	1,022
College graduate or more	1,015	249	81.5	306	32	75	301	644
Family employment status[5]								
2 or more persons worked full year	979	257	87.2	294	33	93	301	1,184
Only 1 person worked full year	2,767	169	68.5	246	24	80	190	597
Some part-year work	2,282	84	49.7	169	20	66	205	452
No person worked	4,781	86	51.1	168	27	55	200	430
Worst perceived health status of any family member[6]								
Excellent	1,429	140	66.0	212	27	75	263	452
Good	3,630	136	66.5	205	30	76	205	578
Fair	3,110	108	52.3	206	24	70	230	557
Poor	2,640	110	50.8	216	20	42	155	430
Most severe limitation in usual activity of any family member								
None	4,190	142	58.3	244	29	75	230	761
Some limitation	865	152	65.8	*231	*40	*103	*404	*625
Cannot perform usual activity	5,754	103	57.6	179	24	59	193	401
Family's bed days[3]								
0	3,349	88	53.6	164	24	47	143	402
1-5	2,100	129	64.2	201	34	66	225	620
6-10	1,364	144	57.8	250	26	81	339	597
11-20	1,098	151	61.1	247	28	90	200	851
More than 20	2,897	135	59.5	227	25	74	250	500

Table 45—continued

Out-of-pocket expenditures for dental visits for multiple-person families with members 65 years of age and over, by selected characteristics: United States, 1980

[Rate per family year. Civilian noninstitutionalized population with civilian family head]

Characteristic	All families		Families with visits					
	Number in thousands	Mean expenditures	Percent	Mean expenditures	Expenditures at selected percentiles			
					25th	50th	75th	90th
Family health care coverage								
All members covered full year..........	8,879	$130	59.1	$220	$29	$71	$246	$578
Private insurance only...............	*258	*467	*69.1	*676	*45	*131	*1,144	*1,968
Medicaid only......................	*15	*0	*100.0	*0	*0	*0	*0	*0
Medicare only......................	*574	*53	*48.0	*111	*30	*75	*151	*250
Medicare and other public programs....	*459	*24	*39.8	*61	*0	*0	*25	*456
Medicare and private insurance........	7,380	133	61.2	217	30	75	251	578
Other public and private mixes........	*91	*120	*51.5	*234	*0	*20	*83	*851
Other mixes of public programs........	-	-	-	-	-	-	-	-
Source unknown.....................	*102	*20	*36.4	*55	*0	*30	*139	*139
All members covered, some part year....	701	*133	64.0	*207	*37	*65	*171	*597
Some members not covered.............	1,159	61	50.8	*120	*10	*40	*125	*430
All members not covered..............	*71	*27	*53.2	*52	*6	*66	*78	*78

1Average size during period of family's existence rounded to nearest integer; exactly half an integer rounded upward.
2There were too few Hispanic families of races other than white for separate tabulation.
3Annual rate.
4Includes only families with heads 17 years of age and over.
5Excludes families with all members under 14 years of age.
6Excludes families with all members with health status unknown.

NOTE: Multiple-person families are families with average size 1.5 or greater.

152

Table 46

Out-of-pocket expenditures for dental visits for 1-person families, by selected characteristics: United States, 1980

[Rate per family year. Civilian noninstitutionalized population with civilian family head]

Characteristic	All families		Families with visits		Expenditures at selected percentiles			
	Number in thousands	Mean expenditures	Percent	Mean expenditures	25th	50th	75th	90th
Total................................	26,233	$57	43.1	$132	$18	$45	$130	$321
Sex								
Male.................................	11,866	47	38.7	122	15	37	103	302
Female...............................	14,367	65	46.8	138	20	50	146	356
Race and ethnicity[1]								
White................................	22,811	57	45.0	126	20	45	125	318
Hispanic...........................	,818	*59	37.2	*158	*0	*25	*275	*430
Non-Hispanic.......................	21,993	57	45.3	125	20	45	125	312
Black................................	2,711	*29	28.0	*102	*10	*32	*88	*242
Other................................	*712	*165	*41.7	*396	*34	*87	*670	*926
Family dynamics								
Unchanging, full year................	22,570	58	45.3	127	18	44	123	313
Change in composition or existed less than full year......................	3,662	51	29.5	172	21	60	179	412
Poverty status in 1980								
Below 150 percent poverty level......	9,379	36	31.6	114	10	36	122	270
Below poverty level................	5,252	33	28.5	115	0	30	137	250
Poverty level to 149 percent......	4,128	40	35.5	113	12	46	120	270
150-199 percent......................	2,974	42	35.9	116	22	38	102	313
200-299 percent......................	5,563	74	41.9	176	26	58	173	468
300-499 percent......................	5,426	71	57.3	123	20	45	125	288
500 percent or more..................	2,891	81	63.7	128	13	35	105	397
Family income in 1980[2]								
Less than $10,000....................	14,468	45	34.1	133	15	45	127	340
$10,000-$19,999......................	8,280	70	51.5	135	21	48	132	318
$20,000-$34,999......................	2,664	68	57.8	117	20	38	103	270
$35,000 or more......................	820	93	70.0	*133	*5	*34	*116	*570
Education[3]								
None or elementary school............	4,782	26	21.9	120	4	41	100	250
Some high school.....................	3,996	43	28.9	148	15	40	155	356
High school graduate.................	7,413	50	47.7	105	20	45	107	267
Some college.........................	4,842	69	52.1	133	22	50	154	367
College graduate or more.............	5,122	95	59.2	160	20	43	132	425

Table 46--continued

Out-of-pocket expenditures for dental visits for 1-person families, by selected characteristics: United States, 1980

[Rate per family year. Civilian noninstitutionalized population with civilian family head]

Characteristic	All families		Families with visits					
	Number in thousands	Mean expenditures	Percent	Mean expenditures	Expenditures at selected percentiles			
					25th	50th	75th	90th
Employment status[4]								
Worked full year.............	10,374	$60	52.0	$116	$18	$40	$116	$287
Worked part year.............	7,129	66	40.0	164	20	45	131	542
Never worked.................	8,703	45	35.3	128	15	50	137	286
Perceived health status[5]								
Excellent....................	11,226	56	47.3	118	16	40	108	295
Good.........................	9,642	74	44.1	167	22	57	200	430
Fair.........................	3,691	31	35.1	89	14	35	84	170
Poor.........................	1,568	*13	26.1	*51	*0	*9	*60	*190
Limitation in usual activity								
None.........................	21,977	61	45.1	135	20	44	130	350
Some limitation..............	731	*52	39.4	*131	*10	*40	*180	*255
Cannot perform usual activity	3,525	33	31.7	105	4	50	102	225
Bed days[2]								
0............................	12,629	52	42.3	124	20	44	125	312
1-5..........................	6,587	57	46.5	123	19	42	102	246
6-10.........................	2,671	71	43.2	165	20	60	250	430
11-20........................	1,924	*92	47.1	194	20	50	186	545
More than 20.................	2,422	34	35.6	96	0	33	90	255
Family health care coverage								
All members covered full year........	20,491	56	45.0	125	15	45	127	294
Private insurance only...............	10,523	67	52.8	127	20	42	125	298
Medicaid only........................	*317	*2	*34.1	*7	*0	*0	*4	*46
Medicare only........................	1,262	*33	18.0	*184	*23	*78	*185	*296
Medicare and other public programs...	993	*23	21.1	*109	*0	*15	*195	*225
Medicare and private insurance.......	4,819	54	42.9	126	25	60	123	294
Other public and private mixes.......	1,361	*55	41.8	*133	*2	*40	*200	*471
Other mixes of public programs.......	*186	*131	*72.6	*180	*20	*27	*321	*425
Source unknown.......................	1,030	*21	34.1	*63	*0	*15	*58	*160

154

All members covered, some part year.....	3,223	52	37.2	141	20	39	85	542
Some members not covered.....	*24	*0	*0.0	-	-	-	-	-
All members not covered.....	2,495	68	35.9	189	22	45	215	430

[1]There were too few Hispanic families of races other than white for separate tabulation.
[2]Annual rate.
[3]Includes only families with heads 17 years of age and over.
[4]Excludes families with all members under 14 years of age.
[5]Excludes families with all members with health status unknown.

NOTE: 1-person families are families with average size less than 1.5. For 1-person families with more than 1 distinct individual, characteristics are those of head or of family as in Table 1.

Table 47

Out-of-pocket expenditures for dental visits for 1-person families under 65 years of age, by selected characteristics: United States, 1980

[Rate per family year. Civilian noninstitutionalized population with civilian family head]

Characteristic	All families		Families with visits		Expenditures at selected percentiles			
	Number in thousands	Mean expenditures	Percent	Mean expenditures	25th	50th	75th	90th
Total........................	18,519	$62	46.3	$133	$16	$40	$125	$350
Age								
Under 25 years..............	5,208	54	45.0	121	15	42	115	350
25–44 years.................	7,630	73	50.2	145	20	43	137	318
45–64 years.................	5,680	53	42.3	126	12	36	112	440
Sex								
Male........................	10,082	49	41.4	118	15	35	102	287
Female......................	8,437	77	52.1	147	20	47	152	425
Race and ethnicity[1]								
White.......................	15,786	61	48.7	126	18	40	122	350
Hispanic....................	680	*66	35.1	*189	*0	*53	*318	*430
Non-Hispanic................	15,106	61	49.3	124	19	40	120	350
Black.......................	2,128	*32	29.7	*106	*10	*32	*83	*250
Other.......................	*605	*178	*41.8	*427	*40	*139	*670	*2,006
Family dynamics								
Unchanging, full year.......	15,487	64	49.4	129	16	39	115	350
Change in composition or existed less than full year........	3,032	51	30.5	168	19	60	179	460
Poverty status in 1980								
Below 150 percent...........	5,181	45	35.1	127	2	34	120	406
Below poverty level.........	3,031	38	31.2	120	0	30	111	340
Poverty level to 149 percent.......	2,149	55	40.5	135	4	35	131	420
150–199 percent.............	1,855	37	37.3	*99	*20	*34	*102	*236
200–299 percent.............	4,250	75	40.7	185	25	56	200	468
300–499 percent.............	4,643	69	57.3	120	20	44	115	288
500 percent or more.........	2,590	79	64.8	121	10	35	105	302
Family income in 1980[2]								
Less than $10,000...........	8,222	52	36.9	141	14	35	120	406
$10,000–$19,999.............	7,113	69	50.4	136	20	45	158	339
$20,000–$34,999.............	2,529	67	59.0	113	20	38	103	270
$35,000 or more.............	*656	*87	*70.2	*123	*5	*25	*105	*570

Education[3]								
None or elementary school..............	1,770	*30	24.5	*122	*4	*25	*90	*482
Some high school.......................	2,546	48	30.7	157	10	24	82	542
High school graduate...................	5,759	51	47.0	109	20	42	107	275
Some college...........................	4,037	67	52.3	128	22	46	154	360
College graduate or more...............	4,329	92	58.2	158	20	38	132	425
Employment status[4]								
Worked full year.......................	9,963	61	52.1	118	17	39	125	287
Worked part year.......................	6,265	68	41.6	164	20	44	131	542
Never worked...........................	2,264	46	34.5	*134	*4	*36	*107	*482
Perceived health status[5]								
Excellent..............................	8,913	57	48.3	118	15	35	108	312
Good...................................	6,852	80	47.3	168	20	52	200	471
Fair...................................	1,866	*35	43.6	*80	*12	*30	*67	*107
Poor...................................	803	*11	23.3	*46	*0	*0	*9	*20
Limitation in usual activity								
None...................................	16,928	65	47.3	137	20	41	131	360
Some limitation........................	*209	*29	*44.9	*64	*0	*6	*155	*255
Cannot perform usual activity..........	1,383	*28	33.9	*84	*0	*20	*80	*103
Bed days[2]								
0......................................	8,291	56	45.4	124	18	39	107	318
1-5....................................	5,721	56	47.5	119	18	41	102	246
6-10...................................	2,013	86	47.4	181	25	90	258	482
11-20..................................	1,222	*111	56.1	*198	*20	*50	*193	*468
More than 20...........................	1,273	*34	36.1	*95	*0	*14	*50	*255
Family health care coverage								
All members covered full year..........	12,974	62	50.2	124	15	40	125	302
Private insurance only................	10,511	67	52.9	127	20	42	125	298
Medicaid only.........................	*317	*2	*34.1	*7	*0	*0	*4	*46
Medicare only.........................	*108	*2	*12.9	*15	*15	*15	*15	*15
Medicare and other public programs....	-	-	-	-	-	-	-	-
Medicare and private insurance........	-	-	-	-	-	-	-	-
Other public and private mixes........	1,361	*55	41.8	*133	*2	*40	*200	*471
Other mixes of public programs........	*186	*131	*72.6	*180	*20	*27	*321	*425
Source unknown........................	*491	*6	*25.5	*22	*0	*0	*0	*103
All members covered, some part year....	3,223	52	37.2	141	20	39	85	542
Some members not covered...............	-	-	-	-	-	-	-	-
All members not covered................	2,322	72	37.4	191	22	45	215	430

[1]There were too few Hispanic of races other than white families for separate tabulation.
[2]Annual rate.
[3]Includes only families with heads 17 years of age and over.
[4]Excludes families with all members under 14 years of age.
[5]Excludes families with all members with health status unknown.

NOTE: 1-person families are families with average size less than 1.5. For 1-person families with more than 1 distinct individual, characteristics are those of head or of family as in Table 2.

Table 48

Out-of-pocket expenditures for dental visits for 1-person families under 65 years of age with health care coverage all year, by selected characteristics: United States, 1980

[Rate per family year. Civilian noninstitutionalized population with civilian family head]

Characteristic	All families		Families with visits			Expenditures at selected percentiles			
	Number in thousands	Mean expenditures	Percent	Mean expenditures	25th	50th	75th	90th
Total..............	12,974	$62	50.2	$124	$15	$40	$125	$302
Age								
Under 25 years............	3,166	54	48.0	111	15	45	115	276
25-44 years............	5,206	69	54.5	126	19	39	132	269
45-64 years............	4,601	61	46.7	130	12	38	125	440
Sex								
Male............	6,807	55	43.8	126	12	37	105	276
Female............	6,167	70	57.2	122	15	45	131	340
Race and ethnicity[1]								
White............	11,183	61	52.0	117	15	41	127	298
Hispanic............	*400	*36	*31.1	*117	*0	*53	*275	*318
Non-Hispanic............	10,782	62	52.8	117	15	41	125	288
Black............	1,428	*38	35.7	*106	*4	*29	*80	*250
Other............	*363	*191	*49.1	*389	*34	*40	*169	*2,006
Family dynamics								
Unchanging, full year...........	11,017	66	53.6	123	15	40	120	288
Change in composition or existed less than full year...........	1,957	41	30.7	132	11	41	141	396
Poverty status in 1980								
Below 150 percent............	2,775	48	36.8	129	0	34	120	305
Below poverty level............	1,638	*35	31.4	*111	*0	*28	*108	*186
Poverty level to 149 percent............	1,137	*66	44.4	*148	*4	*35	*131	*471
150-199 percent............	1,072	*32	40.3	*78	*15	*32	*102	*164
200-299 percent............	2,997	77	43.6	176	25	62	158	350
300-499 percent............	3,918	59	58.8	100	19	43	115	267
500 percent or more............	2,212	81	65.2	124	9	34	132	302
Family income in 1980[2]								
Less than $10,000............	4,620	52	39.2	133	13	35	108	255
$10,000-$19,999............	5,656	65	53.2	121	20	46	132	318
$20,000-$34,999............	2,114	68	60.5	113	15	38	132	270
$35,000 or more............	*584	*96	*70.1	*136	*5	*28	*116	*570

Education[3]								
None or elementary school.........	1,328	*33	27.7	*120	*2	*25	*90	*245
Some high school..................	1,538	53	32.0	*166	*10	*32	*72	*396
High school graduate..............	4,047	52	50.9	103	16	39	107	271
Some college......................	2,830	63	57.2	111	20	46	131	288
College graduate or more..........	3,201	91	61.2	148	19	40	132	425
Employment status[4]								
Worked full year..................	7,649	56	55.0	103	15	40	116	271
Worked part year..................	3,554	85	47.0	182	16	43	154	600
Never worked......................	1,769	*41	35.8	*113	*0	*40	*103	*152
Perceived health status[5]								
Excellent.........................	6,353	55	52.5	105	15	38	114	298
Good..............................	4,537	85	52.0	163	20	50	169	396
Fair..............................	1,425	*40	46.7	*86	*12	*28	*67	*107
Poor..............................	*572	*1	*19.5	*5	*0	*0	*9	*20
Limitation in usual activity								
None..............................	11,652	66	51.8	127	15	40	131	312
Some limitation...................	*127	*32	*51.2	*62	*0	*12	*59	*255
Cannot perform usual activity.....	1,195	*33	34.4	*96	*0	*40	*88	*103
Bed days[2]								
0.................................	5,669	63	50.2	124	15	40	125	318
1-5...............................	4,146	52	51.5	100	13	41	102	237
6-10..............................	1,247	70	50.2	*140	*25	*65	*220	*288
11-20.............................	984	*111	54.8	*203	*20	*50	*186	*570
More than 20......................	928	*44	38.7	*114	*0	*14	*67	*561
Family health care coverage								
Private insurance only............	10,511	67	52.9	127	20	42	125	298
Medicaid only.....................	*317	*2	*34.1	*7	*0	*0	*4	*46
Medicare only.....................	*108	*2	*12.9	*15	*15	*15	*15	*15
Medicare and other public programs......	–	–	–	–	–	–	–	–
Medicare and private insurance..........	–	–	–	–	–	–	–	–
Other public and private mixes..........	1,361	*55	41.8	*133	*2	*40	*200	*471
Other mixes of public programs..........	*186	*131	*72.6	*180	*20	*27	*321	*425
Source unknown...................	*491	*6	*25.5	*22	*0	*0	*0	*103

[1]There were too few Hispanic families of races other than white for separate tabulation.
[2]Annual rate.
[3]Includes only families with heads 17 years of age and over.
[4]Excludes families with all members under 14 years of age.
[5]Excludes families with all members with health status unknown.

NOTE: 1-person families are families with average size less than 1.5. For 1-person families with more than 1 distinct individual, characteristics are those of head or of family as in Table 2.

159

Table 49

Out-of-pocket expenditures for dental visits for 1-person families under 65 years of age without health care coverage all year, by selected characteristics: United States, 1980

[Rate per family year. Civilian noninstitutionalized population with civilian family head]

Characteristic	All families		Families with visits		Expenditures at selected percentiles			
	Number in thousands	Mean expenditures	Percent	Mean expenditures	25th	50th	75th	90th
Total............	5,545	$60	37.3	$162	$21	$39	$157	$535
Age								
Under 25 years.......	2,042	56	40.4	138	15	33	108	360
25-44 years..........	2,424	*82	40.9	*200	25	45	200	593
45-64 years..........	1,079	*21	23.5	*90	*0	*23	*80	*314
Sex								
Male.................	3,275	36	36.6	98	20	35	80	339
Female...............	2,270	96	38.3	251	25	58	306	710
Race and ethnicity[1]								
White................	4,603	62	40.7	151	20	35	96	430
Hispanic.............	*280	*109	*40.8	*268	*0	*25	*430	*960
Non-Hispanic.........	4,323	59	40.7	144	20	35	95	406
Black................	*700	*19	*17.4	*108	*23	*70	*180	*195
Other................	*242	*159	*30.8	*517	*200	*670	*926	*926
Family dynamics								
Unchanging, full year.......	4,470	*58	39.0	149	20	35	95	482
Change in composition or existed less than full year.......	1,075	*71	30.2	*234	*43	*73	*242	*618
Poverty status in 1980								
Below 150 percent.............	2,405	41	33.1	*125	*12	*33	*166	*420
Below poverty level.........	1,394	*41	31.0	*132	*12	*35	*167	*356
Poverty level to 149 percent.....	1,012	*42	36.2	*117	*15	*33	*155	*420
150-199 percent...............	784	*44	33.2	*133	*25	*35	*108	*430
200-299 percent..............	1,253	*72	33.6	*214	*24	*47	*306	*593
300-499 percent..............	*725	*120	*48.9	*245	*24	*45	*80	*710
500 percent or more..........	*379	*64	*62.4	*103	*20	*50	*85	*95
Family income in 1980[2]								
Less than $10,000.............	3,602	52	34.0	152	18	35	195	482
$10,000-$19,999...............	1,457	*85	39.8	*215	*24	*45	*180	*710
$20,000-$34,999...............	*415	*58	*51.1	*113	*24	*64	*85	*670
$35,000 or more...............	*71	*14	*71.5	*19	*0	*15	*50	*50

Education[3]

None or elementary school	*443	*[...]	*[...]	*[...]	*23	*25	*482	*482
Some high school	1,008	*41	28.8	*143	*0	*24	*155	*542
High school graduate	1,713	49	38.0	*130	*26	*47	*95	*356
Some college	1,208	*75	40.9	*184	*25	*50	*200	*593
College graduate or more	1,127	*95	49.5	*192	*20	*34	*65	*420

Employment status[4]

Worked full year	2,314	*77	42.6	*182	20	39	180	535
Worked part year	2,711	46	34.5	132	24	45	95	430
Never worked	*495	*66	*29.9	*222	*20	*36	*242	*960

Perceived health status[5]

Excellent	2,559	*62	37.7	*164	20	35	85	420
Good	2,314	69	38.1	182	22	56	306	593
Fair	*441	*19	*33.6	*56	*27	*35	*77	*166
Poor	*231	*35	*32.7	*108	*0	*0	*0	*482

Limitation in usual activity

None	5,276	63	37.6	168	22	45	167	535
Some limitation	*82	*25	*35.0	*70	*0	*0	*155	*155
Cannot perform usual activity	*188	*0	*31.2	*0	*0	*0	*0	*0

Bed days[2]

0	2,622	43	34.9	123	20	37	77	314
1-5	1,575	*69	36.8	*187	*24	*47	*96	*535
6-10	766	*112	42.9	*261	*30	*200	*430	*710
11-20	*237	*111	*61.1	*181	*22	*180	*356	*420
More than 20	*345	*8	*29.2	*26	*0	*0	*30	*111

Family health care coverage

All members covered, some part year	3,223	52	37.2	141	20	39	85	542
Some members not covered	-	-	-	-	-	-	-	-
All members not covered	2,322	72	37.4	191	22	45	215	430

[1]There were too few Hispanic families of races other than white for separate tabulation.
[2]Annual rate.
[3]Includes only families with heads 17 years of age and over.
[4]Excludes families with all members under 14 years of age.
[5]Excludes families with all members with health status unknown.

NOTE: 1-person families are families with average size less than 1.5. For 1-person families with more than 1 distinct individual, characteristics are those of head or of family as in Table 2.

161

Table 50

Out-of-pocket expenditures for dental visits for 1-person families 65 years of age and over, by selected characteristics: United States, 1980

[Rate per family year. Civilian noninstitutionalized population with civilian family head]

| Characteristic | All families | | Families with visits | | | | | |
| | Number in thousands | Mean expenditures | Percent | Mean expenditures | Expenditures at selected percentiles | | | |
					25th	50th	75th	90th
Total................	7,714	$45	35.5	$127	$20	$57	$146	$283
Sex								
Male..................	1,784	*38	23.5	*163	*23	*57	*180	*408
Female................	5,930	47	39.2	120	20	57	139	280
Race and ethnicity[1]								
White.................	7,025	47	36.6	127	22	58	143	286
Hispanic..............	*138	*22	*47.6	46	*0	*0	*0	*225
Non-Hispanic..........	6,887	47	36.4	129	23	58	143	286
Black.................	582	*18	21.7	*83	*15	*30	*195	*209
Other.................	*106	*90	*41.2	*219	*0	*15	*757	*757
Family dynamics								
Unchanging, full year.......	7,083	45	36.5	123	20	57	146	280
Change in composition or existed less than full year......	630	*48	24.9	*194	*21	*52	*254	*333
Poverty status in 1980								
Below 150 percent poverty level......	4,199	25	27.3	92	13	50	122	225
Below poverty level..........	2,220	26	24.8	*105	*10	*36	*190	*250
Poverty level to 149 percent........	1,979	24	30.1	*80	*20	*51	*100	*188
150-199 percent........	1,118	*49	33.7	*146	*24	*58	*143	*313
200-299 percent........	1,313	70	46.0	*151	*35	*64	*150	*367
300-499 percent........	783	82	57.5	*142	*17	*69	*160	*283
500 percent or more........	*300	*105	*53.9	*194	*35	*57	*146	*716
Family income in 1980[2]								
Less than $10,000........	6,246	37	30.4	121	20	56	147	280
$10,000-$19,999........	1,167	74	58.1	128	26	60	132	283
$20,000-$34,999........	*136	*89	*35.5	*250	*35	*37	*37	*934
$35,000 or more........	*165	*118	*69.0	*170	*50	*70	*146	*716
Education								
None or elementary school......	3,012	*24	20.4	119	10	46	115	250
Some high school......	1,451	33	25.7	*129	*22	*73	*190	*280
High school graduate......	1,653	45	49.9	90	20	56	113	225
Some college......	804	82	51.4	*159	*35	*62	*173	*440
College graduate or more......	793	109	65.0	*168	*22	*58	*162	*583

Category								
Employment status								
Worked full year..........	*411	*41	*49.0	*84	*30	*58	*97	*170
Worked part year..........	863	*48	28.6	*166	*26	*57	*101	*295
Never worked..............	6,439	45	35.6	126	20	57	160	286
Perceived health status[3]								
Excellent.................	2,313	52	43.8	119	22	50	100	283
Good......................	2,790	59	36.3	162	27	75	208	313
Fair......................	1,825	28	26.3	*105	*18	*41	*147	*356
Poor......................	765	*16	29.0	*54	*5	*25	*73	*190
Limitation in usual activity								
None......................	5,049	47	37.6	125	20	56	115	283
Some limitation...........	*523	*61	*37.2	*164	*24	*52	*200	*220
Cannot perform usual activity....	2,142	36	30.2	120	21	64	161	313
Bed days[2]								
0.........................	4,338	45	36.3	124	20	58	170	283
1-5.......................	867	*63	39.9	*159	*20	*56	*123	*365
6-10......................	658	*27	30.0	*88	*15	*40	*162	*250
11-20.....................	702	*58	31.4	*183	*22	*48	*95	*545
More than 20..............	1,149	*34	35.0	*97	*25	*60	*101	*188
Family health care coverage								
All members covered full year.....	7,517	46	36.1	127	20	57	146	283
Private insurance only............	*13	*0	*0.0	-	-	-	-	-
Medicaid only.....................	-	-	-	-	-	-	-	-
Medicare only.....................	1,154	*36	18.5	*195	*35	*78	*185	*296
Medicare and other public programs....	993	*23	21.1	*109	*0	*15	*195	*225
Medicare and private insurance........	4,819	54	42.9	126	25	60	123	294
Other public and private mixes........	-	-	-	-	-	-	-	-
Other mixes of public programs........	-	-	-	-	-	-	-	-
Source unknown....................	*538	*36	*41.9	*85	*12	*35	*58	*190
All members covered, some part year....	-	-	-	-	-	-	-	-
Some members not covered..........	*24	*0	*0.0	-	-	-	-	-
All members not covered...........	*172	*18	*14.8	*119	*48	*48	*200	*200

[1]There were too few Hispanic families of races other than white for separate tabulation.
[2]Annual rate.
[3]Excludes families with all members with health status unknown.

NOTE: 1-person families are families with average size less than 1.5. For 1-person families with more than 1 distinct individual, characteristics are those of head or of family as in Table 5.

163

Table 51

Out-of-pocket expenditures for prescription medicines for multiple-person families, by selected characteristics: United States, 1980

[Rate per family year. Civilian noninstitutionalized population with civilian family head]

Characteristic	All families		Families with prescriptions					
	Number in thousands	Mean expenditures	Percent	Mean expenditures	Expenditures at selected percentiles			
					25th	50th	75th	90th
Total........................	58,135	$68	92.6	$74	$12	$37	$90	$180
Family size[1]								
2 persons....................	22,916	78	88.7	88	12	41	110	232
3 persons....................	12,567	61	95.0	64	11	33	79	164
4 persons....................	12,269	64	95.6	67	15	38	81	152
5 or more persons............	10,383	60	94.9	64	11	33	78	146
Age of head								
Under 25 years...............	4,308	27	90.3	30	5	16	45	75
25-44 years..................	25,173	47	93.5	51	11	29	66	114
45-64 years..................	20,129	79	92.2	85	14	45	106	213
65 years and over............	8,525	125	92.1	136	28	85	190	331
Sex of head								
Male.........................	44,874	73	92.7	79	15	43	96	191
Female.......................	13,262	52	92.2	56	5	20	63	150
Race and ethnicity[2] of head								
White........................	51,015	71	93.2	77	14	39	93	188
Hispanic.....................	3,403	47	93.9	50	6	22	64	133
Non-Hispanic.................	47,613	73	93.1	79	14	40	95	194
Black........................	6,090	46	89.7	51	5	20	60	145
Other........................	1,030	36	82.9	43	6	24	55	121
Family structure								
Head and spouse present whole time......	42,556	73	93.2	78	16	44	96	189
Child under 17 years.........	22,442	58	95.2	61	15	36	76	135
No child under 17 years......	20,114	89	90.9	98	17	55	120	248
Head only, no spouse at any time........	13,977	51	90.2	57	5	22	65	153
Child under 17 years.........	8,643	37	92.1	40	3	16	43	108
No child under 17 years......	5,334	73	87.1	84	10	36	92	235
Other........................	1,602	97	99.2	97	8	28	119	262
Family dynamics								
Unchanging, full year........	46,990	70	92.5	75	12	38	91	187
Change in composition or existed less than full year	11,145	62	93.3	67	12	33	84	160

164

Characteristic							
Family poverty status in 1980							
Below 150 percent poverty level	10,938	56	91.1	62	3	22	76	185
Below poverty level	6,047	44	91.0	48	0	12	58	141
Poverty level to 149 percent	4,892	71	91.2	78	10	38	101	213
150-199 percent	6,355	82	93.2	88	15	39	101	223
200-299 percent	12,860	77	93.1	83	15	39	97	202
300-499 percent	17,047	66	92.8	71	15	39	90	165
500 percent or more	10,935	65	92.9	70	14	42	88	167
Family income in 1980[3]							
Less than $10,000	10,629	70	90.6	77	3	24	93	231
$10,000-$19,999	16,728	76	91.3	84	15	39	102	210
$20,000-$34,999	19,706	60	93.5	64	14	35	79	149
$35,000 or more	11,073	70	94.9	73	15	46	93	167
Education of head[4]							
None or elementary school	10,491	92	92.3	99	15	54	134	258
Some high school	9,267	67	92.4	72	8	34	90	193
High school graduate	20,605	62	92.3	68	12	34	80	155
Some college	8,651	62	93.8	66	12	36	82	159
College graduate or more	9,099	62	92.7	67	15	37	85	163
Family employment status[5]							
2 or more persons worked full year	14,607	62	92.9	66	14	36	83	161
Only 1 person worked full year	24,549	63	92.7	68	14	38	84	155
Some part-year work	11,303	64	91.6	70	8	32	83	192
No person worked	7,676	104	93.4	112	7	55	150	303
Worst perceived health status of any family member[6]							
Excellent	16,200	38	87.9	44	9	25	60	102
Good	24,467	60	93.1	65	13	37	84	152
Fair	11,131	89	96.0	93	14	49	122	225
Poor	6,318	138	97.2	142	20	76	189	386
Most severe limitation in usual activity of any family member							
None	43,941	52	91.5	57	11	32	74	136
Some limitation	3,679	72	94.4	77	13	39	103	197
Cannot perform usual activity	10,515	133	96.7	137	22	76	192	367
Family's bed days[3]							
0	11,173	58	81.8	71	9	36	91	176
1-5	14,527	52	91.8	57	10	28	74	145
6-10	8,834	60	94.8	63	10	34	69	163
11-20	9,982	67	96.1	70	15	38	89	168
More than 20	13,619	99	98.4	101	18	50	116	244

Table 51—continued

Out-of-pocket expenditures for prescription medicines for multiple-person families, by selected characteristics: United States, 1980

[Rate per family year. Civilian noninstitutionalized population with civilian family head]

| Characteristic | All families | | Families with prescriptions | | Expenditures at selected percentiles | | | |
	Number in thousands	Mean expenditures	Percent	Mean expenditures	25th	50th	75th	90th
Family health care coverage								
All members covered full year........	42,453	$71	93.6	$76	$13	$38	$93	$192
Private insurance only.............	25,759	57	93.2	62	15	36	76	139
Medicaid only.....................	1,621	*11	91.4	*12	0	0	8	17
Medicare only....................	*574	*140	*90.2	*156	*40	*119	*210	*394
Medicare and other public programs....	*471	*59	*95.9	*61	*0	*25	*111	*153
Medicare and private insurance......	7,475	135	93.7	145	30	93	203	347
Other public and private mixes......	5,853	59	95.8	61	6	25	73	160
Other mixes of public programs......	*135	*42	*98.5	*43	*2	*24	*101	*109
Source unknown...................	*564	*63	*97.6	*65	*0	*6	*111	*202
All members covered, some part year.....	8,669	61	92.2	66	12	35	83	148
Some members not covered.............	4,963	70	90.5	78	12	38	89	193
All members not covered.............	2,051	40	78.3	51	12	29	61	120

[1] Average size during period of family's existence rounded to nearest integer; exactly half an integer rounded upward.
[2] There were too few Hispanic families of races other than white for separate tabulation.
[3] Annual rate.
[4] Includes only families with heads 17 years of age and over.
[5] Excludes families with all members under 14 years of age.
[6] Excludes families with all members with health status unknown.

NOTE: Multiple-person families are families with average size 1.5 or greater.

Table 52

Out-of-pocket expenditures for prescription medicines for multiple-person families with all members under 65 years of age, by selected characteristics: United States, 1980

[Rate per family year. Civilian noninstitutionalized population with civilian family head]

Characteristic	All families		Families with prescriptions		Expenditures at selected percentiles			
	Number in thousands	Mean expenditures	Percent	Mean expenditures	25th	50th	75th	90th
Total................................	47,327	$54	92.6	$59	$11	$32	$75	$139
Family size[1]								
2 persons........................	14,958	54	86.9	62	9	29	75	150
3 persons........................	11,228	52	95.4	54	10	30	72	125
4 persons........................	11,546	60	95.4	62	15	38	79	146
5 or more persons................	9,595	53	94.6	56	11	31	72	118
Age of head								
Under 25 years...................	4,283	27	90.3	30	5	16	45	76
25–44 years......................	24,783	46	93.5	50	11	29	65	113
45–64 years......................	18,261	72	91.8	78	14	41	98	197
Sex of head								
Male.............................	36,477	60	92.8	65	14	36	81	146
Female...........................	10,850	36	91.6	39	3	17	44	105
Race and ethnicity[2] of head								
White............................	41,444	57	93.1	61	12	34	77	140
Hispanic.........................	3,040	43	93.5	46	6	22	58	110
Non-Hispanic.....................	38,405	58	93.0	62	13	35	79	142
Black............................	5,064	41	89.9	45	5	17	50	117
Other............................	819	29	82.8	35	5	20	44	106
Family structure								
Head and spouse present whole time......	34,963	59	93.1	64	14	37	81	143
Child under 17 years.............	21,668	56	95.2	58	15	36	75	126
No child under 17 years..........	13,295	65	89.7	73	13	40	93	175
Head only, no spouse at any time......	11,169	38	89.9	42	4	17	44	109
Child under 17 years.............	8,258	32	91.7	35	2	15	40	92
No child under 17 years..........	2,911	52	84.9	62	8	29	73	156
Other............................	1,194	69	99.7	69	6	25	75	210
Family dynamics								
Unchanging, full year............	37,714	55	92.5	60	11	32	74	143
Change in composition or existed less than full year.............	9,613	52	92.8	56	11	30	75	121

Table 52—continued

Out-of-pocket expenditures for prescription medicines for multiple-person families with all members under 65 years of age, by selected characteristics: United States, 1980

[Rate per family year. Civilian noninstitutionalized population with civilian family head]

| Characteristic | All families | | Families with prescriptions | | | | | |
| | Number in thousands | Mean expenditures | Percent | Mean expenditures | Expenditures at selected percentiles | | | |
					25th	50th	75th	90th
Family poverty status in 1980								
Below 150 percent poverty level	8,770	$40	91.2	$44	$1	$15	$56	$117
Below poverty level	5,083	34	91.1	38	0	8	36	105
Poverty level to 149 percent	3,687	47	91.3	52	8	29	68	147
150–199 percent	4,825	57	92.2	62	14	37	75	131
200–299 percent	10,075	62	93.1	67	14	34	83	152
300–499 percent	14,307	56	93.0	60	14	35	77	136
500 percent or more	9,350	56	92.7	61	13	36	80	139
Family income in 1980[3]								
Less than $10,000	7,496	41	89.6	46	0	12	49	119
$10,000–$19,999	12,555	57	91.1	63	14	34	79	147
$20,000–$34,999	17,279	53	93.5	56	13	32	71	121
$35,000 or more	9,997	64	94.9	68	14	41	87	152
Education of head[4]								
None or elementary school	5,822	58	92.0	63	9	34	86	159
Some high school	7,546	52	92.6	57	8	27	71	147
High school graduate	18,299	55	91.9	60	11	31	73	129
Some college	7,556	52	94.0	56	12	32	73	125
College graduate or more	8,084	55	93.0	59	14	34	76	144
Family employment status[5]								
2 or more persons worked full year	13,629	56	92.6	60	14	34	76	141
Only 1 person worked full year	21,782	56	92.8	60	14	35	76	139
Some part-year work	9,021	52	92.1	56	7	25	69	131
No person worked	2,896	45	91.4	49	0	7	41	135
Worst perceived health status of any family member[6]								
Excellent	14,771	37	88.9	41	9	25	57	97
Good	20,837	50	92.7	54	12	33	73	125
Fair	8,021	70	96.4	73	12	37	98	176
Poor	3,678	115	98.3	117	13	60	143	291

Most severe limitation in usual activity
of any family member

None.............................	39,751	49	91.9	53	11	30	69	122
Some limitation..................	2,814	60	94.3	64	10	33	77	140
Cannot perform usual activity....	4,762	100	97.2	103	13	51	122	263

Family's bed days³

0................................	7,825	44	80.4	55	8	27	73	123
1-5..............................	12,427	43	91.2	47	9	24	60	113
6-10.............................	7,470	46	94.7	48	9	30	60	107
11-20............................	8,884	59	96.0	62	14	36	81	141
More than 20.....................	10,722	78	98.6	80	15	43	98	176

Family health care coverage

All members covered full year....	33,575	54	93.7	58	11	31	73	133
Private insurance only...........	25,502	56	93.2	61	15	36	76	133
Medicaid only....................	1,606	*11	91.3	*12	0	0	8	17
Medicare only....................	-	-	-	-	-	-	-	-
Medicare and other public programs....	*12	*153	*100.0	*153	*153	*153	*153	*153
Medicare and private insurance........	*95	*91	*100.0	*91	*17	*96	*120	*291
Other public and private mixes........	5,762	57	95.9	59	6	25	73	143
Other mixes of public programs........	*135	*42	*98.5	*43	*2	*24	*101	*109
Source unknown........................	.*463	*47	*97.1	*48	*0	*6	*72	*149
All members covered, some part year...	7,968	57	92.3	61	11	33	80	146
Some members not covered..............	3,804	60	90.1	66	11	34	83	172
All members not covered...............	1,980	38	79.0	49	12	27	59	117

¹Average size during period of family's existence rounded to nearest integer; exactly half an integer rounded upward.
²There were too few Hispanic families of races other than white for separate tabulation.
³Annual rate.
⁴Includes only families with heads 17 years of age and over.
⁵Excludes families with all members under 14 years of age.
⁶Excludes families with all members with health status unknown.

NOTE: Multiple-person families are families with average size 1.5 or greater.

Table 53

Out-of-pocket expenditures for prescription medicines for multiple-person families with all members under 65 years of age and all members with health care coverage all year, by selected characteristics: United States, 1980

[Rate per family year. Civilian noninstitutionalized population with civilian family head]

Characteristic	All families		Families with prescriptions					
	Number in thousands	Mean expenditures	Percent	Mean expenditures	Expenditures at selected percentiles			
					25th	50th	75th	90th
Total..................	33,575	$54	93.7	$58	$11	$31	$73	$133
Family size[1]								
2 persons..................	10,994	56	89.1	63	9	29	81	152
3 persons..................	8,010	50	96.0	52	10	28	66	114
4 persons..................	8,464	59	95.9	62	15	36	77	147
5 or more persons..........	6,107	51	95.9	53	11	31	67	115
Age of head								
Under 25 years.............	2,585	28	92.7	30	4	16	45	76
25-44 years................	18,256	45	94.2	48	11	28	64	110
45-64 years................	12,733	73	93.2	79	14	41	97	199
Sex of head								
Male.......................	27,351	60	94.0	63	14	36	80	142
Female.....................	6,224	31	92.2	34	1	14	39	92
Race and ethnicity[2] of head								
White......................	29,902	57	94.3	60	12	33	76	139
Hispanic...................	1,711	42	95.8	44	6	22	56	109
Non-Hispanic...............	28,191	57	94.2	61	13	34	77	141
Black......................	3,139	37	89.6	41	4	15	39	94
Other......................	533	29	82.4	*35	*6	*20	*40	*115
Family structure								
Head and spouse present whole time.....	26,517	59	94.2	63	14	37	80	141
Child under 17 years.......	16,251	55	96.2	57	15	35	73	128
No child under 17 years....	10,266	66	91.2	72	13	39	90	168
Head only, no spouse at any time.....	6,394	35	90.8	38	1	15	40	103
Child under 17 years.......	5,051	29	92.5	31	0	12	33	77
No child under 17 years....	1,343	58	84.8	69	11	29	92	161
Other......................	663	47	99.5	*47	*5	*20	*35	*131
Family dynamics								
Unchanging, full year......	28,266	56	93.8	59	11	32	74	142
Change in composition or existed less than full year.....	5,308	48	93.1	51	10	29	66	112

Characteristic								
Family poverty status in 1980								
Below 150 percent poverty level	4,640	36	93.3	39	0	9	39	106
Below poverty level	2,919	29	92.8	31	0	4	21	82
Poverty level to 149 percent	1,721	48	93.9	51	8	29	65	149
150-199 percent	2,657	64	93.4	68	16	39	82	155
200-299 percent	7,074	58	94.4	61	14	32	73	139
300-499 percent	11,427	56	94.1	60	14	35	77	138
500 percent or more	7,776	55	92.9	60	12	36	76	131
Family income in 1980[3]								
Less than $10,000	4,023	39	92.2	42	0	8	37	106
$10,000-$19,999	7,715	59	92.3	64	15	36	77	142
$20,000-$34,999	13,970	51	93.9	55	13	31	69	121
$35,000 or more	7,867	63	95.5	66	13	40	84	144
Education of head[4]								
None or elementary school	3,188	61	93.2	66	9	34	93	163
Some high school	4,620	49	93.4	52	8	28	60	111
High school graduate	13,366	54	93.8	57	11	30	71	130
Some college	5,757	54	94.5	58	13	33	73	127
College graduate or more	6,625	56	93.4	60	14	32	74	140
Family employment status[5]								
2 or more persons worked full year	10,347	56	93.9	60	14	33	73	142
Only 1 person worked full year	16,128	57	93.5	60	14	36	75	135
Some part-year work	4,933	47	94.5	50	5	23	64	111
No person worked	2,167	44	92.2	48	0	6	49	131
Worst perceived health status of any family member[6]								
Excellent	11,162	38	90.7	42	9	25	59	101
Good	15,029	51	94.0	54	11	32	70	126
Fair	5,209	75	97.3	77	13	43	102	177
Poor	2,155	110	98.2	112	12	48	131	313
Most severe limitation in usual activity of any family member								
None	28,461	49	93.4	53	11	30	68	119
Some limitation	2,067	65	93.3	70	12	35	84	176
Cannot perform usual activity	3,047	96	97.2	99	11	49	115	278
Family's bed days[3]								
0	5,766	47	82.4	57	8	27	73	131
1-5	8,806	44	92.8	47	9	24	60	112
6-10	5,513	44	95.6	46	9	31	61	100
11-20	6,162	62	97.2	64	14	35	84	149
More than 20	7,328	74	99.3	74	15	41	94	169

Table 53—continued

Out-of-pocket expenditures for prescription medicines for multiple-person families with all members under 65 years of age and all members with health care coverage all year, by selected characteristics: United States, 1980

[Rate per family year. Civilian noninstitutionalized population with civilian family head]

Characteristic	All families		Families with prescriptions					
	Number in thousands	Mean expenditures	Percent	Mean expenditures	Expenditures at selected percentiles			
					25th	50th	75th	90th
Family health care coverage								
Private insurance only..................	25,502	$56	93.2	$61	$15	$36	$76	$133
Medicaid only.........................	1,606	*11	91.3	*12	0	0	8	17
Medicare only.........................	*12	–	–	–	–	–	–	–
Medicare and other public programs......		*153	*100.0	*153	*153	*153	*153	*153
Medicare and private insurance..........	*95	*91	*100.0	*91	*17	*96	*120	*291
Other public and private mixes..........	5,762	57	95.9	59	6	25	73	143
Other mixes of public programs..........	*135	*42	*98.5	*43	*2	*24	*101	*109
Source unknown........................	*463	*47	*97.1	*48	*0	*6	*72	*149

[1]Average size during period of family's existence rounded to nearest integer; exactly half an integer rounded upward.
[2]There were too few Hispanic families of races other than white for separate tabulation.
[3]Annual rate.
[4]Includes only families with heads 17 years of age and over.
[5]Excludes families with all members under 14 years of age.
[6]Excludes families with all members with health status unknown.

NOTE: Multiple-person families are families with average size 1.5 or greater.

Table 54

Out-of-pocket expenditures for prescription medicines for multiple-person families with all members under 65 years of age and some or all members without health care coverage all year, by selected characteristics: United States, 1980

[Rate per family year. Civilian noninstitutionalized population with civilian family head]

Characteristic	All families		Families with prescriptions		Expenditures at selected percentiles			
	Number in thousands	Mean expenditures	Percent	Mean expenditures	25th	50th	75th	90th
Total..............	13,752	$55	89.8	$61	$11	$33	$79	$147
Family size[1]								
2 persons...........	3,964	46	80.8	57	9	27	60	148
3 persons...........	3,218	57	93.9	61	11	34	83	152
4 persons...........	3,082	61	94.0	65	16	43	80	139
5 or more persons...	3,488	57	92.4	62	10	30	83	140
Age of head								
Under 25 years......	1,698	26	86.6	30	6	16	49	80
25-44 years.........	6,527	51	91.4	55	11	31	73	124
45-64 years.........	5,528	69	88.7	78	12	41	105	190
Sex of head								
Male................	9,126	61	89.2	69	14	38	86	159
Female..............	4,627	43	90.8	47	7	22	59	125
Race and ethnicity[2] **of head**								
White...............	11,542	57	89.8	63	11	34	80	147
Hispanic............	1,328	43	90.5	48	7	20	60	133
Non-Hispanic........	10,214	59	89.7	65	12	36	83	147
Black...............	1,924	47	90.4	52	10	25	60	146
Other...............	*286	*30	*83.4	*36	*4	*12	*46	*86
Family structure								
Head and spouse present whole time......	8,446	60	89.7	67	14	38	86	157
Child under 17 years..............	5,417	57	92.4	62	15	37	80	125
No child under 17 years...........	3,029	65	84.8	76	13	41	105	191
Head only, no spouse at any time......	4,775	42	88.7	47	7	22	59	114
Child under 17 years..............	3,207	39	90.5	43	7	20	59	112
No child under 17 years...........	1,568	48	84.9	56	7	26	56	126
Other...............	*532	*95	*100.0	*95	*7	*38	*92	*233
Family dynamics								
Unchanging, full year.............	9,448	54	88.5	61	11	33	77	147
Change in composition or existed less than full year.............	4,304	58	92.5	62	11	32	83	142

173

Table 54—continued

Out-of-pocket expenditures for prescription medicines for multiple-person families with all members under 65 years of age and some or all members without health care coverage all year, by selected characteristics: United States, 1980

[Rate per family year. Civilian noninstitutionalized population with civilian family head]

Characteristic	All families		Families with prescriptions					
	Number in thousands	Mean expenditures	Percent	Mean expenditures	Expenditures at selected percentiles			
					25th	50th	75th	90th
Family poverty status in 1980								
Below 150 percent poverty level	4,130	$44	88.9	$49	$6	$21	$62	$133
Below poverty level	2,164	42	88.7	47	3	20	59	125
Poverty level to 149 percent	1,966	47	89.1	52	10	29	68	147
150—199 percent	2,168	49	90.8	54	10	33	74	114
200—299 percent	3,000	73	90.2	81	14	35	98	176
300—499 percent	2,880	53	88.5	60	14	36	74	126
500 percent or more	1,574	61	92.1	67	14	47	95	157
Family income in 1980[3]								
Less than $10,000	3,473	43	86.6	50	4	20	59	133
$10,000—$19,999	4,840	54	89.1	61	12	33	80	147
$20,000—$34,999	3,310	58	92.0	63	14	38	77	123
$35,000 or more	2,130	70	92.8	76	15	48	107	175
Education of head[4]								
None or elementary school	2,634	54	90.5	60	10	34	80	145
Some high school	2,926	58	91.3	64	10	27	90	185
High school graduate	4,934	57	87.0	66	12	31	75	126
Some college	1,800	46	92.5	49	11	32	73	125
College graduate or more	1,459	52	91.3	57	14	37	83	152
Family employment status[5]								
2 or more persons worked full year	3,282	54	88.6	61	15	36	82	141
Only 1 person worked full year	5,654	55	90.9	60	12	35	80	147
Some part-year work	4,087	58	89.2	65	8	30	78	146
No person worked	*729	*46	*89.2	*51	*0	*18	*40	*165
Worst perceived health status of any family member[6]								
Excellent	3,609	32	83.0	39	9	25	55	90
Good	5,808	49	89.3	55	12	34	75	125
Fair	2,812	61	94.6	64	10	31	91	176
Poor	1,524	122	98.5	123	18	75	147	267

174

Most severe limitation in usual activity
of any family member

None.....................	11,290	47	88.1	54	11	32	74	126
Some limitation..........	747	47	96.9	49	7	21	64	118
Cannot perform usual activity...	1,715	108	97.2	111	20	58	139	235

Family's bed days[3]

0........................	2,059	35	74.9	47	7	27	73	112
1-5......................	3,620	39	87.5	45	10	25	60	116
6-10.....................	1,957	52	92.0	56	8	27	58	169
11-20....................	2,722	52	93.3	55	14	37	80	121
More than 20.............	3,394	88	97.2	91	16	45	108	195

Family health care coverage

All members covered, some part year.....	7,968	57	92.3	61	11	33	80	146
Some members not covered............	3,804	60	90.1	66	11	34	83	172
All members not covered.............	1,980	38	79.0	49	12	27	59	117

[1]Average size during period of family's existence rounded to nearest integer; exactly half an integer rounded upward.
[2]There were too few Hispanic families of races other than white for separate tabulation.
[3]Annual rate.
[4]Includes only families with heads 17 years of age and over.
[5]Excludes families with all members under 14 years of age.
[6]Excludes families with all members with health status unknown.

NOTE: Multiple-person families are families with average size 1.5 or greater.

Table 55

Out-of-pocket expenditures for prescription medicines for multiple-person families with members 65 years of age and over, by selected characteristics: United States, 1980

[Rate per family year. Civilian noninstitutionalized population with civilian family head]

Characteristic	All families		Families with prescriptions					
	Number in thousands	Mean expenditures	Percent	Mean expenditures	Expenditures at selected percentiles			
					25th	50th	75th	90th
Total..........................	10,809	$128	92.9	$138	$28	$84	$193	$345
Family size[1]								
2 persons.......................	7,958	124	92.1	135	27	87	190	326
3 persons.......................	1,339	135	91.7	148	33	79	206	419
4 persons.......................	724	135	98.8	136	14	69	144	366
5 or more persons..............	788	148	97.7	152	30	102	209	397
Family age								
All members 65 years and over...	4,141	141	93.6	151	32	100	198	367
Some members under 65..........	6,668	120	92.5	129	23	76	182	335
Sex of head								
Male............................	8,397	129	92.3	140	31	91	193	335
Female..........................	2,412	124	94.9	131	13	67	194	378
Race and ethnicity[2] of head								
White...........................	9,571	136	93.5	145	30	89	199	367
Hispanic......................	*363	*78	*97.2	*80	*5	*37	*159	*191
Non-Hispanic..................	9,208	138	93.4	148	32	91	204	378
Black..........................	1,027	72	88.8	81	10	53	110	220
Other..........................	*211	*61	*83.2	*73	*24	*24	*121	*168
Family structure								
Head and spouse present whole time......	7,593	134	93.3	144	33	94	196	337
Child under 17 years...........	774	127	93.6	136	15	57	189	398
No child under 17 years........	6,819	135	93.3	145	36	96	197	332
Head only, no spouse at any time.......	2,808	104	91.1	114	13	58	165	326
Child under 17 years...........	*384	*138	*99.4	*139	*42	*97	*209	*267
No child under 17 years........	2,424	99	89.8	110	12	54	163	342
Other..........................	*408	*179	*97.5	*184	*34	*134	*239	*468
Family dynamics								
Unchanging, full year..........	9,276	128	92.4	139	27	85	191	345
Change in composition or existed less than full year......	1,533	127	96.1	132	32	79	206	338

Family poverty status in 1980

Below 150 percent poverty level	2,169	122	90.8	135	29	97	204	318
Below poverty level	964	96	90.7	106	22	65	168	261
Poverty level to 149 percent	1,205	143	90.8	158	40	126	228	367
150-199 percent	1,530	161	96.2	168	21	93	196	453
200-299 percent	2,785	131	92.9	141	24	85	170	428
300-499 percent	2,740	118	92.2	128	31	77	170	321
500 percent or more	1,585	116	93.8	124	38	77	173	276

Family income in 1980[3]

Less than $10,000	3,133	138	93.1	148	29	96	209	342
$10,000-$19,999	4,173	134	92.1	145	24	94	203	409
$20,000-$34,999	2,427	109	93.2	117	28	70	168	298
$35,000 or more	1,076	119	94.6	126	34	77	170	271

Education of head[4]

None or elementary school	4,669	133	92.7	144	25	97	209	367
Some high school	1,721	129	91.5	141	19	76	188	350
High school graduate	2,306	123	95.4	129	29	69	179	318
Some college	1,095	127	92.8	137	18	72	172	402
College graduate or more	1,015	114	90.8	126	44	100	163	300

Family employment status[5]

2 or more persons worked full year	979	142	96.0	148	32	83	200	370
Only 1 person worked full year	2,767	115	91.3	126	18	70	187	335
Some part-year work	2,282	111	89.7	124	24	72	197	301
No person worked	4,781	140	94.7	148	33	97	193	394

Worst perceived health status of any family member[6]

Excellent	1,429	55	77.8	71	13	46	99	168
Good	3,630	118	95.1	124	31	77	169	312
Fair	3,110	137	94.9	145	27	99	204	332
Poor	2,640	170	95.6	178	36	108	267	442

Most severe limitation in usual activity of any family member

None	4,190	88	87.9	100	18	65	134	243
Some limitation	865	111	94.9	117	37	106	175	271
Cannot perform usual activity	5,754	160	96.3	166	33	105	232	409

Family's bed days[3]

0	3,349	92	85.2	108	18	69	149	281
1-5	2,100	111	95.3	116	32	76	158	267
6-10	1,364	140	95.5	147	25	93	212	391
11-20	1,098	130	96.8	134	26	94	208	294
More than 20	2,897	176	97.4	181	37	111	247	457

Table 55--continued

Out-of-pocket expenditures for prescription medicines for multiple-person families with members 65 years of age and over, by selected characteristics: United States, 1980

[Rate per family year. Civilian noninstitutionalized population with civilian family head]

Characteristic	All families		Families with prescriptions					
	Number in thousands	Mean expenditures	Percent	Mean expenditures	Expenditures at selected percentiles			
					25th	50th	75th	90th
Family health care coverage								
All members covered full year............	8,879	$133	93.4	$142	$29	$92	$199	$350
Private insurance only...............	*258	*156	*89.3	*175	*47	*126	*261	*493
Medicaid only......................	*15	*0	*100.0	*0	*0	*0	*0	*0
Medicare only.....................	*574	*140	*90.2	*156	*40	*119	*210	*394
Medicare and other public programs....	*459	*56	*95.8	*59	*0	*25	*100	*150
Medicare and private insurance.......	7,380	136	93.6	145	31	93	204	347
Other public and private mixes.......	*91	*174	*88.7	*196	*63	*73	*501	*501
Other mixes of public programs........	-	-	-	-	-	-	-	-
Source unknown..................	*102	*140	*100.0	*140	*4	*123	*280	*434
All members covered, some part year.....	701	105	91.9	114	23	57	144	281
Some members not covered.............	1,159	106	91.6	115	15	58	143	285
All members not covered..............	*71	*95	*59.6	*160	*138	*138	*172	*300

1Average size during period of family's existence rounded to nearest integer; exactly half an integer rounded upward.
2There were too few Hispanic families of races other than white for separate tabulation.
3Annual rate.
4Includes only families with heads 17 years of age and over.
5Excludes families with all members under 14 years of age.
6Excludes families with all members with health status unknown.

NOTE: Multiple-person families are families with average size 1.5 or greater.

Table 56

Out-of-pocket expenditures for prescription medicines for 1-person families, by selected characteristics: United States, 1980

[Rate per family year. Civilian noninstitutionalized population with civilian family head]

Characteristic	All families		Families with prescriptions					
	Number in thousands	Mean expenditures	Percent	Mean expenditures	Expenditures at selected percentiles			
					25th	50th	75th	90th
Total......	26,233	$38	70.0	$54	$7	$24	$67	$133
Sex								
Male......	11,866	19	56.2	34	4	13	40	84
Female......	14,367	54	81.3	66	10	34	80	162
Race and ethnicity[1]								
White......	22,811	38	70.1	55	8	25	69	133
Hispanic......	818	16	62.0	*26	*0	*16	*37	*63
Non-Hispanic......	21,993	39	70.4	56	8	26	71	139
Black......	2,711	43	72.9	59	6	20	59	175
Other......	*712	*9	*53.0	*17	*8	*15	*25	*39
Family dynamics								
Unchanging, full year......	22,570	40	72.8	54	7	24	67	130
Change in composition or existed less than full year......	3,662	29	52.6	56	7	24	72	153
Poverty status in 1980								
Below 150 percent poverty level......	9,379	47	72.7	64	7	27	79	163
Below poverty level......	5,252	38	69.4	55	4	18	62	153
Poverty level to 149 percent......	4,128	57	76.8	75	11	43	103	177
150-199 percent......	2,974	45	67.2	67	9	32	79	215
200-299 percent......	5,563	34	68.2	50	10	28	67	114
300-499 percent......	5,426	30	71.0	42	7	18	54	95
500 percent or more......	2,891	26	65.5	40	4	17	58	114
Family income in 1980[2]								
Less than $10,000......	14,468	45	71.1	64	8	31	77	163
$10,000-$19,999......	8,280	31	69.9	44	8	20	53	100
$20,000-$34,999......	2,664	26	66.8	38	5	17	56	101
$35,000 or more......	820	21	60.1	*34	*3	*13	*33	*108
Education[3]								
None or elementary school......	4,782	59	78.5	75	9	31	107	221
Some high school......	3,996	38	65.2	58	7	26	76	145
High school graduate......	7,413	36	70.4	51	7	23	64	118
Some college......	4,842	27	68.3	40	6	21	50	84
College graduate or more......	5,122	33	66.9	49	8	23	62	116

179

Table 56—continued

Out-of-pocket expenditures for prescription medicines for 1-person families, by selected characteristics: United States, 1980

[Rate per family year. Civilian noninstitutionalized population with civilian family head]

Characteristic	All families		Families with prescriptions					
	Number in thousands	Mean expenditures	Percent	Mean expenditures	Expenditures at selected percentiles			
					25th	50th	75th	90th
Employment status[4]								
Worked full year.........	10,374	$24	66.0	$36	$7	$17	$45	$81
Worked part year.........	7,129	30	63.8	46	6	20	59	108
Never worked.............	8,703	62	79.8	78	11	41	103	193
Perceived health status[5]								
Excellent................	11,226	21	62.2	34	7	17	47	83
Good.....................	9,642	37	69.8	53	7	25	66	133
Fair.....................	3,691	68	85.1	80	9	45	107	211
Poor.....................	1,568	94	89.5	105	10	47	132	377
Limitation in usual activity								
None.....................	21,977	32	66.9	47	7	22	62	116
Some limitation..........	731	62	84.4	73	17	36	98	175
Cannot perform usual activity	3,525	73	85.7	85	7	38	108	265
Bed days[2]								
0........................	12,629	31	58.0	54	7	25	73	133
1-5......................	6,587	29	71.1	41	6	17	58	98
6-10.....................	2,671	44	87.8	50	9	24	57	123
11-20....................	1,924	56	89.4	63	12	23	62	159
More than 20.............	2,422	77	94.3	82	10	42	103	222
Family health care coverage								
All members covered full year.......	20,491	42	73.8	57	7	24	71	148
Private insurance only...	10,523	25	66.6	38	6	17	47	86
Medicaid only............	*317	*5	*76.6	*6	*0	*4	*9	*23
Medicare only...........	1,262	73	66.1	110	31	79	163	298
Medicare and other public programs....	993	22	84.1	27	0	6	24	95
Medicare and private insurance.......	4,819	74	83.4	89	19	59	125	212
Other public and private mixes......	1,361	51	81.9	62	5	27	72	132
Other mixes of public programs.......	*186	*12	*68.7	*18	*0	*9	*16	*44
Source unknown...........	1,030	47	90.8	52	1	21	57	167

All members covered, some part year.....	3,223	26	60.1	43	5	16	42	79
Some members not covered.............	*24	*156	*100.0	*156	*40	*252	*252	*252
All members not covered.............	2,495	22	51.0	42	10	30	63	105

[1]There were too few Hispanic families of races other than white for separate tabulation.
[2]Annual rate.
[3]Includes only families with heads 17 years of age and over.
[4]Excludes families with all members under 14 years of age.
[5]Excludes families with all members with health status unknown.

NOTE: 1-person families are families with average size less than 1.5. For 1-person families with more than 1 distinct individual, characteristics are those of head or of family as in Table 1.

Table 57

Out-of-pocket expenditures for prescription medicines for 1-person families under 65 years of age, by selected characteristics: United States, 1980

[Rate per family year. Civilian noninstitutionalized population with civilian family head]

Characteristic	All families		Families with prescriptions		Expenditures at selected percentiles			
	Number in thousands	Mean expenditures	Percent	Mean expenditures	25th	50th	75th	90th
Total..................	18,519	$27	65.3	$41	$6	$17	$50	$93
Age								
Under 25 years..........	5,208	16	61.8	27	6	14	39	63
25–44 years.............	7,630	19	62.8	29	4	14	36	75
45–64 years.............	5,680	47	72.0	65	9	30	75	149
Sex								
Male....................	10,082	14	53.2	26	3	12	31	72
Female..................	8,437	42	79.8	52	9	26	63	113
Race and ethnicity[1]								
White...................	15,786	25	65.0	39	6	17	50	86
Hispanic................	680	15	58.0	*26	*0	*16	*31	*84
Non-Hispanic............	15,106	26	65.3	39	6	17	50	87
Black...................	2,128	42	72.3	59	7	20	59	177
Other...................	*605	*8	*48.8	*17	*8	*15	*24	*39
Family dynamics								
Unchanging, full year...	15,487	28	69.5	40	6	16	49	87
Change in composition or existed less than full year...	3,032	20	44.3	45	7	19	56	103
Poverty status in 1980								
Below 150 percent.......	5,181	31	65.2	48	5	16	51	105
Below poverty level.....	3,031	27	61.9	44	0	14	36	99
Poverty level to 149 percent.....	2,149	37	69.9	53	8	32	66	116
150–199 percent.........	1,855	24	57.9	41	5	19	52	84
200–299 percent.........	4,250	29	66.1	44	8	21	50	100
300–499 percent.........	4,643	23	68.7	34	6	15	42	78
500 percent or more.....	2,590	22	63.4	34	4	16	50	97
Family income in 1980[2]								
Less than $10,000.......	8,222	29	64.4	46	6	19	56	101
$10,000–$19,999.........	7,113	26	67.2	39	7	17	44	82
$20,000–$34,999.........	2,529	23	66.9	35	5	16	50	81
$35,000 or more.........	*656	*9	*50.1	*18	*0	*12	*21	*62

Education[3]

None or elementary school	1,770	35	69.0	50	6	14	56	117
Some high school	2,546	29	61.6	46	6	20	56	100
High school graduate	5,759	28	67.6	42	6	17	50	101
Some college	4,037	22	66.7	32	5	16	43	74
College graduate or more	4,329	25	62.1	40	7	17	52	81

Employment status[4]

Worked full year	9,963	23	65.4	35	6	17	43	81
Worked part year	6,265	27	62.6	43	6	18	50	99
Never worked	2,264	42	72.6	58	3	19	59	118

Perceived health status[5]

Excellent	8,913	17	59.3	28	5	14	35	78
Good	6,852	28	66.4	43	6	19	50	101
Fair	1,866	43	80.8	53	7	35	66	117
Poor	803	84	85.7	*98	*14	*47	*105	*400

Limitation in usual activity

None	16,928	24	64.1	38	*6	17	46	83
Some limitation	*209	*69	*74.9	*92	*14	*75	*82	*322
Cannot perform usual activity	1,383	48	79.3	61	3	15	64	181

Bed days[2]

0	8,291	17	50.2	34	5	15	46	86
1–5	5,721	24	69.1	34	5	15	44	83
6–10	2,013	41	86.7	48	9	24	46	115
11–20	1,222	42	87.2	48	11	19	49	80
More than 20	1,273	63	91.8	69	7	36	72	197

Family health care coverage

All members covered full year	12,974	28	69.4	40	5	16	47	94
Private insurance only	10,511	25	66.5	38	6	17	47	86
Medicaid only	*317	*5	*76.6	*6	*0	*4	*9	*23
Medicare only	*108	*97	*53.8	*180	*35	*59	*197	*527
Medicare and other public programs	–	–	–	–	–	–	–	–
Medicare and private insurance	–	–	–	–	–	–	–	–
Other public and private mixes	1,361	51	81.9	62	5	27	72	132
Other mixes of public programs	*186	*12	*68.7	*18	*0	*9	*16	*44
Source unknown	*491	*33	*94.0	*35	*0	*3	*32	*80
All members covered, some part year	3,223	26	60.1	43	5	16	42	79
Some members not covered	–	–	–	–	–	–	–	–
All members not covered	2,322	20	50.0	39	10	27	63	87

[1] There were too few Hispanic of races other than white families for separate tabulation.
[2] Annual rate.
[3] Includes only families with heads 17 years of age and over.
[4] Excludes families with all members under 14 years of age.
[5] Excludes families with all members with health status unknown.

NOTE: 1-person families are families with average size less than 1.5. For 1-person families with more than 1 distinct individual, characteristics are those of head or of family as in Table 2.

183

Table 58

Out-of-pocket expenditures for prescription medicines for 1-person families under 65 years of age with health care coverage all year, by selected characteristics: United States, 1980

[Rate per family year. Civilian noninstitutionalized population with civilian family head]

Characteristic	All families		Families with prescriptions					
	Number in thousands	Mean expenditures	Percent	Mean expenditures	Expenditures at selected percentiles			
					25th	50th	75th	90th
Total..................	12,974	$28	69.4	$40	$5	$16	$47	$94
Age								
Under 25 years..........	3,166	17	63.0	27	5	12	37	66
25-44 years.............	5,206	18	66.6	26	4	13	34	74
45-64 years.............	4,601	47	76.9	62	8	25	66	149
Sex								
Male....................	6,807	13	57.8	23	2	11	31	72
Female..................	6,167	44	82.2	54	8	23	62	118
Race and ethnicity[1]								
White...................	11,183	26	69.2	38	5	16	46	88
Hispanic................	*400	*20	*70.9	*28	*0	*17	*31	*84
Non-Hispanic............	10,782	26	69.1	38	5	16	47	89
Black...................	1,428	47	76.2	61	5	20	59	177
Other...................	*363	*8	*48.7	*17	*11	*15	*20	*39
Family dynamics								
Unchanging, full year...	11,017	30	73.8	41	5	16	49	93
Change in composition or existed less than full year....	1,957	16	44.4	36	6	17	37	99
Poverty status in 1980								
Below 150 percent.......	2,775	37	72.3	51	1	14	45	118
Below poverty level.....	1,638	37	71.2	52	0	9	31	164
Poverty level to 149 percent....	1,137	36	73.7	49	4	15	49	118
150-199 percent.........	1,072	31	63.2	*49	*5	*19	*62	*132
200-299 percent.........	2,997	34	70.9	48	8	22	53	104
300-499 percent.........	3,918	20	70.1	28	6	14	37	74
500 percent or more.....	2,212	21	65.3	33	4	16	54	81
Family income in 1980[2]								
Less than $10,000.......	4,620	35	69.4	51	4	16	56	115
$10,000-$19,999........	5,656	26	71.4	36	7	16	41	82
$20,000-$34,999........	2,114	23	69.3	33	5	17	54	81
$35,000 or more.........	*584	*10	*49.2	*19	*3	*12	*14	*62

Education[3]

None or elementary school	1,328	38	73.1	52	4	13	49	128
Some high school	1,538	31	69.0	44	4	18	53	103
High school graduate	4,047	28	71.5	40	6	16	49	95
Some college	2,830	24	68.8	35	6	21	46	78
College graduate or more	3,201	25	66.3	38	7	15	49	86

Employment status[4]

Worked full year	7,649	24	68.4	35	7	16	44	81
Worked part year	3,554	27	65.4	42	4	14	50	100
Never worked	1,769	47	81.2	58	1	16	59	118

Perceived health status[5]

Excellent	6,353	18	62.8	29	6	14	37	79
Good	4,537	30	71.7	42	5	16	50	101
Fair	1,425	36	83.0	43	4	22	65	115
Poor	*572	*101	*88.2	*115	*8	*44	*132	*400

Limitation in usual activity

None	11,652	26	68.0	38	6	16	46	84
Some limitation	*127	*55	*95.7	*58	*14	*66	*82	*151
Cannot perform usual activity	1,195	47	80.2	59	1	13	59	197

Bed days[2]

0	5,669	18	56.0	33	4	14	46	84
1-5	4,146	24	69.5	34	5	13	43	84
6-10	1,247	48	93.0	51	9	23	52	115
11-20	984	41	90.6	45	11	19	38	80
More than 20	928	65	96.1	68	3	31	70	235

Family health care coverage

Private insurance only	10,511	25	66.5	38	6	17	47	86
Medicaid only	*317	*5	*76.6	*6	*0	*4	*9	*23
Medicare only	*108	*97	*53.8	*180	*35	*59	*197	*527
Medicare and other public programs	-	-	-	-	-	-	-	-
Medicare and private insurance	-	-	-	-	-	-	-	-
Other public and private mixes	1,361	51	81.9	62	5	27	72	132
Other mixes of public programs	*186	*12	*68.7	*18	*0	*9	*16	*44
Source unknown	*491	*33	*94.0	*35	*0	*3	*32	*80

[1]There were too few Hispanic families of races other than white for separate tabulation.
[2]Annual rate.
[3]Includes only families with heads 17 years of age and over.
[4]Excludes families with all members under 14 years of age.
[5]Excludes families with all members with health status unknown.

NOTE: 1-person families are families with average size less than 1.5. For 1-person families with more than 1 distinct individual, characteristics are those of head or of family as in Table 2.

Table 59

Out-of-pocket expenditures for prescription medicines for 1-person families under 65 years of age without health care coverage all year, by selected characteristics: United States, 1980

[Rate per family year. Civilian noninstitutionalized population with civilian family head]

| Characteristic | All families | | Families with prescriptions | | | | | |
	Number in thousands	Mean expenditures	Percent	Mean expenditures	25th	50th	75th	90th
					Expenditures at selected percentiles			
Total..................	5,545	$23	55.9	$42	$7	$21	$54	$87
Age								
Under 25 years..........	2,042	16	59.9	26	6	15	39	63
25–44 years.............	2,424	20	54.6	37	5	19	51	75
45–64 years.............	1,079	45	51.3	*87	*29	*58	*99	*117
Sex								
Male....................	3,275	15	43.8	34	5	12	32	69
Female..................	2,270	36	73.3	49	13	30	63	99
Race and ethnicity[1]								
White...................	4,603	23	55.0	41	7	22	57	80
Hispanic................	*280	*9	*39.6	*22	*0	*14	*37	*41
Non-Hispanic............	4,323	24	56.0	42	7	23	58	80
Black...................	*700	*33	*64.3	*52	*10	*20	*63	*117
Other...................	*242	*8	*49.0	*17	*5	*24	*27	*39
Family dynamics								
Unchanging, full year...	4,470	23	58.7	38	6	19	50	79
Change in composition or existed less than full year...	1,075	27	44.1	*61	*13	*37	*73	*119
Poverty status in 1980								
Below 150 percent.......	2,405	25	57.2	44	8	26	62	105
Below poverty level.....	1,394	15	51.0	*30	*5	*16	*59	*74
Poverty level to 149 percent.....	1,012	39	65.7	*59	*12	*40	*66	*116
150–199 percent.........	784	14	50.7	*27	*5	*19	*41	*63
200–299 percent.........	1,253	16	54.6	*29	*8	*19	*39	*73
300–499 percent.........	*725	*40	*61.4	*65	*8	*16	*69	*119
500 percent or more.....	*379	*25	*52.3	*47	*1	*7	*25	*119
Family income in 1980[2]								
Less than $10,000.......	3,602	22	57.9	38	8	23	52	78
$10,000–$19,999.........	1,457	*26	51.0	*52	*10	*22	*64	*87
$20,000–$34,999.........	*415	*26	*55.2	*47	*5	*8	*25	*119
$35,000 or more.........	*71	*7	*57.4	*12	*0	*24	*24	*24

Education[3]

None or elementary school	*443	*23	*56.6	*41	*10	*32	*63	*105
Some high school	1,008	25	50.2	*50	*14	*32	*58	*99
High school graduate	1,713	28	58.4	49	9	23	57	116
Some college	1,208	15	61.7	*24	*3	*11	*34	*70
College graduate or more	1,127	*24	50.0	*47	*9	*23	*62	*79

Employment status[4]

Worked full year	2,314	20	55.2	36	6	19	40	81
Worked part year	2,711	26	59.0	45	8	20	56	80
Never worked	*495	*25	*41.5	*61	*23	*32	*62	*105

Perceived health status[5]

Excellent	2,559	13	50.6	27	5	13	27	74
Good	2,314	24	56.1	43	8	23	52	89
Fair	*441	*67	*73.5	*91	*15	*46	*79	*322
Poor	*231	*42	*79.6	*53	*33	*50	*64	*73

Limitation in usual activity

None	5,276	21	55.5	38	7	19	50	80
Some limitation	*82	*90	*42.6	*212	*26	*322	*322	*322
Cannot perform usual activity	*188	*57	*73.4	*78	*33	*58	*73	*94

Bed days[2]

0	2,622	14	37.8	38	5	18	46	105
1–5	1,575	23	68.1	34	6	15	59	76
6–10	766	32	76.6	*41	*11	*24	*41	*69
11–20	*237	*46	*73.1	*62	*8	*25	*63	*109
More than 20	*345	*58	*80.1	*72	*33	*58	*73	*94

Family health care coverage

All members covered, some part year	3,223	26	60.1	43	5	16	42	79
Some members not covered	-	-	-	-	-	-	-	-
All members not covered	2,322	20	50.0	39	10	27	63	87

[1] There were too few Hispanic families of races other than white for separate tabulation.
[2] Annual rate.
[3] Includes only families with heads 17 years of age and over.
[4] Excludes families with all members under 14 years of age.
[5] Excludes families with all members with health status unknown.

NOTE: 1-person families are families with average size less than 1.5. For 1-person families with more than 1 distinct individual, characteristics are those of head or of family as in Table 2.

Table 60

Out-of-pocket expenditures for prescription medicines for 1-person families 65 years of age and over, by selected characteristics: United States, 1980

[Rate per family year. Civilian noninstitutionalized population with civilian family head]

Characteristic	All families		Families with prescriptions		Expenditures at selected percentiles			
	Number in thousands	Mean expenditures	Percent	Mean expenditures	25th	50th	75th	90th
Total............................	7,714	$66	81.1	$81	$14	$50	$108	$193
Sex								
Male............................	1,784	48	73.0	66	9	36	91	167
Female..........................	5,930	71	83.5	85	16	54	116	208
Race and ethnicity[1]								
White...........................	7,025	68	81.6	84	16	53	116	203
Hispanic......................	*138	*20	*81.9	*24	*0	*19	*48	*49
Non-Hispanic..................	6,887	69	81.6	85	16	56	118	208
Black...........................	582	44	75.2	59	*4	*27	*95	*175
Other...........................	*106	*14	*76.8	*18	*7	*25	*28	*38
Family dynamics								
Unchanging, full year...........	7,083	65	80.0	81	15	51	107	193
Change in composition or existed less than full year............	630	76	92.7	82	12	40	149	252
Poverty status in 1980								
Below 150 percent poverty level..	4,199	65	81.8	80	10	48	116	193
Below poverty level............	2,220	53	79.7	67	8	27	84	180
Poverty level to 149 percent...	1,979	79	84.2	94	17	63	135	214
150-199 percent.................	1,118	81	82.6	98	17	51	128	273
200-299 percent.................	1,313	52	74.9	69	24	50	97	160
300-499 percent.................	783	68	84.2	81	16	56	108	173
500 percent or more.............	*300	*66	*83.3	*79	*31	*79	*114	*191
Family income in 1980[2]								
Less than $10,000...............	6,246	66	79.9	83	12	50	116	212
$10,000-$19,999.................	1,167	62	86.4	71	18	50	99	162
$20,000-$34,999.................	*136	*66	*63.2	*105	*20	*94	*149	*191
$35,000 or more.................	*165	*65	*99.9	*66	*31	*33	*98	*153

Education

None or elementary school........	3,012	74	84.2	87	11	48	130	246
Some high school.................	1,451	53	71.6	75	9	44	96	190
High school graduate.............	1,653	63	80.0	79	19	51	97	161
Some college.....................	804	55	76.4	*71	*20	*47	*84	*173
College graduate or more.........	793	74	93.5	80	31	57	114	175

Employment status

Worked full year.................	*411	*39	*80.7	*48	*12	*19	*79	*82
Worked part year.................	863	50	71.8	69	10	40	107	177
Never worked.....................	6,439	70	82.3	84	16	51	117	211

Perceived health status[3]

Excellent........................	2,313	39	73.7	54	15	36	75	116
Good.............................	2,790	59	78.1	75	16	54	103	191
Fair.............................	1,825	93	89.6	104	16	68	162	255
Poor.............................	765	105	93.5	112	10	48	152	352

Limitation in usual activity

None.............................	5,049	56	76.5	74	15	49	100	177
Some limitation..................	*523	*59	*88.2	*67	*18	*31	*99	*153
Cannot perform usual activity....	2,142	89	89.9	99	11	56	143	288

Bed days[2]

0................................	4,338	58	72.7	80	16	53	108	208
1–5..............................	867	67	84.2	80	16	50	100	159
6–10.............................	658	51	90.9	*57	*10	*22	*80	*177
11–20............................	702	81	93.3	87	16	48	117	255
More than 20.....................	1,149	92	97.1	95	16	54	130	224

Family health care coverage

All members covered full year....	7,517	66	81.4	81	14	50	108	193
Private insurance only...........	*13	*41	*100.0	*41	*41	*41	*41	*41
Medicaid only....................	—	—	—	—	—	—	—	—
Medicare only....................	1,154	70	67.3	104	28	79	157	290
Medicare and other public programs	993	22	84.1	27	0	6	24	95
Medicare and private insurance...	4,819	74	83.4	89	19	59	125	212
Other public and private mixes...	—	—	—	—	—	—	—	—
Other mixes of public programs...	—	—	—	—	—	—	—	—
Source unknown...................	*538	*61	*87.8	*69	*15	*31	*104	*211
[1]All members covered, some part year...	—	—	—	—	—	—	—	—
Some members not covered.........	*24	*156	*100.0	*156	*40	*252	*252	*252
All members not covered..........	*172	*47	*64.1	*73	*11	*99	*105	*152

[1]There were too few Hispanic families of races other than white for separate tabulation.
[2]Annual rate.
[3]Excludes families with all members with health status unknown.

NOTE: 1-person families are families with average size less than 1.5. For 1-person families with more than 1 distinct individual, characteristics are those of head or of family as in Table 5.

189

Table 61

Out-of-pocket expenditures for all health care for multiple-person families, by selected characteristics: United States, 1980

[Rate per family year. Civilian noninstitutionalized population with civilian family head]

Characteristic	All families		Families using health care					
	Number in thousands	Mean expenditures	Percent	Mean expenditures	Expenditures at selected percentiles			
					25th	50th	75th	90th
Total....................	58,135	$575	98.8	$582	$156	$350	$699	$1,310
Family size[1]								
2 persons....................	22,916	525	97.5	539	135	310	611	1,128
3 persons....................	12,567	513	99.2	517	155	347	673	1,098
4 persons....................	12,269	611	100.0	611	195	395	761	1,472
5 or more persons...........	10,383	718	99.7	720	181	408	872	1,614
Age of head								
Under 25 years...............	4,308	355	98.5	360	53	192	421	790
25-44 years..................	25,173	547	99.0	552	151	330	654	1,210
45-64 years..................	20,129	623	99.0	629	182	404	800	1,402
65 years and over............	8,525	658	97.6	674	191	403	751	1,463
Sex of head								
Male.........................	44,874	624	98.9	631	190	391	767	1,385
Female.......................	13,262	408	98.3	415	56	216	481	894
Race and ethnicity[2] of head								
White........................	51,015	599	98.9	606	177	372	730	1,351
Hispanic.....................	3,403	543	98.2	553	87	263	617	1,500
Non-Hispanic.................	47,613	603	98.9	609	184	377	735	1,351
Black........................	6,090	392	98.0	400	35	159	410	921
Other........................	1,030	483	98.6	490	80	210	626	1,249
Family structure								
Head and spouse present whole time......	42,556	614	99.1	619	195	395	765	1,361
Child under 17 years.........	22,442	652	99.8	653	205	418	821	1,500
No child under 17 years......	20,114	571	98.4	581	186	367	700	1,187
Head only, no spouse at any time......	13,977	429	97.6	440	56	210	466	847
Child under 17 years.........	8,643	413	98.8	418	32	180	421	765
No child under 17 years......	5,334	456	95.7	476	88	245	526	940
Other........................	1,602	820	99.4	825	135	418	1,211	1,745
Family dynamics								
Unchanging, full year........	46,990	551	98.8	558	157	341	675	1,199
Change in composition or existed less than full year......	11,145	677	98.7	686	149	404	815	1,621

Family poverty status in 1980								
Below 150 percent poverty level	10,938	394	97.9	402	27	186	450	1,008
Below poverty level	6,047	287	98.2	293	5	91	356	765
Poverty level to 149 percent	4,892	525	97.5	539	103	285	560	1,186
150–199 percent	6,355	691	99.3	696	149	317	688	1,484
200–299 percent	12,860	566	98.8	572	173	372	697	1,310
300–499 percent	17,047	601	98.9	607	196	385	744	1,322
500 percent or more	10,935	660	99.1	666	211	418	828	1,496
Family income in 1980[3]								
Less than $10,000	10,629	414	97.8	423	23	176	464	1,002
$10,000–$19,999	16,728	557	98.4	566	152	336	636	1,210
$20,000–$34,999	19,706	578	99.1	583	191	365	731	1,260
$35,000 or more	11,073	753	99.7	755	264	501	966	1,600
Education of head[4]								
None or elementary school	10,491	534	97.3	548	135	339	674	1,322
Some high school	9,267	478	98.6	484	106	274	581	1,096
High school graduate	20,605	567	98.9	574	159	344	677	1,213
Some college	8,651	586	99.6	588	176	377	739	1,343
College graduate or more	9,099	730	99.6	733	221	440	869	1,578
Family employment status[5]								
2 or more persons worked full year	14,607	611	99.3	615	202	389	784	1,418
Only 1 person worked full year	24,549	601	98.6	609	182	374	708	1,338
Some part-year work	11,303	486	98.4	493	100	284	605	1,121
No person worked	7,676	555	98.5	563	58	294	666	1,344
Worst perceived health status of any family member[6]								
Excellent	16,200	484	98.3	492	146	312	601	1,072
Good	24,467	545	98.9	551	155	347	685	1,221
Fair	11,131	604	98.9	611	166	359	728	1,376
Poor	6,318	873	99.1	881	183	489	995	1,797
Most severe limitation in usual activity of any family member								
None	43,941	524	98.7	531	150	328	652	1,176
Some limitation	3,679	650	99.7	652	157	353	787	1,497
Cannot perform usual activity	10,515	761	98.8	770	205	462	944	1,732
Family's bed days[3]								
0	11,173	358	95.8	373	110	248	484	852
1–5	14,527	440	99.0	445	138	306	557	981
6–10	8,834	515	99.6	518	160	339	683	1,172
11–20	9,982	605	99.5	608	188	402	743	1,300
More than 20	13,619	914	99.9	915	223	518	1,105	2,136

Table 61--continued

Out-of-pocket expenditures for all health care for multiple-person families, by selected characteristics: United States, 1980

[Rate per family year. Civilian noninstitutionalized population with civilian family head]

Characteristic	All families			Families using health care				
				Mean expenditures	Expenditures at selected percentiles			
	Number in thousands	Mean expenditures	Percent		25th	50th	75th	90th
Family health care coverage								
All members covered full year............	42,453	$573	99.1	$578	$168	$361	$705	$1,273
Private insurance only.............	25,759	610	99.2	615	203	386	746	1,340
Medicaid only..................	1,621	*91	98.5	*92	0	4	63	269
Medicare only..................	*574	*457	*95.9	*477	*222	*406	*620	*930
Medicare and other public programs....	*471	*233	*100.0	*233	*5	*108	*224	*699
Medicare and private insurance........	7,475	672	98.6	681	227	452	876	1,558
Other public and private mixes.......	5,853	476	99.8	477	111	283	556	1,046
Other mixes of public programs........	*135	*359	*100.0	*359	*170	*256	*489	*651
Source unknown.................	*564	*443	*100.0	*443	*5	*56	*487	*921
All members covered, some part year.....	8,669	523	98.6	531	135	314	625	1,263
Some members not covered...........	4,963	734	97.7	751	119	357	876	1,673
All members not covered............	2,051	451	94.6	477	96	228	496	1,086

[1] Average size during period of family's existence rounded to nearest integer; exactly half an integer rounded upward.
[2] There were too few Hispanic families of races other than white for separate tabulation.
[3] Annual rate.
[4] Includes only families with heads 17 years of age and over.
[5] Excludes families with all members under 14 years of age.
[6] Excludes families with all members with health status unknown.

NOTE: Multiple-person families are families with average size 1.5 or greater.

Table 62

Out-of-pocket expenditures for all health care for multiple-person families with all members under 65 years of age, by selected characteristics: United States, 1980

[Rate per family year. Civilian noninstitutionalized population with civilian family head]

Characteristic	All families		Families using health care					
	Number in thousands	Mean expenditures	Percent	Mean expenditures	Expenditures at selected percentiles			
					25th	50th	75th	90th
Total............................	47,327	$550	99.0	$556	$150	$334	$673	$1,249
Family size[1]								
2 persons......................	14,958	481	97.3	494	112	267	534	1,008
3 persons......................	11,228	470	99.5	472	152	325	619	1,055
4 persons......................	11,546	591	100.0	591	193	381	743	1,383
5 or more persons..............	9,595	703	99.7	705	172	404	845	1,573
Age of head								
Under 25 years.................	4,283	355	98.5	360	53	186	421	790
25-44 years...................	24,783	543	99.0	549	150	329	646	1,188
45-64 years...................	18,261	605	99.0	611	178	388	776	1,354
Sex of head								
Male...........................	36,477	600	99.1	605	186	378	745	1,341
Female.........................	10,850	383	98.5	389	43	192	434	800
Race and ethnicity[2] of head								
White..........................	41,444	576	99.0	581	170	354	695	1,289
Hispanic.......................	3,040	552	98.4	562	86	263	636	1,500
Non-Hispanic...................	38,405	577	99.1	583	176	357	699	1,281
Black..........................	5,064	346	98.5	351	35	150	397	821
Other..........................	819	514	98.2	523	88	206	745	1,341
Family structure								
Head and spouse present whole time.....	34,963	592	99.3	597	190	381	748	1,322
Child under 17 years...........	21,668	640	99.8	642	204	413	807	1,458
No child under 17 years........	13,295	514	98.5	522	172	335	640	1,064
Head only, no spouse at any time.....	11,169	411	97.9	420	44	183	445	795
Child under 17 years...........	8,258	409	98.8	414	28	166	405	761
No child under 17 years........	2,911	417	95.4	437	70	212	481	824
Other..........................	1,194	608	100.0	608	106	317	891	1,621
Family dynamics								
Unchanging, full year..........	37,714	534	99.1	539	153	329	650	1,154
Change in composition or existed less than full year..........	9,613	611	98.6	620	136	358	773	1,497

Table 62—continued

Out-of-pocket expenditures for all health care for multiple-person families with all members under 65 years of age, by selected characteristics: United States, 1980

[Rate per family year. Civilian noninstitutionalized population with civilian family head]

Characteristic	All families		Families using health care					
	Number in thousands	Mean expenditures	Percent	Mean expenditures	Expenditures at selected percentiles			
					25th	50th	75th	90th
Family poverty status in 1980								
Below 150 percent poverty level	8,770	$366	98.5	$372	$18	$154	$409	$975
Below poverty level	5,083	272	99.1	275	3	75	328	765
Poverty level to 149 percent	3,687	496	97.8	507	95	247	515	1,161
150-199 percent	4,825	671	99.1	677	151	311	651	1,426
200-299 percent	10,075	537	98.9	543	171	354	669	1,148
300-499 percent	14,307	576	99.1	581	192	373	721	1,281
500 percent or more	9,350	634	99.2	639	205	406	800	1,432
Family income in 1980[3]								
Less than $10,000	7,496	331	98.2	337	7	110	355	825
$10,000-$19,999	12,555	528	98.4	536	146	315	572	1,135
$20,000-$34,999	17,279	558	99.3	562	183	355	702	1,205
$35,000 or more	9,997	728	99.7	730	258	488	924	1,578
Education of head[4]								
None or elementary school	5,822	475	97.6	486	101	279	614	1,300
Some high school	7,546	424	98.9	429	95	266	508	1,016
High school graduate	18,299	546	98.9	552	152	328	649	1,106
Some college	7,556	559	99.6	561	176	366	704	1,259
College graduate or more	8,084	723	99.5	727	218	440	824	1,578
Family employment status[5]								
2 or more persons worked full year	13,629	593	99.3	597	190	377	750	1,354
Only 1 person worked full year	21,782	586	98.8	593	177	362	694	1,302
Some part-year work	9,021	465	98.6	472	84	248	548	1,075
No person worked	2,896	344	99.6	345	0	66	328	922
Worst perceived health status of any family member[6]								
Excellent	14,771	478	98.4	486	146	310	591	1,056
Good	20,837	534	98.9	540	153	335	664	1,186
Fair	8,021	612	99.7	614	147	344	707	1,392
Poor	3,678	794	100.0	794	154	449	894	1,706

Most severe limitation in usual activity of any family member

None	39,751	523	98.9	529	150	326	648	1,154
Some limitation	2,814	625	100.0	625	125	318	758	1,521
Cannot perform usual activity	4,762	729	99.1	735	184	428	925	1,717

Family's bed days[3]

0	7,825	360	96.2	374	110	239	484	894
1–5	12,427	424	99.1	428	125	287	535	956
6–10	7,470	491	99.7	493	153	314	604	1,163
11–20	8,884	584	99.5	588	188	381	729	1,186
More than 20	10,722	848	100.0	848	204	477	989	1,949

Family health care coverage

All members covered full year	33,575	553	99.3	557	160	344	675	1,178
Private insurance only	25,502	604	99.2	608	203	384	738	1,301
Medicaid only	1,606	*89	98.5	*90	0	3	61	253
Medicare only	-	-	-	-	-	-	-	-
Medicare and other public programs	*12	*156	*100.0	*156	*156	*156	*156	*156
Medicare and private insurance	*95	*360	*100.0	*360	*200	*274	*702	*922
Other public and private mixes	5,762	476	100.0	476	111	281	555	1,046
Other mixes of public programs	*135	*359	*100.0	*359	*170	*256	*489	*651
Source unknown	*463	*447	*100.0	*447	*5	*56	*278	*714
All members covered, some part year	7,968	506	98.8	513	125	306	619	1,252
Some members not covered	3,804	679	98.4	690	122	358	815	1,616
All members not covered	1,980	424	94.4	449	95	230	496	1,086

[1] Average size during period of family's existence rounded to nearest integer; exactly half an integer rounded upward.
[2] There were too few Hispanic families of races other than white for separate tabulation.
[3] Annual rate.
[4] Includes only families with heads 17 years of age and over.
[5] Excludes families with all members under 14 years of age.
[6] Excludes families with all members with health status unknown.

NOTE: Multiple-person families are families with average size 1.5 or greater.

Table 63

Out-of-pocket expenditures for all health care for multiple-person families with all members under 65 years of age and all members with health care coverage all year, by selected characteristics: United States, 1980

[Rate per family year. Civilian noninstitutionalized population with civilian family head]

Characteristic	All families		Families using health care					
	Number in thousands	Mean expenditures	Percent	Mean expenditures	Expenditures at selected percentiles			
					25th	50th	75th	90th
Total.................	33,575	$553	99.3	$557	$160	$344	$675	$1,178
Family size[1]								
2 persons.................	10,994	523	98.1	533	131	291	568	1,029
3 persons.................	8,010	470	99.9	471	155	334	619	1,046
4 persons.................	8,464	595	99.9	595	204	395	756	1,422
5 or more persons.........	6,107	658	100.0	658	180	416	801	1,496
Age of head								
Under 25 years...........	2,585	322	99.5	324	46	168	365	682
25–44 years..............	18,256	550	99.2	555	157	339	652	1,155
45–64 years..............	12,733	604	99.5	607	192	404	782	1,332
Sex of head								
Male.....................	27,351	604	99.4	608	194	383	744	1,289
Female...................	6,224	329	99.0	332	23	174	403	735
Race and ethnicity[2] of head								
White....................	29,902	578	99.4	581	182	365	700	1,238
Hispanic.................	1,711	536	99.4	539	81	234	656	1,286
Non-Hispanic.............	28,191	580	99.4	584	188	372	702	1,234
Black....................	3,139	309	98.8	312	32	133	336	704
Other....................	533	608	98.3	619	92	378	955	1,373
Family structure								
Head and spouse present whole time......	26,517	592	99.6	594	200	386	746	1,264
Child under 17 years.....	16,251	633	100.0	633	216	417	809	1,401
No child under 17 years..	10,266	527	99.0	532	180	344	641	1,044
Head only, no spouse at any time.........	6,394	387	98.2	394	24	172	392	711
Child under 17 years.....	5,051	337	98.8	341	14	153	352	644
No child under 17 years..	1,343	574	96.0	597	115	247	574	1,355
Other....................	663	609	100.0	609	93	224	758	1,621
Family dynamics								
Unchanging, full year..........	28,266	544	99.4	547	163	340	663	1,148
Change in composition or existed less than full year.........	5,308	604	98.9	611	135	365	758	1,426

196

Family poverty status in 1980

Below 150 percent poverty level	4,640	345	98.9	349	5	117	352	804
Below poverty level	2,919	222	99.5	223	0	35	269	550
Poverty level to 149 percent	1,721	556	98.0	567	102	287	523	1,135
150-199 percent	2,657	656	99.3	661	184	317	667	1,525
200-299 percent	7,074	529	99.6	531	178	375	670	1,096
300-499 percent	11,427	569	99.2	573	194	365	702	1,215
500 percent or more	7,776	641	99.5	644	205	406	807	1,379

Family income in 1980[3]

Less than $10,000	4,023	324	98.7	329	0	77	311	746
$10,000-$19,999	7,715	523	99.4	526	154	333	572	1,069
$20,000-$34,999	13,970	540	99.2	545	184	350	692	1,146
$35,000 or more	7,867	723	100.0	723	255	477	909	1,561

Education of head[4]

None or elementary school	3,188	451	98.9	456	111	287	581	1,091
Some high school	4,620	389	99.7	390	106	259	501	929
High school graduate	13,366	523	99.0	528	161	339	641	1,059
Some college	5,757	566	99.6	568	174	362	717	1,259
College graduate or more	6,625	769	99.8	770	234	448	895	1,652

Family employment status[5]

2 or more persons worked full year	10,347	605	99.7	607	202	390	756	1,365
Only 1 person worked full year	16,128	588	99.1	593	188	373	687	1,213
Some part-year work	4,933	419	99.2	423	93	272	541	965
No person worked	2,167	353	100.0	353	0	56	304	909

Worst perceived health status of any family member[6]

Excellent	11,162	510	99.1	515	160	329	643	1,091
Good	15,029	537	99.3	541	161	347	665	1,185
Fair	5,209	592	99.8	594	152	348	704	1,264
Poor	2,155	787	100.0	787	154	414	816	1,741

Most severe limitation in usual activity of any family member

None	28,461	528	99.3	531	160	339	653	1,122
Some limitation	2,067	700	100.0	700	130	345	815	1,542
Cannot perform usual activity	3,047	693	99.3	697	182	407	816	1,793

Family's bed days[3]

0	5,766	387	97.8	395	119	258	522	935
1-5	8,806	430	99.3	433	141	309	544	956
6-10	5,513	486	99.7	487	161	332	600	1,073
11-20	6,162	574	99.8	575	192	402	738	1,234
More than 20	7,328	866	100.0	866	227	486	971	2,070

Table 63--continued

Out-of-pocket expenditures for all health care for multiple-person families with all members under 65 years of age and all members with health care coverage all year, by selected characteristics: United States, 1980

[Rate per family year. Civilian noninstitutionalized population with civilian family head]

| Characteristic | All families | | Families using health care | | | | | |
| | Number in thousands | Mean expenditures | Percent | Mean expenditures | Expenditures at selected percentiles | | | |
					25th	50th	75th	90th
Family health care coverage								
Private insurance only.................	25,502	$604	99.2	$608	$203	$384	$738	$1,301
Medicaid only.........................	1,606	*89	98.5	*90	0	3	61	253
Medicare only.........................	-	-	-	-	-	-	-	-
Medicare and other public programs.....	*12	*156	*100.0	*156	*156	*156	*156	*156
Medicare and private insurance.........	*95	*360	*100.0	*360	*200	*274	*702	*922
Other public and private mixes.........	5,762	476	100.0	476	111	281	555	1,046
Other mixes of public programs.........	*135	*359	*100.0	*359	*170	*256	*489	*651
Source unknown........................	*463	*447	*100.0	*447	*5	*56	*278	*714

[1] Average size during period of family's existence rounded to nearest integer; exactly half an integer rounded upward.
[2] There were too few Hispanic families of races other than white for separate tabulation.
[3] Annual rate.
[4] Includes only families with heads 17 years of age and over.
[5] Excludes families with all members under 14 years of age.
[6] Excludes families with all members with health status unknown.

NOTE: Multiple-person families are families with average size 1.5 or greater.

Table 64

Out-of-pocket expenditures for all health care for multiple-person families with all members under 65 years of age and some or all members without health care coverage all year, by selected characteristics: United States, 1980

[Rate per family year. Civilian noninstitutionalized population with civilian family head]

Characteristic	All families			Families using health care				
					Expenditures at selected percentiles			
	Number in thousands	Mean expenditures	Percent	Mean expenditures	25th	50th	75th	90th
Total..............	13,752	$542	98.0	$553	$119	$306	$669	$1,353
Family size[1]								
2 persons.........	3,964	363	95.1	381	73	200	449	925
3 persons.........	3,218	470	98.5	477	144	320	624	1,155
4 persons.........	3,082	578	100.0	578	166	352	695	1,288
5 or more persons..	3,488	781	99.2	787	165	386	962	1,742
Age of head								
Under 25 years.....	1,698	405	97.0	417	57	209	461	936
25-44 years.......	6,527	523	98.3	532	117	300	619	1,311
45-64 years.......	5,528	607	98.0	620	146	356	767	1,433
Sex of head								
Male..............	9,126	586	98.1	597	166	356	756	1,458
Female............	4,627	456	97.8	466	67	212	518	1,016
Race and ethnicity[2] of head								
White.............	11,542	570	98.0	581	146	324	688	1,395
Hispanic..........	1,328	574	97.0	592	101	289	593	1,557
Non-Hispanic......	10,214	569	98.2	580	150	328	695	1,353
Black.............	1,924	407	98.0	415	42	182	560	1,134
Other.............	*286	*337	*98.1	*344	*49	*147	*453	*1,194
Family structure								
Head and spouse present whole time......	8,446	594	98.2	604	173	357	755	1,507
Child under 17 years........	5,417	662	99.2	668	183	396	793	1,615
No child under 17 years......	3,029	471	96.5	488	151	305	613	1,157
Head only, no spouse at any time......	4,775	444	97.5	455	67	206	495	876
Child under 17 years........	3,207	522	98.7	529	78	223	522	1,252
No child under 17 years......	1,568	283	94.9	298	47	169	372	800
Other.............	*532	*608	*100.0	*608	*176	*419	*937	*1,353
Family dynamics								
Unchanging, full year.............	9,448	506	98.0	517	115	288	609	1,172
Change in composition or existed less than full year......	4,304	621	98.2	632	143	358	815	1,567

Table 64—continued

Out-of-pocket expenditures for all health care for multiple-person families with all members under 65 years of age and some or all members without health care coverage all year, by selected characteristics: United States, 1980

[Rate per family year. Civilian noninstitutionalized population with civilian family head]

Characteristic	All families		Families using health care					
	Number in thousands	Mean expenditures	Percent	Mean expenditures	Expenditures at selected percentiles			
					25th	50th	75th	90th
Family poverty status in 1980								
Below 150 percent poverty level	4,130	$390	98.1	$397	$45	$185	$446	$1,097
Below poverty level	2,164	341	98.6	346	20	117	419	1,016
Poverty level to 149 percent	1,966	443	97.6	455	91	228	498	1,227
150-199 percent	2,168	688	98.7	697	142	296	636	1,402
200-299 percent	3,000	556	97.1	572	160	329	667	1,408
300-499 percent	2,880	605	98.5	614	181	397	811	1,448
500 percent or more	1,574	600	98.0	613	210	409	766	1,507
Family income in 1980[3]								
Less than $10,000	3,473	339	97.8	347	30	151	428	925
$10,000-$19,999	4,840	536	96.9	553	122	285	576	1,288
$20,000-$34,999	3,310	634	99.7	636	182	385	761	1,448
$35,000 or more	2,130	744	98.5	755	274	521	940	1,657
Education of head[4]								
None or elementary school	2,634	504	96.0	524	92	270	671	1,433
Some high school	2,926	480	97.6	492	78	274	570	1,270
High school graduate	4,934	609	98.8	616	115	305	695	1,408
Some college	1,800	536	99.4	540	183	385	630	1,205
College graduate or more	1,459	518	98.1	528	178	342	688	1,119
Family employment status[5]								
2 or more persons worked full year	3,282	553	98.0	564	178	329	691	1,346
Only 1 person worked full year	5,654	581	98.1	592	151	344	723	1,507
Some part-year work	4,087	520	97.9	531	78	228	564	1,195
No person worked	*729	*315	*98.4	*320	*3	*92	*442	*925
Worst perceived health status of any family member[6]								
Excellent	3,609	378	96.3	393	101	254	484	876
Good	5,808	524	97.9	535	119	300	660	1,221
Fair	2,812	647	99.5	651	142	341	787	1,664
Poor	1,524	805	100.0	805	157	510	1,082	1,674

Most severe limitation in usual activity
of any family member

None..........................	11,290	512	97.8	524	118	292	613	1,315
Some limitation...............	747	417	100.0	417	69	266	482	1,082
Cannot perform usual activity..	1,715	793	98.8	803	188	498	1,055	1,674

Family's bed days[3]

0..............................	2,059	284	91.7	310	86	209	419	723
1-5............................	3,620	409	98.6	415	93	248	521	930
6-10...........................	1,957	505	99.4	507	119	253	611	1,507
11-20..........................	2,722	608	98.7	617	180	357	691	1,119
More than 20...................	3,394	809	100.0	809	154	454	1,078	1,849

Family health care coverage

All members covered, some part year.....	7,968	506	98.8	513	125	306	619	1,252
Some members not covered......	3,804	679	98.4	690	122	358	815	1,616
All members not covered.......	1,980	424	94.4	449	95	230	496	1,086

[1]Average size during period of family's existence rounded to nearest integer; exactly half an integer rounded upward.
[2]There were too few Hispanic families of races other than white for separate tabulation.
[3]Annual rate.
[4]Includes only families with heads 17 years of age and over.
[5]Excludes families with all members under 14 years of age.
[6]Excludes families with all members with health status unknown.

NOTE: Multiple-person families are families with average size 1.5 or greater.

Table 65

Out-of-pocket expenditures for all health care for multiple-person families with members 65 years of age and over, by selected characteristics: United States, 1980

[Rate per family year. Civilian noninstitutionalized population with civilian family head]

Characteristic	All families		Families using health care					
	Number in thousands	Mean expenditures	Percent	Mean expenditures	Expenditures at selected percentiles			
					25th	50th	75th	90th
Total........................	10,809	$685	97.9	$700	$196	$415	$828	$1,560
Family size[1]								
2 persons....................	7,958	609	97.7	623	192	392	711	1,327
3 persons....................	1,339	870	96.8	899	216	617	1,049	2,005
4 persons....................	724	939	100.0	939	216	604	1,494	2,169
5 or more persons............	788	904	100.0	904	285	582	1,110	1,898
Family age								
All members 65 years and over...	4,141	674	98.1	687	203	404	753	1,418
Some members under 65........	6,668	692	97.8	708	194	432	913	1,684
Sex of head								
Male.........................	8,397	732	98.1	746	208	452	914	1,720
Female.......................	2,412	521	97.2	536	138	361	641	1,211
Race and ethnicity[2] of head								
White........................	9,571	699	98.1	712	212	441	867	1,639
Hispanic.....................	*363	*468	*97.2	*482	*136	*258	*567	*1,079
Non-Hispanic.................	9,208	708	98.1	721	216	447	911	1,644
Black........................	1,027	622	95.6	650	50	259	576	1,325
Other........................	*211	*362	*100.0	*362	*80	*323	*482	*1,249
Family structure								
Head and spouse present whole time...	7,593	712	98.4	724	216	471	867	1,639
Child under 17 years........	774	971	100.0	971	259	757	1,223	2,169
No child under 17 years.....	6,819	683	98.2	696	212	452	803	1,441
Head only, no spouse at any time...	2,808	501	96.6	518	128	341	599	1,166
Child under 17 years........	*384	*494	*100.0	*494	*138	*285	*441	*1,521
No child under 17 years.....	2,424	502	96.1	523	102	355	601	1,112
Other........................	*408	*1,438	*97.5	*1,475	*297	*1,142	*2,145	*3,037
Family dynamics								
Unchanging, full year........	9,276	618	97.7	633	186	403	757	1,353
Change in composition or existed less than full year...	1,533	1,087	99.2	1,095	318	604	1,397	2,604

Family poverty status in 1980								
Below 150 percent poverty level	2,169	504	95.1	530	108	323	560	1,160
Below poverty level	964	365	93.2	392	64	267	468	812
Poverty level to 149 percent	1,205	615	96.6	637	202	375	641	1,198
150–199 percent	1,530	754	100.0	754	138	400	790	1,530
200–299 percent	2,785	669	98.7	678	194	424	1,007	1,745
300–499 percent	2,740	729	97.9	745	222	463	849	1,494
500 percent or more	1,585	817	98.4	831	326	524	1,075	1,758
Family income in 1980[3]								
Less than $10,000	3,133	611	96.6	632	135	341	620	1,289
$10,000–$19,999	4,173	643	98.3	654	183	415	753	1,521
$20,000–$34,999	2,427	720	98.0	735	239	479	985	1,778
$35,000 or more	1,076	984	100.0	984	339	666	1,199	1,737
Education of head[4]								
None or elementary school	4,669	607	96.9	627	176	397	722	1,352
Some high school	1,721	712	97.5	730	160	390	786	1,639
High school graduate	2,306	735	98.3	748	261	490	929	1,720
Some college	1,095	776	99.9	777	194	482	1,088	1,590
College graduate or more	1,015	782	100.0	782	273	440	1,007	1,790
Family employment status[5]								
2 or more persons worked full year	979	875	100.0	875	339	690	1,121	1,737
Only 1 person worked full year	2,767	717	97.1	739	200	415	828	1,521
Some part-year work	2,282	569	97.9	581	156	388	716	1,294
No person worked	4,781	683	97.9	697	190	405	802	1,644
Worst perceived health status of any family member[6]								
Excellent	1,429	544	97.4	559	150	325	643	1,256
Good	3,630	610	98.9	617	192	408	781	1,344
Fair	3,110	584	96.9	603	208	398	757	1,372
Poor	2,640	983	98.0	1,004	261	567	1,109	2,021
Most severe limitation in usual activity of any family member								
None	4,190	534	96.9	551	153	354	678	1,249
Some limitation	865	732	98.6	742	256	408	997	1,327
Cannot perform usual activity	5,754	788	98.5	800	224	487	1,000	1,756
Family's bed days[3]								
0	3,349	353	95.0	372	128	282	481	731
1–5	2,100	538	98.4	547	205	388	688	1,203
6–10	1,364	649	99.1	655	250	533	985	1,289
11–20	1,098	775	100.0	775	215	472	1,000	1,704
More than 20	2,897	1,158	99.6	1,163	312	734	1,521	2,455

Table 65—continued

Out-of-pocket expenditures for all health care for multiple-person families with members 65 years of age and over, by selected characteristics: United States, 1980

[Rate per family year. Civilian noninstitutionalized population with civilian family head]

| Characteristic | All families | | Families using health care | | | | | |
| | Number in thousands | Mean expenditures | Percent | Mean expenditures | Expenditures at selected percentiles | | | |
					25th	50th	75th	90th
Family health care coverage								
All members covered full year..........	8,879	$648	98.3	$659	$212	$434	$828	$1,521
Private insurance only...............	*258	*1,192	*95.1	*1,253	*390	*801	*1,560	*2,441
Medicaid only........................	*15	*285	*100.0	*285	*285	*285	*285	*285
Medicare only........................	*574	*457	*95.9	*477	*222	*406	*620	*930
Medicare and other public programs....	*459	*235	*100.0	*235	*5	*108	*224	*699
Medicare and private insurance.......	7,380	676	98.6	685	230	453	877	1,590
Other public and private mixes.......	*91	*503	*88.7	*567	*266	*529	*708	*1,484
Other mixes of public programs.......	–	–	–	–	–	–	–	–
Source unknown....................	*102	*424	*100.0	*424	*6	*329	*920	*1,112
All members covered, some part year.....	701	715	96.2	743	138	344	687	1,491
Some members not covered.............	1,159	915	95.4	959	91	339	997	2,005
All members not covered..............	*71	*1,198	*100.0	*1,198	*96	*138	*519	*7,860

[1]Average size during period of family's existence rounded to nearest integer; exactly half an integer rounded upward.
[2]There were too few Hispanic families of races other than white for separate tabulation.
[3]Annual rate.
[4]Includes only families with heads 17 years of age and over.
[5]Excludes families with all members under 14 years of age.
[6]Excludes families with all members with health status unknown.

NOTE: Multiple-person families are families with average size 1.5 or greater.

Table 66

Out-of-pocket expenditures for all health care for 1-person families, by selected characteristics: United States, 1980

[Rate per family year. Civilian noninstitutionalized population with civilian family head]

Characteristic	All families		Families using health care					
	Number in thousands	Mean expenditures	Percent	Mean expenditures	Expenditures at selected percentiles			
					25th	50th	75th	90th
Total..........................	26,233	$287	90.4	$317	$43	$131	$313	$665
Sex								
Male...........................	11,866	200	85.0	236	26	82	197	492
Female.........................	14,367	358	94.9	377	71	181	383	750
Race and ethnicity[1]								
White..........................	22,811	280	90.9	308	46	136	327	665
Hispanic.......................	818	*313	84.2	*372	*25	*65	*224	*598
Non-Hispanic...................	21,993	279	91.2	306	47	139	329	665
Black..........................	2,711	307	87.2	352	25	120	254	510
Other..........................	*712	*424	*87.3	*486	*40	*89	*181	*762
Family dynamics								
Unchanging, full year..........	22,570	268	91.9	291	45	134	307	644
Change in composition or existed less than full year..........	3,662	402	81.0	496	31	108	349	846
Poverty status in 1980								
Below 150 percent poverty level......	9,379	303	90.0	337	29	120	284	675
Below poverty level............	5,252	248	88.6	280	18	91	234	528
Poverty level to 149 percent...	4,128	374	91.9	407	47	167	346	729
150-199 percent................	2,974	259	88.0	294	45	118	286	556
200-299 percent................	5,563	329	87.8	375	61	147	349	794
300-499 percent................	5,426	235	93.9	250	48	126	291	579
500 percent or more............	2,891	277	92.7	298	47	154	368	720
Family income in 1980[2]								
Less than $10,000..............	14,468	313	89.4	350	40	127	298	692
$10,000-$19,999................	8,280	256	91.3	280	50	135	333	613
$20,000-$34,999................	2,664	226	91.2	247	43	139	296	556
$35,000 or more................	820	333	96.8	344	17	151	508	778
Education[3]								
None or elementary school......	4,782	279	89.0	314	29	121	326	690
Some high school...............	3,996	337	83.7	402	47	122	248	716
High school graduate...........	7,413	280	92.3	303	44	130	302	528
Some college...................	4,842	237	92.1	258	42	130	339	672
College graduate or more.......	5,122	314	92.8	338	48	152	367	723

205

Table 66--continued

Out-of-pocket expenditures for all health care for 1-person families, by selected characteristics: United States, 1980

[Rate per family year. Civilian noninstitutionalized population with civilian family head]

Characteristic	All families		Families using health care					
	Number in thousands	Mean expenditures	Percent	Mean expenditures	Expenditures at selected percentiles			
					25th	50th	75th	90th
Employment status[4]								
Worked full year	10,374	$193	89.9	$215	$43	$122	$254	$500
Worked part year	7,129	364	87.9	414	40	123	303	735
Never worked	8,703	335	93.2	360	47	156	377	846
Perceived health status[5]								
Excellent	11,226	214	89.0	240	40	107	244	471
Good	9,642	330	89.3	370	47	143	355	716
Fair	3,691	328	94.5	347	65	161	353	750
Poor	1,568	437	97.6	448	32	135	464	1,005
Limitation in usual activity								
None	21,977	241	89.7	268	43	126	282	598
Some limitation	731	445	92.1	483	70	248	510	1,383
Cannot perform usual activity	3,525	539	94.4	571	42	157	437	1,109
Bed days[2]								
0	12,629	175	85.7	204	35	110	250	470
1-5	6,587	187	91.4	205	43	126	249	460
6-10	2,671	362	97.8	370	66	165	439	839
11-20	1,924	632	99.0	638	70	192	485	1,394
More than 20	2,422	783	97.8	801	42	281	757	1,986
Family health care coverage								
All members covered full year	20,491	277	92.0	301	46	142	329	662
Private insurance only	10,523	220	90.8	243	46	128	266	538
Medicaid only	*317	*23	*86.6	*26	*0	*7	*30	*86
Medicare only	1,262	409	80.5	508	79	215	460	1,472
Medicare and other public programs	993	176	95.9	184	1	35	174	492
Medicare and private insurance	4,819	412	96.1	428	104	237	452	867
Other public and private mixes	1,361	323	92.1	350	40	154	387	723
Other mixes of public programs	*186	*214	*91.6	*233	*24	*68	*355	*447
Source unknown	1,030	185	97.5	189	7	80	239	417

All members covered, some part year.....	3,223	219	87.8	249	31	89	190	630
Some members not covered...............	*24	*3,736	*100.0	*3,736	*856	*856	*7,243	*7,243
All members not covered................	2,495	*422	80.3	*526	44	105	286	692

[1]There were too few Hispanic families of races other than white for separate tabulation.
[2]Annual rate.
[3]Includes only families with heads 17 years of age and over.
[4]Excludes families with all members under 14 years of age.
[5]Excludes families with all members with health status unknown.

NOTE: 1-person families are families with average size less than 1.5. For 1-person families with more than 1 distinct individual, characteristics are those of head or of family as in Table 1.

Table 67

Out-of-pocket expenditures for all health care for 1-person families under 65 years of age, by selected characteristics: United States, 1980

[Rate per family year. Civilian noninstitutionalized population with civilian family head]

Characteristic	All families		Families using health care					
	Number in thousands	Mean expenditures	Percent	Mean expenditures	Expenditures at selected percentiles			
					25th	50th	75th	90th
Total.................	18,519	$250	89.2	$280	$39	$112	$264	$576
Age								
Under 25 years.................	5,208	195	87.8	222	37	97	238	447
25–44 years.................	7,630	272	89.7	303	36	101	250	558
45–64 years.................	5,680	272	90.0	302	45	135	333	723
Sex								
Male.................	10,082	178	84.5	211	25	75	170	413
Female.................	8,437	336	94.9	354	65	160	360	715
Race and ethnicity[1]								
White.................	15,786	228	89.8	254	40	112	264	556
Hispanic.................	680	*360	82.8	*435	*25	*70	*224	*960
Non-Hispanic.................	15,106	222	90.1	247	41	114	264	532
Black.................	2,128	*354	86.5	*409	32	121	270	787
Other.................	*605	*457	*85.0	*538	*40	*89	*180	*762
Family dynamics								
Unchanging, full year.................	15,487	244	91.5	267	40	117	260	538
Change in composition or existed less than full year.................	3,032	280	77.5	362	27	90	270	682
Poverty status in 1980								
Below 150 percent.................	5,181	304	86.7	350	25	91	242	641
Below poverty level.................	3,031	261	84.8	308	14	78	224	528
Poverty level to 149 percent.................	2,149	*364	89.5	*407	44	120	270	669
150-199 percent.................	1,855	*206	84.1	*245	41	85	197	386
200-299 percent.................	4,250	248	87.5	284	48	121	313	641
300-499 percent.................	4,643	206	93.6	220	42	107	265	490
500 percent or more.................	2,590	256	92.9	276	43	151	331	712
Family income in 1980[2]								
Less than $10,000.................	8,222	297	86.8	342	30	102	246	641
$10,000-$19,999.................	7,113	204	90.5	225	46	119	282	527
$20,000-$34,999.................	2,529	218	91.7	237	42	134	292	524
$35,000 or more.................	*656	*286	*96.0	*299	*7	*103	*329	*712

Education[3]

None or elementary school	1,770	153	82.3	186	14	80	184	532
Some high school	2,546	*388	81.0	*479	44	103	197	661
High school graduate	5,759	219	91.4	240	41	107	260	467
Some college	4,037	215	91.9	234	41	119	294	647
College graduate or more	4,329	286	91.8	311	39	134	286	666

Employment status[4]

Worked full year	9,963	194	89.9	216	43	121	252	500
Worked part year	6,265	336	87.8	383	39	115	284	707
Never worked	2,264	264	90.7	291	20	86	223	669

Perceived health status[5]

Excellent	8,913	197	88.2	223	34	94	229	464
Good	6,852	299	88.5	338	42	126	327	682
Fair	1,866	250	92.8	269	45	135	266	483
Poor	803	424	98.3	432	23	80	407	1,005

Limitation in usual activity

None	16,928	227	89.0	255	40	116	259	532
Some limitation	*209	*508	*90.2	*564	*33	*292	*510	*2,662
Cannot perform usual activity	1,383	*488	91.6	*533	24	86	290	1,005

Bed days[2]

0	8,291	153	83.6	183	29	88	218	435
1-5	5,721	172	90.6	190	40	108	231	429
6-10	2,013	365	98.2	371	72	159	393	813
11-20	1,222	*616	98.5	*626	71	151	291	970
More than 20	1,273	701	96.9	724	29	245	707	2,004

Family health care coverage

All members covered full year	12,974	225	91.2	247	40	119	266	558
Private insurance only	10,511	220	90.8	242	46	128	265	538
Medicaid only	*317	*23	*86.6	*26	*0	*7	*30	*86
Medicare only	*108	*394	*84.3	*468	*95	*97	*847	*1,986
Medicare and other public programs	–	–	–	–	–	–	–	–
Medicare and private insurance								
Other public and private mixes	1,361	323	92.1	350	40	154	387	723
Other mixes of public programs	*186	*214	*91.6	*233	*24	*68	*355	*447
Source unknown	*491	*164	*100.0	*164	*0	*29	*103	*245
All members covered, some part year	3,223	219	87.8	249	31	89	190	630
Some members not covered	–	–	–	–	–	–	–	–
All members not covered	2,322	*433	80.4	*539	44	104	284	692

[1]There were too few Hispanic of races other than white families for separate tabulation.
[2]Annual rate.
[3]Includes only families with heads 17 years of age and over.
[4]Excludes families with all members under 14 years of age.
[5]Excludes families with all members with health status unknown.

NOTE: 1-person families are families with average size less than 1.5. For 1-person families with more than 1 distinct individual, characteristics are those of head or of family as in Table 2.

Table 68

Out-of-pocket expenditures for all health care for 1-person families under 65 years of age with health care coverage all year, by selected characteristics: United States, 1980

[Rate per family year. Civilian noninstitutionalized population with civilian family head]

| Characteristic | All families | | Families using health care | | | | | |
| | Number in thousands | Mean expenditures | Percent | Mean expenditures | Expenditures at selected percentiles | | | |
					25th	50th	75th	90th
Total....................	12,974	$225	91.2	$247	$40	$119	$266	$558
Age								
Under 25 years..........	3,166	162	90.0	180	37	102	245	442
25-44 years.............	5,206	222	91.4	243	37	103	242	471
45-64 years.............	4,601	272	91.7	296	46	141	355	723
Sex								
Male....................	6,807	180	87.5	205	25	83	183	442
Female..................	6,167	275	95.2	289	71	170	359	645
Race and ethnicity[1]								
White...................	11,183	211	91.6	230	41	121	275	556
Hispanic................	*400	*122	*84.5	*145	*29	*80	*199	*387
Non-Hispanic............	10,782	214	91.9	233	41	123	275	556
Black...................	1,428	235	88.8	265	25	119	238	787
Other...................	*363	*613	*85.6	*716	*35	*71	*180	*762
Family dynamics								
Unchanging, full year...	11,017	235	93.6	251	41	123	270	538
Change in composition or existed less than full year...	1,957	169	77.3	218	23	86	240	639
Poverty status in 1980								
Below 150 percent.......	2,775	217	89.4	243	14	86	238	528
Below poverty level.....	1,638	231	87.9	263	7	80	187	528
Poverty level to 149 percent....	1,137	197	91.5	215	32	97	254	641
150-199 percent.........	1,072	148	85.4	173	41	85	214	375
200-299 percent.........	2,997	272	90.4	301	55	127	337	641
300-499 percent.........	3,918	194	93.9	207	42	116	265	482
500 percent or more.....	2,212	263	92.4	285	43	154	329	712
Family income in 1980[2]								
Less than $10,000.......	4,620	237	88.6	268	27	102	245	500
$10,000-$19,999.........	5,656	207	92.9	223	49	121	289	527
$20,000-$34,999.........	2,114	224	90.8	247	43	154	292	556
$35,000 or more.........	*584	*303	*95.5	*317	*7	*112	*329	*746

210

	C1	C2	C3	C4	C5	C6	C7	C8
Education[3]								
None or elementary school	1,328	175	87.3	200	11	85	192	626
Some high school	1,538	238	86.4	276	33	103	206	429
High school graduate	4,047	186	92.7	201	41	116	289	467
Some college	2,830	214	91.9	233	43	134	295	598
College graduate or more	3,201	299	92.7	322	40	137	285	666
Employment status[4]								
Worked full year	7,649	191	91.8	209	50	128	249	482
Worked part year	3,554	271	89.5	303	29	103	335	720
Never worked	1,769	277	91.9	301	14	99	223	727
Perceived health status[5]								
Excellent	6,353	171	90.7	189	39	105	233	463
Good	4,537	271	90.4	299	43	134	328	645
Fair	1,425	190	92.2	207	44	126	248	447
Poor	*572	*542	*100.0	*542	*20	*121	*669	*1,411
Limitation in usual activity								
None	11,652	214	91.1	235	41	121	264	528
Some limitation	*127	*264	*96.5	*274	*70	*292	*442	*510
Cannot perform usual activity	1,195	329	91.4	*360	24	97	333	1,005
Bed days[2]								
0	5,669	168	86.4	195	29	95	245	451
1-5	4,146	169	91.6	184	43	117	233	436
6-10	1,247	285	99.1	288	85	159	359	727
11-20	984	*425	98.4	*432	71	151	282	746
More than 20	928	528	99.6	530	25	296	626	1,554
Family health care coverage								
Private insurance only	10,511	220	90.8	242	46	128	265	538
Medicaid only	*317	*23	*86.6	*26	*0	*7	*30	*86
Medicare only	*108	*394	*84.3	*468	*95	*97	*847	*1,986
Medicare and other public programs	-	-	-	-	-	-	-	-
Medicare and private insurance	-	-	-	-	-	-	-	-
Other public and private mixes	1,361	323	92.1	350	40	154	387	723
Other mixes of public programs	*186	*214	*91.6	*233	*24	*68	*355	*447
Source unknown	491	*164	*100.0	*164	*0	*29	*103	*245

[1]There were too few Hispanic families of races other than white for separate tabulation.
[2]Annual rate.
[3]Includes only families with heads 17 years of age and over.
[4]Excludes families with all members under 14 years of age.
[5]Excludes families with all members with health status unknown.

NOTE: 1-person families are families with average size less than 1.5. For 1-person families with more than 1 distinct individual, characteristics are those of head or of family as in Table 2.

Table 69

Out-of-pocket expenditures for all health care for 1-person families under 65 years of age without health care coverage all year, by selected characteristics: United States, 1980

[Rate per family year. Civilian noninstitutionalized population with civilian family head]

Characteristic	All families		Families using health care					
	Number in thousands	Mean expenditures	Percent	Mean expenditures	Expenditures at selected percentiles			
					25th	50th	75th	90th
Total........................	5,545	$309	84.7	$364	$37	$94	$245	$661
Age								
Under 25 years................	2,042	246	84.3	291	40	89	203	509
25-44 years..................	2,424	*379	86.0	*440	32	95	257	704
45-64 years..................	1,079	271	82.6	328	45	104	284	532
Sex								
Male.........................	3,275	176	78.3	224	22	64	147	363
Female.......................	2,270	501	94.0	532	62	143	377	976
Race and ethnicity[1]								
White........................	4,603	270	85.3	316	35	86	229	630
Hispanic.....................	*280	*701	*80.3	*873	*8	*70	*960	*1,884
Non-Hispanic.................	4,323	242	85.6	282	37	89	215	487
Black........................	*700	*595	*81.6	*729	*37	*123	*291	*1,051
Other........................	*242	*224	*84.1	*266	*78	*94	*275	*1,019
Family dynamics								
Unchanging, full year........	4,470	267	86.4	309	37	93	215	532
Change in composition or existed less than full year.......	1,075	*484	77.9	*621	39	106	339	1,107
Poverty status in 1980								
Below 150 percent............	2,405	*404	83.7	*483	37	104	257	692
Below poverty level........	1,394	*296	81.1	*365	15	72	224	509
Poverty level to 149 percent..	1,012	*552	87.1	*633	50	132	345	707
150-199 percent..............	784	*286	82.3	*348	*42	*83	*197	*487
200-299 percent..............	1,253	192	80.6	238	32	108	190	665
300-499 percent..............	*725	*267	92.2	*290	*45	*94	*291	*704
500 percent or more..........	*379	*216	95.9	*226	*41	*88	*397	*715
Family income in 1980[2]								
Less than $10,000............	3,602	374	84.6	442	40	104	257	692
$10,000-$19,999..............	1,457	191	81.1	235	37	95	230	439
$20,000-$34,999..............	415	*184	96.2	*192	*28	*82	*180	*408
$35,000 or more..............	*71	*151	*100.0	*151	*0	*5	*464	*464

212

Education[3]								
None or elementary school	*443	*87	*67.1	*129	*45	*62	*184	'*418
Some high school	1,008	*616	72.9	*845	*45	*89	*197	*1,107
High school graduate	1,713	297	88.5	335	41	95	236	397
Some college	1,208	215	91.8	235	28	73	294	707
College graduate or more	1,127	248	89.0	278	36	126	286	509
Employment status[4]								
Worked full year	2,314	201	83.7	240	30	86	257	630
Worked part year	2,711	420	85.5	492	45	117	229	707
Never worked	*495	*216	*86.4	*249	*20	*72	*256	*532
Perceived health status[5]								
Excellent	2,559	*260	82.2	316	29	78	165	464
Good	2,314	*354	84.7	*419	42	117	294	707
Fair	*441	*443	*94.8	*467	*65	*150	*351	*1,394
Poor	*231	*133	*94.0	*142	*45	*73	*224	*377
Limitation in usual activity								
None	5,276	257	84.5	304	39	96	256	630
Some limitation	*82	*889	*80.3	*1,106	*0	*1,107	*2,662	*2,662
Cannot perform usual activity	*188	*1,500	*92.7	*1,618	*15	*64	*80	*224
Bed days[2]								
0	2,622	119	77.4	153	27	73	145	377
1-5	1,575	180	87.9	205	39	102	215	397
6-10	766	*494	96.9	*510	*51	*164	*439	*1,019
11-20	*237	*1,411	98.7	*1,429	*44	*168	*485	*1,418
More than 20	*345	*1,168	*89.5	*1,306	*58	*150	*1,164	*2,577
Family health care coverage								
All members covered, some part year	3,223	219	87.8	249	31	89	190	630
Some members not covered	–	–	–	–	–	–	–	–
All members not covered	2,322	*433	80.4	*539	44	104	284	692

[1] There were too few Hispanic families of races other than white for separate tabulation.
[2] Annual rate.
[3] Includes only families with heads 17 years of age and over.
[4] Excludes families with all members under 14 years of age.
[5] Excludes families with all members with health status unknown.

NOTE: 1-person families are families with average size less than 1.5. For 1-person families with more than 1 distinct individual, characteristics are those of head or of family as in Table 2.

Table 70

Out-of-pocket expenditures for all health care for 1-person families 65 years of age and over, by selected characteristics: United States, 1980

[Rate per family year. Civilian noninstitutionalized population with civilian family head]

Characteristic	All families		Families using health care					
					Expenditures at selected percentiles			
	Number in thousands	Mean expenditures	Percent	Mean expenditures	25th	50th	75th	90th
Total........................	7,714	$374	93.3	$401	$68	$206	$407	$848
Sex								
Male.........................	1,784	325	88.1	369	34	153	346	1,156
Female.......................	5,930	389	94.8	410	75	219	410	844
Race and ethnicity[1]								
White........................	7,025	396	93.4	424	76	219	430	956
Hispanic.....................	*138	*81	*91.5	*89	*25	*49	*225	*239
Non-Hispanic.................	6,887	403	93.5	431	81	221	438	966
Black........................	582	134	89.8	149	*14	*101	*209	*411
Other........................	*106	*234	*100.0	*234	*26	*60	*181	*1,156
Family dynamics								
Unchanging, full year........	7,083	320	92.8	344	68	192	382	794
Change in composition or existed less than full year........	630	987	97.9	1,009	42	267	666	2,166
Poverty status in 1980								
Below 150 percent poverty level.........	4,199	303	94.1	322	47	165	339	690
Below poverty level..........	2,220	230	93.8	246	31	113	254	516
Poverty level to 149 percent...........	1,979	384	94.5	407	68	225	430	867
150-199 percent..............	1,118	345	94.5	365	75	221	438	718
200-299 percent..............	1,313	590	88.6	665	129	249	481	1,673
300-499 percent..............	783	408	95.4	427	101	267	563	856
500 percent or more..........	*300	*452	*91.7	*493	*133	*379	*666	*1,377
Family income in 1980[2]								
Less than $10,000............	6,246	333	92.8	359	60	180	367	794
$10,000-$19,999..............	1,167	*572	95.9	*597	132	269	511	1,073
$20,000-$34,999..............	*136	*372	*81.6	*456	*64	*265	*531	*1,383
$35,000 or more..............	*165	*517	*100.0	*517	*166	*508	*666	*1,262

Education

None or elementary school	3,012	354	93.0	380	46	154	359	794
Some high school	1,451	247	88.5	279	62	165	303	716
High school graduate	1,653	491	95.5	514	82	222	434	887
Some college	804	351	93.3	376	86	246	513	808
College graduate or more	793	467	98.3	475	166	346	599	1,193

Employment status

Worked full year	*411	*183	*89.6	*204	*63	*173	*265	*467
Worked part year	863	*568	89.1	*638	82	222	359	1,073
Never worked	6,439	360	94.1	383	65	208	417	856

Perceived health status[3]

Excellent	2,313	281	92.0	306	65	177	325	685
Good	2,790	407	91.2	446	60	206	430	856
Fair	1,825	408	96.3	423	81	224	475	1,023
Poor	765	451	97.0	465	62	249	476	1,033

Limitation in usual activity

None	5,049	286	92.0	310	63	179	346	685
Some limitation	*523	*420	*92.9	*452	*108	*248	*515	*1,383
Cannot perform usual activity	2,142	572	96.2	594	73	241	517	1,189

Bed days[2]

0	4,338	217	89.6	242	65	161	307	513
1-5	867	286	96.3	297	101	222	346	637
6-10	658	353	96.5	365	45	207	492	856
11-20	702	659	100.0	659	65	335	760	1,730
More than 20	1,149	874	98.8	885	73	293	848	1,859

Family health care coverage

All members covered full year	7,517	366	93.6	391	66	206	404	844
Private insurance only	*13	*666	*100.0	*666	*666	*666	*666	*666
Medicaid only	—	—	—	—	—	—	—	—
Medicare only	1,154	410	80.2	512	75	221	460	1,472
Medicare and other public programs	993	176	95.9	184	1	174	174	492
Medicare and private insurance	4,819	412	96.1	428	104	237	452	867
Other public and private mixes	—	—	—	—	—	—	—	—
Other mixes of public programs	—	—	—	—	—	—	—	—
Source unknown	*538	*204	*95.3	*214	*30	*131	*329	*417
All members covered, some part year	—	—	—	—	—	—	—	—
Some members not covered	*24	*3,736	*100.0	*3,736	*856	*856	*7,243	*7,243
All members not covered	*172	*272	*78.7	*346	*54	*105	*489	*1,212

[1]There were too few Hispanic families of races other than white for separate tabulation.
[2]Annual rate.
[3]Excludes families with all members with health status unknown.

NOTE: 1-person families are families with average size less than 1.5. For 1-person families with more than 1 distinct individual, characteristics are those of head or of family as in Table 5.

Appendixes

Contents

List of Appendix Tables

Appendix I.
Technical Notes on Methods

Survey Background

The National Medical Care Utilization and Expenditure Survey (NMCUES) was a panel survey designed to collect data about the U.S. civilian noninstitutionalized population in 1980. During the course of the survey, information was obtained on health, access to and use of medical services, associated charges and sources of payment, and health insurance coverage. Information was collected in such a way that data can be provided at the family level as well as for individuals. The survey contained both a household sample and a Medicaid case sample. This report is based on the household sample. NMCUES was cosponsored by the National Center for Health Statistics and the Health Care Financing Administration. Data collection was provided under contract by the Research Triangle Institute and its subcontractors, National Opinion Research Center and SysteMetrics, Inc.

The basic survey plan for NMCUES drew heavily on two surveys, the National Health Interview Survey (NHIS), conducted annually by the National Center for Health Statistics, and the National Medical Care Expenditure Survey (NMCES), cosponsored by the National Center for Health Services Research and the National Center for Health Statistics.

NHIS is a continuing, multipurpose, cross-sectional survey first conducted in 1957. The main purpose of NHIS is to collect information on illness, disability, and the use of medical care. Although some information on medical expenditures and insurance payments has been collected in NHIS, the cross-sectional nature of the survey design is not well suited for providing annual data on expenditures and payments.

NMCES was a panel survey in which a sample of households was interviewed six times over an 18-month period in 1977 and 1978. NMCES was specifically designed to provide comprehensive data on how health services were used and paid for in the United States in 1977.

NMCUES is similar to NMCES in survey design and questionnaire wording, so analysis of some of the changes during the period 1977–80 is possible. Both NMCUES and NMCES used question wording that was similar to NHIS in areas common to the three surveys. Together, NMCES and NMCUES provide extensive information on illness, disability, use of medical care, costs of medical care, sources of payment for medical care, and health insurance coverage at two points in time.

Sample Design

The NMCUES sample of housing units and group quarters, hereafter jointly referred to as dwelling units, is a concatenation of two independently selected national samples, one provided by the Research Triangle Institute and the other by the National Opinion Research Center. The sample designs used by these two organizations are similar with respect to principal design features; both can be characterized as stratified, four-stage area probability designs. The principal differences between the two designs are the type of stratification variables and the specific definitions of sampling units at each stage. The salient design features of the two sample surveys are summarized in the following sections.

The target population for NMCUES consisted of all persons who were members of the U.S. civilian noninstitutionalized population at any time from January 1, 1980, through December 31, 1980. All persons living in a sample dwelling unit at the time of the first interview contact became part of the national sample. Unmarried students 17–22 years of age who lived away from home were included in the sample when a parent or guardian was included in the sample. In addition, persons who died or were institutionalized between January 1 and the date of the first interview were included in the sample if they were related to persons living in the sampled dwelling units. All of these persons were considered "key" persons, and data were collected for them for the full 12 months of 1980 or for the proportion of time that they were part of the U.S. civilian noninstitutionalized population. In addition, babies born to key persons were considered key persons, and data were collected for them from the time of birth. Relatives from outside the original population (that is, institutionalized, in the Armed Forces, or outside the United States between January 1 and the first interview) who moved in with key persons after the first interview were also considered key persons, and data were collected for them from the time they joined the key person. Relatives who moved in with key persons after the first interview but were part of the civilian noninstitutionalized population on January 1, 1980, were classified as "nonkey" persons. Data were collected for nonkey persons for the time that they lived with a key person but, because they had a chance of selection in the initial sample, their data are not used for general person-level analysis. However, data for nonkey persons are used in family analysis because nonkey persons contributed to the family's utilization of and expenditures for health care during the time they were part of the family.

Persons included in the sample were grouped into "reporting units" for data collection purposes. Reporting units were defined as all persons related to each other by blood, marriage, adoption, or foster care status and living in the same dwelling unit. The combined NMCUES sample consisted of 7,244 eligible reporting units, of which 6,599 agreed to participate in the survey. In total, data were obtained on 17,123 key persons. The Research Triangle Institute sample yielded 8,326 key persons, and the National Opinion Research Center sample yielded 8,797.

Research Triangle Institute Sample Design

A primary sampling unit (PSU) is defined as a county, a group of contiguous counties, or parts of counties with a combined minimum 1970 population size of 20,000. A total of 1,686 disjoint PSU's exhaust the land area of the 50 States and Washington, D.C. The PSU's are classified as one of two types. The 16 largest standard metropolitan statistical areas (SMSA's) are designated as self-representing PSU's, and the remaining 1,670 PSU's in the primary sampling frame are designated as non-self-representing PSU's.

PSU's are grouped into strata whose members tend to be relatively alike within strata and relatively unlike between strata. PSU's derived from the 16 largest SMSA's had sufficient population in 1970 to be treated as primary strata. The 1,659 non-self-representing PSU's from the continental United States were stratified into 59 primary strata with approximately equal populations. Each of these primary strata had a 1970 population of about 3⅓ million. One supplementary primary stratum of 11 PSU's, with a 1970 population of about 1 million, was added to the Research Triangle Institute primary frame to include Alaska and Hawaii.

The total first-stage sample for Research Triangle Institute consisted of 59 PSU's, of which 16 were self-representing PSU's. The non-self-representing PSU's were obtained by selecting one PSU from each of the 43 non-self-representing primary strata. These PSU's were selected with probability proportional to 1970 population size.

In each of the 59 sample PSU's, the entire PSU was divided into smaller disjoint area units called secondary sampling units (SSU's). Each SSU consisted of one or more enumeration districts or block groups defined by the 1970 census. Within each PSU, SSU's were ordered and then partitioned to form secondary strata of approximately equal size. Two secondary strata were formed in the non-self-representing PSU drawn from Alaska and Hawaii, and four secondary strata were formed in each of the remaining 42 non-self-representing PSU's. Thus, the non-self-representing PSU's were partitioned into a total of 170 secondary strata. In a similar manner, the 16 self-representing PSU's were partitioned into 144 secondary strata.

In the second stage of selection, one SSU was selected from each of the 144 secondary strata covering the self-representing PSU's, and two SSU's were selected from each of the remaining secondary strata. All second-stage sampling was with replacement and with probability proportional to the SSU's total noninstitutionalized population. The total number of sample SSU's was $2 \times 170 + 144 = 484$.

For the third stage of selection, each SSU was first divided into smaller disjoint geographic areas, and one area within the SSU was selected with probability proportional to the total number of housing units in 1970. Next, one or more disjoint segments of at least 60 housing units were formed in the selected area. One segment was selected from each SSU with probability proportional to the segment housing unit count. In response to the sponsoring agencies' request that the expected household sample size be reduced, a systematic sample of one-sixth of the segments was deleted from the sample. Thus, the total third-stage sample was reduced to 404 segments.

For the fourth stage of selection, all of the dwelling units within the segment were listed, and a systematic sample of dwelling units was selected. The procedures used to determine the sampling rate for segments guaranteed that all dwelling units had an approximately equal overall probability of selection. All of the reporting units within the selected dwelling units were included in the sample.

National Opinion Research Center Sample Design

The land area of the 50 States and Washington, D.C., was also divided into disjoint PSU's for the National Opinion Research Center sample design. A PSU consisted of SMSA's, parts of SMSA's, counties, parts of counties, or independent cities. Grouping of counties into a single PSU occurred when individual counties had a 1970 population of less than 10,000. The PSU's were classified into two groups according to metropolitan status—SMSA or not SMSA. These two groups were individually ordered and then partitioned into zones with a 1970 census population size of approximately 1 million.

A single PSU was selected within each zone with a probability proportional to its 1970 population. It should be noted that this procedure allowed a PSU to be selected more than one time. For instance, an SMSA primary sampling unit with a population of 3 million could be selected as many as four times. The full general-purpose sample contained 204 PSU's. These 204 PSU's were systematically allocated to four subsamples of 51 PSU's. The final set of 76 sample PSU's was chosen by randomly selecting two complete subsamples of 51 PSU's. One subsample was included in its entirety, and 25 of the PSU's in the other subsample were selected systematically for inclusion in NMCUES.

For the second stage, each PSU selected in the first stage was partitioned into a disjoint set of SSU's defined by block groups, enumeration districts, or a combination of the two types of census units. Within each sample PSU, the SSU's were ordered and then partitioned into 18 zones such that each zone contained approximately the same number of households. One SSU had the opportunity to be selected more than once, as was the case in the PSU selection. If a PSU had been hit more than once in the first stage, the second-stage selection process was repeated as many times as there were first-stage hits. The 405 SSU's were identified by selecting 5 SSU's from each of the 51 PSU's in the subsample that was included in its entirety and 6 SSU's from each of the 25 PSU's in the group for which only one-half of the PSU's were included.

The SSU's selected in the second stage were then subdivided into area segments with a minimum size of 100 housing units each. One segment was then selected with probability proportional to the estimated number of housing units. The final-stage sample, in which a selection of housing units was made, was essentially the same as that used by the Research Triangle Institute.

Collection of Data

Field operations for NMCUES were performed by the Research Triangle Institute and the National Opinion Research Center under specifications established by the sponsoring agencies. Persons in the sample dwelling units were interviewed at approximately 3-month intervals beginning in February 1980 and ending in March 1981. The core questionnaire was administered during each of the five rounds of interviews to collect data on health, health care, health care charges, sources of payment, and health insurance coverage. A summary of responses was used to update information reported in previous rounds. Supplements to the core questionnaire were used during the first, third, and fifth rounds of interviews to collect data that were not expected to change during the year or that were needed only once. Approximately 80 percent of the third and fourth rounds of interviews were conducted by telephone; all remaining interviews were conducted in person. The respondent for the interview was required to be a household member 17 years of age or older. A proxy respondent not residing in the household was permitted only if all eligible household members were unable to respond because of health, language, or mental condition.

Imputation

Nonresponse in panel surveys such as NMCUES occurs when sample individuals refuse to participate in the survey (total nonresponse), when initially participating individuals drop out of the survey (attrition nonresponse), or when data for specific items on the questionnaire are not collected (item nonresponse). In general, response rates for NMCUES were excellent. Approximately 90 percent of the sample reporting units agreed to participate in the survey, and approximately 94 percent of the individuals in the participating reporting units supplied complete annual information. Even though the overall response rates are quite high for NMCUES, the estimates of means and proportions may be biased if nonrespondents have different health care experiences than respondents or if there is a substantial response rate differential across subgroups of the target population. Furthermore, totals will tend to be underestimated unless allowance is made for the loss of data because of nonresponse.

Two methods commonly used to compensate for survey nonresponse are data imputation and the adjustment of sampling weights. For NMCUES, imputation was used to compensate for attrition and item nonresponse, and weight adjustment was used to compensate for total nonresponse. The calculation of the weight adjustment factors is discussed in the section on sampling weights.

A specialized form of the sequential hot-deck imputation method was used for attrition imputation. First, each sample person with incomplete annual data (recipient) was linked to a sample person with similar demographic and socioeconomic characteristics who had complete annual data (donor). Second, the time periods for which the recipient had missing data were divided into two categories, imputed eligible days and imputed ineligible days. Imputed eligible days were those days for which the donor was eligible (that is, in scope), and imputed ineligible days were those days for which the donor was ineligible (that is, out of scope). For the recipient's imputed eligible days, the donor's medical care experiences (such as medical provider visits, dental visits, or hospital stays) were imputed into the recipient's record. Finally, the results of the attrition imputation were used to make the final determination of a person's respondent status. If more than two-thirds of the person's total eligible days (both reported and imputed) were imputed, then the person was considered to be a total nonrespondent, and all data for the person were removed from the analytic data file.

The data collection methodology and field quality control procedures for NMCUES were designed so that the data would be as accurate and complete as possible subject to budget considerations. However, individuals cannot report data that are unknown to them, or they may choose not to report the data even if known. This latter situation is especially true for data relating to expenditures, income, and other sensitive topics. Because of the size and complexity of the NMCUES data base, it was not feasible, from the standpoint of cost, to replace all missing data for all data items. The 12-month data files, for example, contain approximately 1,400 data items per person. With this in mind, the NMCUES approach was to designate a subset of the total items on the data base for imputation of the missing data. Thus, for 5 percent of the NMCUES data items, the responses were edited and missing data imputed by a combination of logic and hot-deck procedures to produce revised variables for use in analysis. Items for which imputations were made cover the following data areas.

- Visit charges.
- Source of payment codes and amounts.
- Annual disability days.
- Health insurance premium amount.
- Length of hospital stay.
- Total weeks worked in 1980.
- Average hours worked per week.
- Educational level.
- Hispanic ethnicity.
- Income.
- Age and birth date.
- Race.
- Sex.
- Health insurance coverage.
- Visit dates.

These items were selected as the most important variables for statistical analyses.

Construction of Longitudinal Families

At the time of the initial interview, a group of persons sharing a common housing unit was designated a family if they were related to each other by blood, marriage, adoption, or a formal foster care relationship. An unmarried student 17–22 years of age living away from home was also considered a part of the family, even though his or her residence was in a different location. When, on subsequent interviews, this initial sampled social unit was found to have had changes in membership, it became necessary to find a decision rule (or set of decision rules) for deciding when a family continued, when it ended, and when a new family began.

The decision rule chosen was initially referred to as a principal-predecessor-principal-successor rule (Dicker and Casady, 1982; Whitmore, Cox, and Folsom, 1982; Moser et al., 1983). The term came from the understanding that, at any given point in time, a family may have several predecessor families from which its members came and several successor families into which its members would go. The decisionmaking problem, therefore, was to objectively select only one predecessor family (the principal predecessor) and only one successor family (the principal successor) as representing the family through successive stages in time. If no principal successor family could be found, the initial family had ended. If no principal predecessor family could be found, the current family (at the time of the interview) was a new family. Later discussions in the literature referred to the above rule under a different name. It came to be called a "reciprocal, majority population rule" (McMillen, 1984; Dicker, 1984) because the principal-predecessor-principal-successor rule came to be understood as a rule that linked families on the basis of cross-family majorities. Thus, if two families (as defined above) exist at different but adjacent points in time, they are the same family if and only if a majority of the eligible members of the first family are found in the second family and a majority of the eligible members of the second family are also found in the first family. The reciprocity of the comparison is crucial. A unidirectional majority—either from the first family to the second family or from the second to the first—is not sufficient for the two families to be defined as the same.

Several aspects of the rule as applied in this survey need further elaboration. First, the rule was applied to all families in the longitudinal universe (not only to those in the initial sample) that had cross-membership connections with initially sampled families. Second, only persons eligible over time to be in both families being compared were counted when calculating cross-family majorities. For example, persons in family 1 who died or otherwise left the universe were not eligible for membership in family 2 and were not counted. Likewise, persons who entered family 2 from outside the universe during the interval between interviews, such as a newborn baby or a soldier returning to civilian status, could not have been in family 1 (that is, were not eligible for inclusion in that family) and also were not counted. Third, the reciprocal majority population rule, as stated above, links only two families adjacent in time. However, transitivity between linkages is implied in the rule. This means that given three families (families A, B, and C) existing at three different points in time, if family A is the same as family B and family B is the same as family C, then family A is also the same as family C. A longitudinal family, therefore, is either one or a series of point-interval families linked by the reciprocal majority population rule. Fourth, the final sample of families was limited to initially sampled families and all other families derived from these families that had at least one initially sampled person (a key individual) in them on their beginning date. Thus, the collection of families examined for family construction purposes was divided into key families (a family with a key individual), which were in the sample and given a positive sampling weight, and nonkey families (a family without a key individual), which were not in the sample and given a sampling weight of zero. One reason for not including nonkey families in the sample is that very little data for them were available. Moreover, assumptions were often required to construct these families. (For more details on this methodology, see Dicker and Casady, 1982, and Whitmore, Cox, and Folsom, 1982.)

The dynamic sample of longitudinal families derived from this process tended to have characteristics that are generally sociologically believed to define the beginning and ending of families. For example, an even merger of two individuals through marriage always produced a new family. Similarly, an even split in a two-person family as the result of divorce or separation always ended the family. On the other hand, an uneven split in a larger family would not necessarily end such a family. In most cases, the original family continued as the larger part of the split. For example, if an adult child left a family of three persons or more to set up a separate household, in most cases the original family continued as the same but smaller family. Such an outcome appears to be in agreement with the sociological consensus that the loss of a single family member, other than the head or spouse, does not usually end the original family. The majority of uneven splits arise from this type of situation.

By the same reciprocal majority rule, however, a separation of husband and wife in a situation where children remained with one of the spouses in most cases continued the old family, now reconstituted as a single-spouse family with children. This result may not appear to be the sociologically preferred one. However, a more detailed review of the class of events of which this is a special case suggests that this result is in line both with the results based on sampling criteria for other members of the class and with sociological expectations of what the result should be for those class members. For example, given a head-spouse family with children, the loss of a head or spouse because of death or institutionalization is rarely thought of sociologically as an event ending the family. Rather, the social consensus appears to be that the original family continues, although in a recognizably changed state. The same may be said for the situation in which a head or spouse enters the military or goes overseas and is absent from the family for long periods. The family is not defined as ended but as continuing with an absent spouse. In this survey, all of the above events are defined as out-of-scope sampling events that cannot affect the identity of the family over time. Therefore, families would not end because of their occurrence. Only when the separating head or spouse remains within the noninstitutionalized U.S. population (the universe of inference) does the dilemma arise from sampling and sociological considerations as

to whether the original family has ended. This inscope event, however, is similar in its effect on family functioning as the four previously mentioned out-of-scope events. In all of these situations, the family loses a significant role player. As a consequence, important family role obligations go unfulfilled (or only partially fulfilled). It seemed appropriate, therefore, to treat all of these events in the same manner (as a functionally equivalent happening) for the purpose of constucting longitudinal families. Given the lack of a sociological consensus for treating the above class of events, the reciprocal majority population rule produces an appropriate, if not consensual, decision. When the separating head or spouse or adult child remains within the universe, the reciprocal majority population rule must also be applied to find out if he or she has formed a new family. The decision will depend on whether the person joins a previously existing family in the universe and the size of the family joined.

An uneven merger of two preexisting families also presents some decisionmaking problems from a sociological perspective. Such mergers occur when one or more related persons join another set of related persons or when a marriage occurs and one or more of the marriage partners bring children from a previous marriage (or another related person) with them. The first type of situation presents few problems. Most of these cases involve the entering or reentering of continuing families by elderly parents, adult children, or other relatives. Usually these new family members constitute the smaller of the two merging families. The larger of the two families entering the merger generally has reciprocal majority linkages to the newly merged family. (The smaller family never has.) The two reciprocally linked families are considered one continuing family. Occasionally, an uneven merger may produce a totally new family if the merged family cannot be linked to any preexisting family. The above result appears to be in line with the general sociological consensus that a family's identity is not changed by the addition or return of elderly parents, adult children, etc. Of course, if the additional family members come from out of scope (that is, if they are newborn children, come out of an institution, or return from the military or from overseas), they do not affect the identity of the family. These instances probably represent the majority of uneven mergers. However, there is less sociological consensus as to what the merged family represents when an uneven merger results from a marriage. The reciprocal majority population rule treats this situation in the same manner as the preceding one. For situations in which a single spouse enters an already existing larger family, the result appears appropriate. Where both spouses bring large families into the marriage, the result may be questionable. However, these latter situations represent a very small number of cases.

Construction and Use of Family Weights

Initial Family Weights

The target population of the household survey (HHS) was civilian noninstitutionalized families existing in the United States at any time during 1980. The universe of families existing on any specific day during 1980 was potentially different from that existing on any other day of the year. Conceptually, one could have conducted a census of the eligible population of the United States on January 1, 1980. By following this initial universe of families throughout the year, every unique longitudinal family unit could be identified and labeled. These longitudinal family units are defined by a beginning date, an ending date, and a set of persons who qualify as eligible (civilian and noninstitutionalized) family members. In addition to all family units that can be linked to the initial January 1 family universe, there are persons and families who were ineligible on January 1, 1980, but subsequently returned to the civilian noninstitutionalized population without merging with families containing individuals who were eligible on January 1. Such individuals and families were eligible for the sample but did not have a chance of entering it. Poststratification weight adjustments partially compensated for this undercoverage.

The family weights for longitudinal families in the household sample were developed from the sampling weights for the initially sampled families, which were called originating base reporting units (OBRU's). For each HHS longitudinal family, the key family members all belonged to the same OBRU. Hence, the initial family weight for the jth key HHS longitudinal family was computed as follows.

$$WF_1(j) = [n(j)/g(j)] \, w_o(j),$$

where $n(j)$ is the number of key individuals in family j on its beginning date, $g(j)$ is the total number of members of family j on its beginning date, and $w_o(j)$ is the OBRU initial sampling weight for the key members of family j. Thus, the initial family weight is the OBRU sampling weight adjusted for person-level multiplicity. Essentially, this formula means that the sampling weight of a family beginning on January 1, 1980, is the same as the household sampling weight, regardless of when the family ended or family membership changed in the subsequent 12 months. However, if a family began on some day after January 1, 1980, the household sampling weight was adjusted to take into account the fact that the new family may have had multiple chances of getting into the sample. However, as previously pointed out, positive sampling weights were developed only for key longitudinal families. Further details of the methodology for HHS longitudinal sampling weights are provided by Whitmore, Cox, and Folsom (1982).

Adjustment for Undercoverage and Nonresponse

Poststratification adjustment of the initial HHS family weights to the family counts based on the March Supplement to the 1980 Current Population Survey (CPS) was used to reduce the variance of estimators and the bias from undercoverage. These counts, however, were from estimates based on an updating of the 1970 census. Therefore, NMCUES family counts and estimates may not agree with family counts and estimates based on the 1980 census. The poststratification adjustments and a weighting class adjustment were also used to reduce the bias from nonresponse of longitudinal families.

A key HHS longitudinal family was classified as responding if it satisfied the following three requirements.

1. At least one key family member was classified as a respondent; that is, at least one key family member responded for at least one-third of his or her eligible days in the survey.

2. The total number of responding (known eligible) days during the family's existence summed over all family members is at least one-third of the total number of eligible days during the family's existence summed over all members of the family.

3. The family contained no students who were listed only on the parents' round 1 secondary reporting unit roster and for whom no other data collection instrument was ever received.

This definition of a responding family was felt to be consistent with the definition of person-level response and was used to create the HHS family response indicator variable. Only about 0.1 percent of all longitudinal families were declared to be nonresponding because of condition 3. Imputation of a full year of data for these students was problematic. Hence, inclusion of condition 3 in the definition of a responding family was felt to be cost effective.

The initial multiplicity-adjusted family weight was computed for all longitudinal families from the initial OBRU weight. A poststratification adjustment was then made for nonresponse of families linked to nonresponding OBRU's, producing an adjusted weight. A weighting class adjustment was performed for nonresponding longitudinal families generated by responding OBRU's. This adjusted weight was then truncated to produce a new family weight. The final adjustment was a poststratification and smoothing to the March Current Population Survey family counts to produce the final HHS longitudinal family weight, FWEIGHT. An alternative family weight, AWEIGHT, which was adjusted for each family's eligible days, was also computed from FWEIGHT to facilitate analytic tabulations. AWEIGHT, a time-adjusted family weight, is equal to FWEIGHT times the proportion of 1980 for which the family existed. (Computationally, it equals FWEIGHT times the family's survey eligibility days divided by 366, the total number of days in 1980.) The time-adjusted family weights, AWEIGHT, sum to the average daily number of HHS-eligible longitudinal families in the United States in 1980.

Estimators

This family weighting scheme produces the adjusted family weight, FWEIGHT, which can be used directly for estimation of annual health care utilization and expenditure. For example, if $Y(j)$ represents the total expenditure of the jth HHS longitudinal family for a particular medical service in 1980, then

$$\Sigma FWEIGHT(j)Y(j)$$

estimates the total expenditure of all civilian noninstitutionalized families in the United States for this medical service in 1980, where the summation extends over all longitudinal families in the NMCUES HHS sample.

Rates of utilization and expenditure are, however, of more interest than population totals. The rates of annual utilization and expenditure per family for a given family domain, say domain d, are defined at the population level by

$$R(d) = [\sum_{j=1}^{J} X_d(j)Y(j)]/[\sum_{j=1}^{J} X_d(j)PE(j)],$$

where $j = 1,..., J$ indexes the population of all key longitudinal families that ever existed in 1980 (that is, all longitudinal families that had a chance for selection as key NMCUES families);

$X_d(j) = 1$ if family j belongs to domain d, 0 otherwise;

$Y(j) =$ total utilization or expenditure for family j during the portion of 1980 that family j was eligible for NMCUES; and

$PE(j) =$ proportion of 1980 that family j was eligible for NMCUES, or (FAMEND − FAMBEG + 1)/366, where FAMEND = family ending date (days of 1980 numbered 1 through 366) and FAMBEG = family beginning date.

The family aggregates, $Y(j)$, can be viewed as sums of associated person-level visit counts or expenditures for key and nonkey individuals belonging to family j during the time period in which they were members of the family. The denominator of $R(d)$ is the average daily number of families of type d that existed during 1980. The bracketed portion of the numerator of $R(d)$ is simply the total number of health care visits or the total expenditures of a specified type experienced by

NMCUES eligible persons while they belonged to families of type d.

Unbiased estimators for the numerator and denominator of $R(d)$ lead to the ratio estimator $r(d)$, for which the equation is:

$$r(d) = [\Sigma FWEIGHT(j)X_d(j)Y(j)] / [\Sigma FWEIGHT(j)X_d(j)PE(j)],$$

where the summation extends over all longitudinal families in the sample. Of course, it is necessary to compute $X_d(j)$ and $PE(j)$ only for responding families because FWEIGHT is zero for all other families. Two alternative formulations of this estimator that may be more convenient for some computations are:

$$r(d) = [\Sigma AWEIGHT(j)X_d(j)Y(j)/PE(j)] / [\Sigma AWEIGHT(j)X_d(j)],$$

and

$$r(d) = [\Sigma FWEIGHT(j)X_d(j)Y(j)] / [\Sigma AWEIGHT(j)X_d(j)],$$

where the summations extend over all longitudinal families and AWEIGHT(j), as previously noted, is the final time-adjusted weight for family j; that is,

$$AWEIGHT(j) = FWEIGHT(j) \, PE(j).$$

Throughout this report, all estimates are based on the first of these two alternative formulations. All counts of expenditures for health care employ as the measure of expenditure

$$\Sigma AWEIGHT(j)X_d(j)Y(j)/PE(j),$$

and all counts of families employ as the number of families in question

$$\Sigma AWEIGHT(j)X_d(j).$$

The consequences of this procedure are described in the Introduction to this report.

To be more specific, the statistics presented in the detailed tables of this report are estimated as follows.

The *number of families* with given characteristic(s) is estimated as

$$\Sigma AWEIGHT(j)X_d(j),$$

where $X_d(j) = 1$ if family j has the characteristic(s) in question and 0 otherwise.

Note that this estimator estimates the number of family years experienced by families with the given characteristic(s) or, equivalently, the average number of families with the given characteristic(s) that would have been found at a randomly chosen point in time in 1980. It is, in general, less than the cumulative total of distinct longitudinal families with the given characteristic(s) that ever existed at any time in 1980, some of which existed for only part of the year.

The *mean* is always the mean rate of expenditure per family year and is estimated as

$$[\Sigma \text{AWEIGHT}(j) X_d(j) Y(j) / PE(j)] / [\Sigma \text{AWEIGHT}(j) X_d(j)].$$

The *percent* of families with use of a given type of care (the third column in each detailed table) is estimated as

$$[\Sigma \text{AWEIGHT}(j) X_d(j) X_u(j)] / [\Sigma \text{AWEIGHT}(j) X_d(j)]$$

where $X_u(j) = 1$ if family j has the utilization characteristic in question (use of a given type of care or a given number of discharges per family year) and 0 otherwise.

Note that this estimator has as its denominator the estimated number of family years experienced by all families in a domain defined by a set of family characteristics and has as its numerator the estimated number of family years experienced by families in the domain that also have the utilization characteristic in question. In other words, the estimator involves a ratio of family years.

Percentiles for each family category are estimated as follows. Each case in the HHS sample with the characteristic(s) of the family category is assigned two statistics: (1) an estimated rate of expenditure per family year, $Y(j)/PE(j)$, and (2) an associated number of family years, $\text{AWEIGHT}(j)$. The cases are sorted by the first statistic, the estimated rate expenditure per family year, and listed from lowest to highest. A cumulative sum of the family years (AWEIGHT's) is then constructed for each entry in the list, as is the grand total of family years for all cases in the list. The expenditure rate per family year at any given percentile is then the expenditure rate associated with the case whose position in the list is such that the cumulative sum of family years at its point in the list is equal to the given percentage of the grand total of family years. For example, the 25th percentile rate of expenditure is the rate of expenditure per family year associated with the case at which the cumulative total of family years equals 25 percent of the grand total of family years.

Special Requirements for Imputation of Family Data

As noted in the previous section, estimation of utilization and expenditure rates requires family aggregate data, say $Y(j)$, where the aggregates can be obtained as sums of associated person-level visit counts or expenditures. To compute the family aggregate $Y(j)$, it is necessary to sum over all members of family j, both key and nonkey. Moreover, computation of annual utilization and expenditure statistics requires a full year of data for every member of each responding family. Hence, in the attrition imputation, a weighted sequential hot-deck procedure was used to produce complete data for individuals who did not respond for the full year. In the attrition task (Cox and Sweetland, 1982), each individual was first classified as either having complete data or having incomplete data, based on whether the individual had responded for all 366 days in 1980. The data records for individuals who had not responded for the full year were completed by attrition imputation, including imputation of eligibility status (eligible or ineligible) for each day in 1980. The major importance of the attrition task is that it provided a full year of data for every individual from which family aggregates, $Y(j)$, can be computed. The concept of a key responding family was defined in such a way, however, that minimal use of data from the attrition task is required. Of course, missing item data can also lead to missing values for the family aggregate, $Y(j)$. Hence, item imputation procedures (Cox et al., 1982) were performed in addition to attrition imputation to assure the availability of complete data for important analytical variables for every eligible day for each family member.

Reliability of Estimates

Standard Errors

The estimates presented in this report are based on a sample of the target population rather than on the entire population. Thus, the values of the estimates may be different from values that would be obtained from a complete census. The difference between a sample estimate and the population value is referred to as the sampling error, and the expected magnitude of the sampling error is measured by the standard error. Estimated standard errors for the estimates in Tables 1–70 are found in Tables I–XXX. These tables also give the sample size for each family type category.

The SESUDAAN (Shah, 1981) standard error estimation software package was used to produce the estimates of standard errors. SESUDAAN is a Taylor Series procedure, developed and released by the Research Triangle Institute. It runs within the Statistical Analysis System (SAS Institute, Inc., 1982).

In addition to sampling errors, the estimates presented in this report are subject to nonsampling errors, such as biased interviewing and reporting, undercoverage, and nonresponse. The standard error does not provide an estimate of nonsampling errors. However, as discussed in preceding sections, every effort was made to minimize these errors.

Confidence Intervals

The estimates in this report are subject to sampling error. The true values are unknown. But the sampling error can be used to determine a range of values such that the true value will be within that range with a known probability. This range is called a confidence interval.

Suppose that $\hat{\theta}$ is an unbiased estimator for the parameter θ, and $S_{\hat{\theta}}$ is a consistent estimator for the standard error of $\hat{\theta}$. Under appropriate central limit theorem assumptions regarding $\hat{\theta}$, the statistic $Z = (\hat{\theta} - \theta)/S_{\hat{\theta}}$ has an approximate standard normal distribution for large samples. Thus, an approximate $(1 - \alpha) \times 100$ percent confidence interval for θ is given by

$$(\hat{\theta} + z_{\alpha/2}S_{\hat{\theta}}, \hat{\theta} + z_{1-\alpha/2}S_{\hat{\theta}})$$

where $z_{\alpha/2}$ and $z_{1-\alpha/2}$ are the appropriate values from a standard normal table.

As an example, Table 1 shows that, of all multiple-person families in the civilian noninstitutionalized population of the United States using inpatient hospital care, the estimated mean out-of-pocket expenditure per family for inpatient hospital care in 1980 was $259. The estimated standard error was $26.1 (See Table I in the Appendixes.) As $Z_{.025} = -1.96$ and $Z_{.975} = 1.96$, a 95-percent confidence interval for the mean out-of-pocket expenditure per family for all multiple-person families using inpatient hospital care in 1980 was $259 $\pm$ (1.96 $\times$ $26.1) or the interval $207.84 to $310.16. Approximately 95 percent of the confidence intervals constructed in this manner will contain the true mean out-of-pocket expenditure for families using inpatient hospital care in 1980.

Confidence intervals for the difference of two parameters can be constructed in a similar manner. Suppose θ_1 and θ_2 are the values of the parameter of interest in two mutually exclusive population subgroups. If $\hat{\theta}_1$ and $\hat{\theta}_2$ are unbiased estimators of θ_1 and θ_2, respectively, then $\hat{d} = \hat{\theta}_1 - \hat{\theta}_2$ is unbiased for $d = \theta_1 - \theta_2$ and

$$\text{Var}(\hat{d}) - \text{Var}(\hat{\theta}_1) + \text{Var}(\hat{\theta}_2) - 2\,\text{Cov}(\hat{\theta}_1, \hat{\theta}_2).$$

Unfortunately, the estimation of $\text{Var}(\hat{d})$ presents a problem because it is not possible for the National Center for Health Statistics to provide the reader with covariance estimates for all possible pairs of subdomains of potential interest. However, if it is reasonable to assume that $\text{Cov}(\hat{\theta}_1, \hat{\theta}_2) = 0$, the standard error of d can be estimated by

$$S_{\hat{d}} = \sqrt{S_{\hat{\theta}_1}^2 + S_{\hat{\theta}_2}^2}$$

Then, under appropriate central limit theorem assumptions regarding d, the statistic $Z_d = (\hat{d} - d)/S_{\hat{d}}$ has an approximate standard normal distribution for large samples, and the interval

$$(\hat{d} + z_{\alpha/2}S_{\hat{d}}, \hat{d} + z_{1-\alpha/2}S_{\hat{d}})$$

is an approximate $(1 - \alpha) \times 100$ percent confidence interval for the difference d.

For example, if one wanted to construct a 95-percent confidence interval for the difference between the mean out-of-pocket expenditure of two-person families using inpatient hospital care (θ_1) and the mean out-of-pocket expenditure of five-person families using inpatient care (θ_2). From Table 1 we have $\hat{\theta}_1 = \$354$ and $\hat{\theta}_2 = \$283$ so that

$$\hat{d} = \hat{\theta}_1 - \hat{\theta}_2$$

$$= \$354 - \$283$$

$$= \$71.$$

From Table I in this appendix, it can be seen that $S_{\hat{\theta}_1} = \$56.3$ and $S_{\hat{\theta}_2} = \$66.3$; therefore,

$$S_{\hat{d}} = \sqrt{S_{\hat{\theta}_1}^2 + S_{\hat{\theta}_2}^2}$$

$$= \sqrt{\$3,169.69 + \$4,395.69}$$

$$= \sqrt{\$7,565.38}$$

$$= \$86.98.$$

Then as $\alpha = .05$, it follows that $z_{\alpha/2} = -1.96$ and $z_{1-\alpha/2} = 1.96$; thus, the 95-percent confidence interval for the difference of interest is ($241.48, $0.0).

The reader should be aware that the assumption that $\text{Cov}(\hat{\theta}_1, \hat{\theta}_2) = 0$ is frequently not true for complex sample surveys. This warning is especially germane for sample designs, such as the NMCUES design, that rely on cluster sampling at one or more stages of sample selection. If $\text{Cov}(\hat{\theta}_1, \hat{\theta}_2)$ is positive, the confidence interval will tend to be too large, and hence the confidence level will be understated. More seriously, if $\text{Cov}(\hat{\theta}_1, \hat{\theta}_2)$ is negative, the confidence interval will tend to be too small, and the confidence level will be overstated.

Hypothesis Testing

The statistics Z and Z_d can be used to test hypotheses. For example, the size α critical region for the composite hypothesis

$$H_0 : d \geq d_0$$

versus

$$H_A : d < d_0$$

is given by

$$Z_{d_0} = \frac{\hat{d} - d_0}{S_{\hat{d}}} \leq z_\alpha.$$

As an example, suppose that before any data were collected one had a reason to believe that the mean out-of-pocket expenditure for inpatient hospital care in families in which all members had excellent health (θ_1) was less than the mean out-of-pocket expenditure for inpatient hospital care in families in which at least one member had poor health (θ_2). Letting $d = \theta_1 - \theta_2$, this can be restated as a formal hypothesis:

$$H_0 : d \geq 0$$

versus

$$H_A : d < 0.$$

Note that what is believed to be the true state of nature is reflected by the one-sided alternative.

It can be seen from Tables 1 and I that

$$\hat{d} = \$170 - \$485 = -\$315$$

and

$$S_{\hat{d}} = \sqrt{\$1,421.29 + \$5,730.49}$$

$$= \$84.57,$$

so that $Z_{d_0} = -3.72$. As there are four categories for the variable of family perceived health status in Table 1, a multiple t test based on the Bonferroni inequality (Levy and Lemeshow, 1980) will be used to assess the significance of the comparison. Comparing four categories, two at a time, and not taking sign into account gives six possible comparisons. Use of the table in Levy and Lemeshow (1980, p. 296), gives a one-tail critical value of -2.39. Therefore, H_0 is rejected in favor of H_A as $Z_{d_0} \leq z_\alpha$.

As discussed earlier, the assumption that $\text{Cov}(\hat{\theta}_1, \hat{\theta}_2) = 0$ must be carefully evaluated. If, in fact, the covariance is positive, the size of the test will be smaller than α; and if the covariance is negative, the size of the test will be larger than α. To conduct a more sophisticated analysis of the NMCUES data the reader is advised to consult with a statistician knowledgeable in the analysis of data from complex sample surveys.

Sampling Errors for Medians

Sampling errors for median use of care were not calculated for this report. However, they can be calculated by using another approach to estimating variances (Landis, Lepkowski, Eklund et al., 1982; McCarthy, 1966). An approximation of the 95-percent confidence interval of the median is given by

$$\tilde{m}\left(1 + 1.96 \sqrt{\frac{\pi}{2}} \sqrt{\ln(CV)^2 + 1}\right)$$
$$\tilde{m}\left(1 - 1.96 \sqrt{\frac{\pi}{2}} \sqrt{\ln(CV)^2 + 1}\right),$$

where CV = coefficient of variation.

227

Table I

Sample size for multiple-person families and standard errors for Tables 1, 11, and 21, by selected characteristics: United States, 1980

| Characteristic | Sample size | Standard errors of mean | | | | | |
| | | Table 1 | | Table 11 | | Table 21 | |
		All families	Families with discharges	All families	Families with care	All families	Families with visits
Total..............	4,845	$8.1	$26.1	$3.7	$14.0	$3.1	$3.0
Family size[1]							
2 persons........	1,988	15.3	56.3	5.8	22.8	4.0	4.0
3 persons........	1,050	8.5	25.7	5.2	19.5	5.3	5.3
4 persons........	984	7.1	21.6	6.7	27.9	6.5	6.5
5 or more persons...	823	24.3	66.3	6.9	23.3	6.0	6.1
Age of head							
Under 25 years......	457	24.7	71.9	5.3	20.8	6.9	7.5
25-44 years.........	2,066	11.9	38.7	4.6	19.6	4.0	3.8
45-64 years.........	1,641	11.8	40.1	6.2	25.1	4.7	5.1
65 years and over...	681	24.7	66.0	9.4	26.9	6.4	7.3
Sex of head							
Male...............	3,994	9.9	32.2	3.8	13.6	3.3	3.3
Female.............	851	18.6	60.0	8.4	37.0	5.8	6.2
Race and ethnicity[2] of head							
White..............	4,256	8.6	27.5	4.0	14.8	3.5	3.4
Hispanic...........	268	24.0	70.3	15.2	70.1	10.6	10.6
Non-Hispanic.......	3,988	8.9	28.6	3.8	13.5	3.6	3.5
Black..............	499	30.0	97.4	5.0	24.4	6.0	6.5
Other..............	90	29.2	91.2	20.5	93.7	24.3	26.4
Family structure							
Head and spouse present whole time......	3,814	7.8	24.8	3.7	14.1	3.6	3.5
Child under 17 years....	1,949	6.4	19.4	5.6	20.8	5.2	5.0
No child under 17 years...	1,865	13.7	49.1	3.6	13.7	4.1	4.3
Head only, no spouse at any time......	909	24.7	84.3	8.9	41.0	5.1	5.6
Child under 17 years....	547	35.1	111.5	7.6	34.2	6.4	6.8
No child under 17 years...	362	31.2	128.9	18.5	83.2	6.7	7.9
Other..............	122	59.4	108.1	23.1	60.0	20.6	21.9
Family dynamics							
Unchanging, full year.......	3,754	9.1	32.9	4.0	16.9	3.5	3.5
Change in composition or existed less than full year........	1,091	23.9	47.7	7.1	20.3	5.8	5.9

Family poverty status in 1980							
Below 150 percent poverty level	817	20.8	58.4	5.9	24.8	4.6	5.2
Below poverty level	428	12.4	32.9	3.0	14.8	6.0	6.6
Poverty level to 149 percent	389	43.6	115.8	12.5	44.6	6.8	7.4
150–199 percent	528	51.6	160.8	10.9	43.7	8.1	8.1
200–299 percent	1,065	9.5	29.3	8.0	28.2	5.4	5.4
300–499 percent	1,486	9.4	35.0	5.5	22.5	5.3	5.4
500 percent or more	949	12.3	49.6	5.0	20.8	6.8	7.3
Family income in 1980[3]							
Less than $10,000	806	24.7	73.8	5.2	24.2	4.6	5.1
$10,000–$19,999	1,409	17.5	54.4	7.8	29.4	4.8	4.8
$20,000–$34,999	1,685	7.6	26.8	4.9	20.8	5.5	5.6
$35,000 or more	945	14.4	50.2	4.2	15.0	6.6	6.6
Education of head[4]							
None or elementary school	823	14.6	40.1	7.8	26.1	4.6	4.8
Some high school	749	23.6	67.2	7.7	29.1	5.1	5.3
High school graduate	1,742	14.3	48.8	5.4	20.9	4.7	4.6
Some college	743	9.8	32.9	4.1	17.8	6.1	6.4
College graduate or more	784	25.7	98.3	9.1	36.6	10.6	10.8
Family employment status[5]							
2 or more persons worked full year	1,249	8.4	32.5	4.5	18.4	5.7	5.7
Only 1 person worked full year	2,079	14.5	46.9	4.5	18.2	4.7	4.6
Some part-year work	925	21.6	56.4	6.3	22.1	5.7	5.9
No person worked	592	21.3	55.5	15.3	46.7	6.8	7.2
Worst perceived health status of any family member[6]							
Excellent	1,371	8.1	37.7	2.6	13.2	4.1	3.9
Good	2,077	11.8	40.4	3.3	13.9	4.4	4.7
Fair	905	20.1	56.8	9.6	32.4	5.5	5.7
Poor	489	43.7	75.7	18.1	41.3	9.7	10.3
Most severe limitation in usual activity of any family member							
None	3,701	8.6	33.1	2.4	11.8	3.4	3.3
Some limitation	289	39.2	99.2	14.7	45.4	13.4	13.7
Cannot perform usual activity	855	22.8	43.9	12.3	29.0	6.1	6.4
Family's bed days[3]							
0	950	2.5	133.2	1.8	153.3	3.0	3.5
1–5	1,240	7.2	42.1	2.8	19.0	4.5	4.6
6–10	733	6.2	18.5	3.9	16.0	6.0	6.0
11–20	826	22.3	53.6	4.5	12.5	5.4	5.6
More than 20	1,096	27.7	44.8	13.6	26.6	7.6	7.7

Table I—continued

Sample size for multiple-person families and standard errors for Tables 1, 11, and 21, by selected characteristics: United States, 1980

| | | | | Standard errors of mean | | | |
| | | Table 1 | | Table 11 | | Table 21 | |
Characteristic	Sample size	All families	Families with discharges	All families	Families with care	All families	Families with visits
Family health care coverage							
All members covered full year	3,570	$8.0	$27.0	$4.1	$15.5	$3.8	$3.8
Private insurance only	2,248	11.6	43.0	3.6	14.8	5.0	5.1
Medicaid only	107	1.9	5.3	1.7	10.0	4.6	5.0
Medicare only	47	*26.9	*81.2	*11.2	*39.4	*16.0	*17.8
Medicare and other public programs	38	*41.6	*98.6	*14.4	*50.6	*12.5	*13.8
Medicare and private insurance	603	16.9	41.7	10.2	27.1	7.1	7.1
Other public and private mixes	476	18.2	54.9	8.9	40.1	7.7	8.1
Other mixes of public programs	11	*4.8	*0.3	*3.2	*2.4	*41.1	*45.4
Source unknown	40	*50.7	*95.3	*136.5	*350.1	*14.1	*15.3
All members covered, some part year	724	15.3	45.6	8.0	30.1	6.0	6.4
Some members not covered	374	61.8	178.1	11.5	40.3	8.0	8.3
All members not covered	177	41.0	300.8	10.6	80.9	10.7	12.4

1 Average size during period of family's existence rounded to nearest integer; exactly half an integer rounded upward.
2 There were too few Hispanic families of races other than white for separate tabulation.
3 Annual rate.
4 Includes only families with heads 17 years of age and over.
5 Excludes families with all members under 14 years of age.
6 Excludes families with all members with health status unknown.

NOTE: Multiple-person families are families with average size 1.5 or greater.

Table II

Sample size for multiple-person families with all members under 65 years of age and standard errors for Tables 2, 12, and 22, by selected characteristics: United States, 1980

| | | | | Standard errors of mean | | | | |
| | | Table 2 | | Table 12 | | Table 22 | |
Characteristic	Sample size	All families	Families with discharges	All families	Families with care	All families	Families with visits
Total..........................	3,985	$8.7	$29.6	$3.9	$16.9	$3.3	$3.4
Family size[1]							
2 persons.....................	1,364	20.9	91.2	6.7	34.4	5.3	5.6
3 persons.....................	939	5.5	17.9	5.1	22.1	5.7	5.8
4 persons.....................	921	7.7	23.3	7.1	30.4	6.6	6.6
5 or more persons.............	761	25.2	71.6	7.2	26.2	6.3	6.5
Age of head							
Under 25 years................	454	24.8	71.9	5.3	20.8	6.8	7.5
25-44 years...................	2,035	12.1	39.7	4.7	19.8	3.9	3.7
45-64 years...................	1,496	12.6	46.2	6.7	29.7	4.9	5.3
Sex of head							
Male..........................	3,272	9.2	32.2	3.9	16.4	3.8	3.8
Female........................	713	20.8	72.0	9.6	48.0	5.8	6.3
Race and ethnicity[2] of head							
White.........................	3,478	9.0	31.2	4.2	17.8	3.8	3.8
Hispanic....................	240	26.9	86.7	16.8	76.6	10.6	11.0
Non-Hispanic................	3,238	9.4	33.0	3.9	16.2	4.0	3.9
Black.........................	429	29.0	91.1	5.1	26.6	6.4	7.2
Other.........................	78	36.6	125.8	25.8	136.2	30.4	33.3
Family structure							
Head and spouse present whole time.....	3,155	6.0	20.7	4.0	16.8	3.9	3.9
Child under 17 years........	1,879	6.4	19.6	5.7	21.7	5.0	4.8
No child under 17 years.....	1,276	11.2	49.4	4.1	20.6	5.6	5.8
Head only, no spouse at any time.....	740	29.8	109.3	10.1	53.6	5.3	5.8
Child under 17 years........	522	36.6	119.5	8.0	39.0	5.6	6.0
No child under 17 years.....	218	47.4	294.5	28.2	173.3	8.8	10.5
Other.........................	90	35.5	81.1	9.4	38.5	24.9	26.3
Family dynamics							
Unchanging, full year.........	3,029	8.9	35.4	4.5	21.6	3.8	3.8
Change in composition or existed less than full year........	956	23.8	48.9	5.4	16.5	6.2	6.4

231

Table II—continued

Sample size for multiple-person families with all members under 65 years of age and standard errors for Tables 2, 12, and 22, by selected characteristics: United States, 1980

| Characteristic | Sample size | Standard errors of mean | | | | | |
| | | Table 2 | | Table 12 | | Table 22 | |
		All families	Families with discharges	All families	Families with care	All families	Families with visits
Family poverty status in 1980							
Below 150 percent poverty level	655	$22.9	$65.1	$5.7	$25.2	$5.2	$5.9
Below poverty level	364	11.5	30.0	3.2	16.1	7.0	7.6
Poverty level to 149 percent	291	51.6	139.4	12.6	50.7	8.5	9.4
150–199 percent	402	54.4	187.9	11.1	47.3	9.6	9.7
200–299 percent	841	12.0	39.7	9.2	38.0	5.4	5.5
300–499 percent	1,259	8.1	31.4	5.9	26.2	5.6	5.8
500 percent or more	828	13.7	60.5	4.3	19.9	7.5	8.0
Family income in 1980[3]							
Less than $10,000	564	27.3	82.3	3.6	17.5	5.4	6.1
$10,000–$19,999	1,073	21.6	75.0	9.5	42.2	5.0	5.1
$20,000–$34,999	1,488	8.3	31.1	5.0	23.0	5.9	5.9
$35,000 or more	860	13.0	48.0	4.2	16.0	7.1	7.2
Education of head[4]							
None or elementary school	465	13.5	32.9	8.6	35.4	6.4	6.8
Some high school	608	10.5	32.4	8.2	35.5	6.0	6.4
High school graduate	1,553	15.5	55.8	5.5	22.4	4.8	4.7
Some college	656	8.8	31.0	3.8	17.4	6.0	6.1
College graduate or more	700	28.7	114.2	10.1	43.2	11.8	11.9
Family employment status[5]							
2 or more persons worked full year	1,172	8.5	35.1	4.3	19.8	5.9	6.0
Only 1 person worked full year	1,864	14.7	49.6	4.6	19.5	4.8	4.8
Some part-year work	744	26.8	72.3	7.4	26.7	6.3	6.5
No person worked	205	18.4	57.0	28.3	137.1	7.8	8.4
Worst perceived health status of any family member[6]							
Excellent	1,258	7.0	32.3	2.3	12.6	4.1	3.9
Good	1,786	13.8	48.4	3.4	14.9	4.6	4.9
Fair	652	27.4	79.4	12.0	40.8	7.5	7.7
Poor	286	51.1	96.3	25.6	70.4	14.1	14.9

Most severe limitation in usual activity of any family member

None................................	3,369	9.5	35.6	2.6	12.8	3.5	3.5
Some limitation.....................	218	42.5	110.9	18.6	55.7	15.5	15.7
Cannot perform usual activity.......	398	28.4	58.9	20.7	57.6	8.4	8.5

Family's bed days[3]

0...................................	684	2.0	99.0	0.9	57.8	3.8	4.3
1-5.................................	1,078	8.1	54.9	2.8	22.4	4.9	5.1
6-10................................	625	6.4	21.5	4.1	19.1	6.6	6.7
11-20...............................	736	23.4	60.2	4.8	14.2	5.9	6.1
More than 20........................	862	29.3	49.8	15.4	34.4	8.6	8.8

Family health care coverage

All members covered full year.......	2,853	9.8	34.3	4.5	19.2	4.4	4.4
Private insurance only..............	2,226	11.8	44.2	3.4	14.8	5.0	5.0
Medicaid only.......................	106	1.9	5.4	0.0	0.0	4.6	4.9
Medicare only.......................	—	—	—	—	—	—	—
Medicare and other public programs....	1	*0.0	—	*0.0	—	*0.0	*0.0
Medicare and private insurance......	8	*47.6	*78.0	*27.5	*75.9	*22.7	*28.2
Other public and private mixes......	469	18.5	55.5	9.4	41.3	8.0	8.4
Other mixes of public programs......	11	*4.8	*0.3	*3.2	*2.4	*41.1	*45.4
Source unknown......................	32	*61.6	*109.5	*165.3	*425.8	*12.7	*13.3
All members covered, some part year.....	669	13.1	41.6	8.0	31.7	6.5	6.9
Some members not covered............	292	61.4	191.7	11.7	41.1	9.9	10.4
All members not covered.............	171	24.5	156.7	10.5	85.5	10.9	12.6

[1]Average size during period of family's existence rounded to nearest integer; exactly half an integer rounded upward.
[2]There were too few Hispanic families of races other than white for separate tabulation.
[3]Annual rate.
[4]Includes only families with heads 17 years of age and over.
[5]Excludes families with all members under 14 years of age.
[6]Excludes families with all members with health status unknown.

NOTE: Multiple-person families are families with average size 1.5 or greater.

233

Table III

Sample size for multiple-person families with all members under 65 years of age and all members with health care coverage all year and standard errors for Tables 3, 13, and 23, by selected characteristics: United States, 1980

Characteristic	Sample size	Table 3		Table 13		Table 23	
		All families	Families with discharges	All families	Families with care	All families	Families with visits
Total.................	2,853	$9.8	$34.3	$4.5	$19.2	$4.4	$4.4
Family size[1]							
2 persons................	1,011	27.1	116.9	8.5	41.8	6.5	6.8
3 persons................	674	3.7	12.7	3.7	15.6	6.7	6.9
4 persons................	680	7.9	23.6	9.2	34.7	7.1	7.1
5 or more persons........	488	10.5	31.6	8.5	30.3	8.5	8.4
Age of head							
Under 25 years...........	270	34.3	112.6	5.7	23.5	8.5	9.0
25-44 years..............	1,514	15.9	52.9	4.4	18.7	5.1	5.0
45-64 years..............	1,069	7.4	27.1	8.3	36.0	6.6	6.9
Sex of head							
Male.....................	2,432	11.7	40.5	4.5	18.8	4.8	4.8
Female...................	421	5.5	20.8	12.9	72.9	7.2	7.6
Race and ethnicity[2] of head							
White....................	2,530	9.8	33.9	4.9	20.3	4.8	4.8
Hispanic.................	132	41.3	110.9	25.2	86.0	16.4	16.6
Non-Hispanic.............	2,398	10.1	35.3	4.3	17.8	4.8	4.9
Black....................	270	44.1	157.2	6.6	40.7	6.4	7.1
Other....................	53	54.4	202.9	40.0	166.1	43.8	50.3
Family structure							
Head and spouse present whole time.....	2,372	7.1	24.4	4.5	18.9	4.8	4.9
Child under 17 years.....	1,389	6.0	17.8	6.9	25.5	6.2	6.1
No child under 17 years..	983	14.4	61.7	4.3	21.1	6.2	6.6
Head only, no spouse at any time.....	431	39.8	160.2	12.9	77.5	6.6	7.2
Child under 17 years.....	328	42.4	160.5	2.3	14.4	6.6	7.1
No child under 17 years..	103	101.9	497.3	60.4	278.8	16.5	18.4
Other....................	50	50.9	99.0	14.1	43.8	40.5	42.5
Family dynamics							
Unchanging, full year....	2,297	8.1	32.3	5.3	24.7	4.8	4.8
Change in composition or existed less than full year......	556	40.8	84.0	6.3	17.9	8.9	9.4

Family poverty status in 1980

Below 150 percent poverty level	345	41.8	113.1	9.4	39.2	7.6	8.5
Below poverty level	207	13.4	37.4	4.7	22.5	9.0	9.8
Poverty level to 149 percent	138	110.3	244.3	23.8	76.8	14.8	15.7
150-199 percent	218	59.3	193.1	10.6	46.2	11.8	12.2
200-299 percent	596	7.6	24.1	11.6	44.9	5.2	5.1
300-499 percent	999	8.9	36.0	6.8	31.2	6.8	7.0
500 percent or more	695	15.9	71.0	4.3	21.8	9.6	10.1

Family income in 1980[3]

Less than $10,000	298	49.9	144.3	4.9	20.7	7.3	8.2
$10,000-$19,999	668	20.8	71.6	12.1	51.9	5.6	5.7
$20,000-$34,999	1,207	7.7	28.9	5.6	24.7	6.7	6.6
$35,000 or more	680	15.7	60.9	3.9	17.0	9.4	9.4

Education of head[4]

None or elementary school	259	15.4	43.8	10.1	35.1	9.0	9.3
Some high school	378	10.3	33.1	4.3	18.2	6.6	7.0
High school graduate	1,139	12.6	45.3	7.0	28.7	5.3	5.3
Some college	500	8.0	29.9	4.4	21.3	6.9	7.3
College graduate or more	574	35.1	131.1	11.9	49.4	14.3	14.4

Family employment status[5]

2 or more persons worked full year	896	9.6	41.9	4.7	21.5	6.8	7.0
Only 1 person worked full year	1,387	18.8	63.7	3.8	16.3	6.1	6.3
Some part-year work	412	7.5	19.3	10.8	36.2	9.5	9.9
No person worked	158	21.6	74.2	37.5	195.2	9.5	10.0

Worst perceived health status of any family member[6]

Excellent	946	8.3	37.9	2.3	12.4	5.1	4.9
Good	1,306	11.0	40.0	4.0	18.2	5.4	5.6
Fair	425	40.9	114.0	14.7	50.8	10.5	10.9
Poor	173	66.5	124.2	38.3	99.9	19.3	20.6

Most severe limitation in usual activity of any family member

None	2,438	10.0	38.1	2.8	13.8	4.4	4.4
Some limitation	160	56.1	138.0	24.9	71.1	19.8	20.1
Cannot perform usual activity	255	31.0	61.1	29.5	80.7	9.8	9.8

Family's bed days[3]

0	507	1.1	57.5	0.6	37.3	5.0	5.5
1-5	761	9.7	72.6	1.9	17.7	5.8	5.9
6-10	472	4.0	13.7	4.9	21.0	7.3	7.5
11-20	516	6.3	15.4	4.8	14.7	7.8	8.0
More than 20	597	41.6	70.5	18.4	38.7	11.3	11.3

Table III—continued

Sample size for multiple-person families with all members under 65 years of age and all members with health care coverage all year and standard errors for Tables 3, 13, and 23, by selected characteristics: United States, 1980

Characteristic	Sample size	Standard errors of mean					
		Table 3		Table 13		Table 23	
		All families	Families with discharges	All families	Families with care	All families	Families with visits
Family health care coverage							
Private insurance only..........	2,226	$11.8	$44.2	$3.4	$14.8	$5.0	$5.0
Medicaid only..................	106	1.9	5.4	0.0	0.0	4.6	4.9
Medicare only.................	-	-	-	-	-	-	-
Medicare and other public programs.....	1	*0.0	-	*0.0	-	*0.0	*0.0
Medicare and private insurance........	8	*47.6	*78.0	*27.5	*75.9	*22.7	*28.2
Other public and private mixes........	469	18.5	55.5	9.4	41.3	8.0	8.4
Other mixes of public programs........	11	*4.8	*0.3	*3.2	*2.4	*41.1	*45.4
Source unknown................	32	*61.6	*109.5	*165.3	*425.8	*12.7	*13.3

[1]Average size during period of family's existence rounded to nearest integer; exactly half an integer rounded upward.
[2]There were too few Hispanic families of races other than white for separate tabulation.
[3]Annual rate.
[4]Includes only families with heads 17 years of age and over.
[5]Excludes families with all members under 14 years of age.
[6]Excludes families with all members with health status unknown.

NOTE: Multiple-person families are families with average size 1.5 or greater.

Table IV

Sample size for multiple-person families with all members under 65 years of age and some members without health care coverage all year and standard errors for Tables 4, 14, and 24, by selected characteristics: United States, 1980

Characteristic	Sample size	Standard errors of mean					
		Table 4		Table 14		Table 24	
		All families	Families with discharges	All families	Families with care	All families	Families with visits
Total...................	1,132	$19.1	$64.5	$5.9	$23.8	$4.8	$5.1
Family size[1]							
2 persons................	353	18.5	77.6	6.0	37.1	7.6	9.1
3 persons................	265	13.9	43.7	15.3	57.3	8.3	8.6
4 persons................	241	19.4	63.2	10.9	55.2	12.2	12.6
5 or more persons........	273	69.8	188.0	12.4	44.2	11.1	11.8
Age of head							
Under 25 years...........	184	30.0	81.3	10.4	37.1	14.0	15.3
25–44 years..............	521	19.8	70.7	10.6	42.4	6.9	7.3
45–64 years..............	427	40.3	142.2	7.0	28.8	7.1	7.7
Sex of head							
Male.....................	840	13.4	47.4	5.9	24.2	5.7	6.1
Female...................	292	47.3	148.3	13.8	58.1	8.9	10.1
Race and ethnicity[2] of head							
White....................	948	22.1	79.3	6.7	26.0	4.9	5.1
Hispanic.................	108	46.0	165.4	23.4	159.1	11.0	13.2
Non-Hispanic.............	840	24.8	90.4	6.5	24.4	5.6	5.8
Black....................	159	27.8	72.5	9.0	31.7	16.0	18.3
Other....................	25	*17.5	*53.7	*12.2	*56.7	*32.6	*38.2
Family structure							
Head and spouse present whole time......	783	14.8	49.8	6.3	25.0	6.2	6.6
Child under 17 years..........	490	21.3	70.1	8.1	30.3	8.5	8.8
No child under 17 years.......	293	11.8	49.7	7.8	40.9	9.4	9.6
Head only, no spouse at any time......	309	44.9	151.6	13.6	59.6	7.7	8.8
Child under 17 years..........	194	66.4	178.7	19.8	73.0	9.1	10.0
No child under 17 years.......	115	12.5	80.0	3.7	27.6	9.4	11.4
Other....................	40	*48.6	*139.6	*9.6	*60.3	*28.5	*29.6
Family dynamics							
Unchanging, full year.....	732	27.0	113.9	6.9	32.9	5.2	5.6
Change in composition or existed less than full year...........	400	19.4	42.9	10.6	30.7	8.5	9.3

Table IV—continued

Sample size for multiple-person families with all members under 65 years of age and some members without health care coverage all year and standard errors for Tables 4, 14, and 24, by selected characteristics: United States, 1980

		\multicolumn{6}{c}{Standard errors of mean}					
		Table 4		Table 14		Table 24	
Characteristic	Sample size	All families	Families with discharges	All families	Families with care	All families	Families with visits
Family poverty status in 1980							
Below 150 percent poverty level	310	$19.8	$52.3	$6.0	$24.9	$7.3	$8.2
Below poverty level	157	19.0	47.1	4.5	23.6	11.3	12.3
Poverty level to 149 percent	153	31.0	92.3	11.3	44.3	12.1	13.6
150–199 percent	184	97.5	341.2	23.2	88.0	15.5	16.0
200–299 percent	245	36.1	130.1	15.3	69.7	11.3	12.6
300–499 percent	260	18.8	59.7	10.2	37.9	9.8	9.9
500 percent or more	133	20.8	76.7	12.6	49.8	13.4	14.2
Family income in 1980[3]							
Less than $10,000	266	17.3	53.0	5.7	30.4	8.9	10.1
$10,000–$19,999	405	45.0	168.8	13.3	59.0	8.3	9.1
$20,000–$34,999	281	32.3	113.2	10.7	50.8	11.5	12.5
$35,000 or more	180	20.2	56.7	13.6	41.7	12.8	13.1
Education of head[4]							
None or elementary school	206	25.1	63.5	13.9	67.1	8.8	10.0
Some high school	230	20.2	56.3	20.4	78.1	10.2	11.4
High school graduate	414	49.2	170.9	7.3	28.5	8.9	9.5
Some college	156	23.0	73.4	8.0	33.9	12.5	11.8
College graduate or more	126	12.5	65.5	13.0	68.3	13.5	14.4
Family employment status[5]							
2 or more persons worked full year	276	17.8	64.8	7.8	32.6	9.2	9.9
Only 1 person worked full year	477	15.1	49.6	12.0	50.5	7.1	7.7
Some part-year work	332	57.4	162.0	8.8	35.3	9.8	10.3
No person worked	47	*34.3	*84.0	*16.3	*62.6	*14.3	*15.8
Worst perceived health status of any family member[6]							
Excellent	312	11.6	49.8	5.8	28.9	6.6	7.5
Good	480	37.3	129.7	6.5	26.8	7.8	8.1
Fair	227	30.0	81.0	18.8	61.6	13.3	13.9
Poor	113	74.9	157.1	29.1	83.3	19.1	19.5

238

Most severe limitation in usual activity of any family member

None......................	931	21.0	77.5	5.6	25.8	5.2	5.5
Some limitation...........	58	33.8	118.3	4.4	15.8	13.8	13.8
Cannot perform usual activity...	143	59.8	138.5	25.4	69.4	16.6	17.1

Family's bed days[3]

0.........................	177	6.7	259.6	2.8	169.3	6.7	8.4
1-5.......................	317	15.8	81.7	7.0	44.7	8.1	9.1
6-10......................	153	20.5	69.5	7.4	43.9	15.1	16.4
11-20.....................	220	75.7	192.7	11.9	34.1	10.0	10.6
More than 20..............	265	37.3	76.2	20.6	49.5	10.6	11.0

Family health care coverage

All members covered, some part year.....	669	13.1	41.6	8.0	31.7	6.5	6.9
Some members not covered........	292	61.4	191.7	11.7	41.1	9.9	10.4
All members not covered.........	171	24.5	156.7	10.5	85.5	10.9	12.6

[1] Average size during period of family's existence rounded to nearest integer; exactly half an integer rounded upward.
[2] There were too few Hispanic families of races other than white for separate tabulation.
[3] Annual rate.
[4] Includes only families with heads 17 years of age and over.
[5] Excludes families with all members under 14 years of age.
[6] Excludes families with all members with health status unknown.

NOTE: Multiple-person families are families with average size 1.5 or greater.

Table V

Sample size for multiple-person families with members 65 years of age and over and standard errors for Tables 5, 15, and 25, by selected characteristics: United States, 1980

| | | Standard errors of mean | | | | | |
| | | Table 5 | | Table 15 | | Table 25 | |
Characteristic	Sample size	All families	Families with discharges	All families	Families with care	All families	Families with visits
Total..............	860	$20.3	$49.2	$7.5	$18.8	$5.5	$6.0
Family size[1]							
2 persons.........	624	20.7	58.2	9.8	28.0	6.1	6.4
3 persons.........	111	62.1	119.0	19.6	31.3	15.7	16.3
4 persons.........	63	67.2	152.1	15.3	36.3	33.8	34.8
5 or more persons..	62	92.0	163.3	24.8	50.4	19.2	19.6
Family age							
All members 65 years and over..........	348	53.6	149.2	17.8	48.3	9.7	10.6
Some members under 65......	512	25.7	58.5	7.8	17.1	6.5	7.0
Sex of head							
Male................	722	30.8	76.9	8.1	20.8	5.9	6.4
Female..............	138	40.3	99.0	17.6	49.9	13.5	14.7
Race and ethnicity[2] of head							
White...............	778	24.1	58.9	8.0	20.4	5.7	6.0
Hispanic............	28	*27.7	*69.2	*11.9	*52.1	*29.9	*30.5
Non-Hispanic........	750	25.1	61.4	8.5	21.3	6.0	6.4
Black...............	70	113.5	420.6	18.6	68.0	18.2	19.3
Other...............	12	*8.1	*31.2	*39.5	*81.0	*11.2	*11.9
Family structure							
Head and spouse present whole time......	659	30.2	79.6	6.3	17.2	6.4	6.9
Child under 17 years...	70	49.5	108.7	23.5	54.4	27.0	26.2
No child under 17 years...	589	32.8	88.9	6.6	18.4	6.8	7.4
Head only, no spouse at any time......	169	36.8	100.1	18.2	55.0	11.7	12.8
Child under 17 years...	25	*45.3	*90.8	*18.5	*34.7	*61.9	*61.9
No child under 17 years...	144	40.9	118.9	20.5	68.2	9.2	9.9
Other...............	32	*192.3	*213.6	*85.0	*108.5	*26.9	*28.0
Family dynamics							
Unchanging, full year........	725	25.8	72.8	5.6	17.0	6.2	7.0
Change in composition or existed less than full year........	135	82.9	128.2	34.1	62.8	10.1	10.4

Family poverty status in 1980

Below 150 percent poverty level	162	48.7	137.5	19.3	61.4	8.6	10.3
Below poverty level	64	44.2	130.0	9.8	37.9	9.0	10.2
Poverty level to 149 percent	98	83.0	201.7	33.2	87.9	12.3	13.1
150–199 percent	126	124.8	310.2	19.2	59.1	10.9	11.0
200–299 percent	224	20.4	46.6	13.4	31.6	12.8	13.3
300–499 percent	227	42.1	111.1	18.0	50.4	10.5	11.3
500 percent or more	121	29.6	78.6	21.1	62.2	12.7	12.6

Family income in 1980[3]

Less than $10,000	242	50.8	147.9	15.9	52.8	7.4	8.2
$10,000–$19,999	336	26.2	60.8	11.2	28.8	10.3	11.1
$20,000–$34,999	197	18.1	45.4	19.9	52.1	11.6	12.8
$35,000 or more	85	78.3	165.6	18.0	42.6	13.4	13.3

Education of head[4]

None or elementary school	358	31.2	79.6	10.9	32.4	7.9	8.3
Some high school	141	115.1	269.2	19.3	55.8	8.5	9.4
High school graduate	189	37.0	88.3	21.2	56.7	10.8	11.7
Some college	87	43.7	125.5	22.1	71.4	25.2	26.6
College graduate or more	84	38.0	104.0	11.1	28.7	15.8	16.3

Family employment status[5]

2 or more persons worked full year	77	37.0	88.5	27.3	68.1	17.8	17.7
Only 1 person worked full year	215	46.1	122.4	10.5	32.6	12.5	13.4
Some part-year work	181	20.3	46.4	11.5	32.8	9.3	10.3
No person worked	387	33.3	81.3	14.9	35.4	8.4	8.9

Worst perceived health status of any family member[6]

Excellent	113	57.9	262.6	13.6	63.1	11.5	13.9
Good	291	11.6	31.7	13.7	46.0	10.9	11.4
Fair	253	15.0	35.8	12.4	35.1	8.8	9.2
Poor	203	67.4	113.0	20.0	37.9	10.6	11.8

Most severe limitation in usual activity of any family member

None	332	11.4	46.5	8.7	37.7	9.0	10.1
Some limitation	71	92.0	249.0	16.4	57.6	16.4	16.7
Cannot perform usual activity	457	33.2	62.6	12.5	26.6	7.8	8.2

Family's bed days[3]

0	266	6.8	395.5	5.6	558.9	7.2	8.3
1–5	162	8.3	26.0	5.8	20.1	12.3	13.3
6–10	108	16.6	31.0	11.2	27.1	12.6	12.7
11–20	90	74.2	128.8	17.3	32.1	16.0	16.3
More than 20	234	62.7	80.6	22.9	32.2	13.3	13.6

Table V--continued

Sample size for multiple-person families with members 65 years of age and over and standard errors for Tables 5, 15, and 25, by selected characteristics: United States, 1980

Characteristic	Sample size	Standard errors of mean					
		Table 5		Table 15		Table 25	
		All families	Families with discharges	All families	Families with care	All families	Families with visits
Family health care coverage							
All members covered full year..........	717	$14.5	$36.9	$8.5	$22.7	$6.8	$7.2
Private insurance only...............	22	*68.7	*115.2	*22.8	*34.1	*84.2	*86.5
Medicaid only.......................	1	*0.0	*0.0	*0.0	*0.0	*0.0	*0.0
Medicare only.......................	47	*26.9	*81.2	*11.2	*39.4	*16.0	*17.8
Medicare and other public programs....	37	*42.7	*98.6	*14.8	*50.6	*12.8	*14.2
Medicare and private insurance.......	595	17.2	42.0	10.3	27.3	7.3	7.2
Other public and private mixes.......	7	*12.7	*19.0	*33.4	*0.0	*35.0	*35.6
Other mixes of public programs........	-	-	-	-	-	-	-
Source unknown.....................	8	*20.2	*42.7	*51.0	*103.4	*51.1	*59.6
All members covered, some part year.....	55	121.7	263.6	27.7	68.2	19.5	20.6
Some members not covered.............	82	172.9	395.6	33.1	93.6	9.8	9.9
All members not covered..............	6	*907.4	*0.0	*82.6	*0.0	*15.9	*22.4

[1]Average size during period of family's existence rounded to nearest integer; exactly half an integer rounded upward.
[2]There were too few Hispanic families of races other than white for separate tabulation.
[3]Annual rate.
[4]Includes only families with heads 17 years of age and over.
[5]Excludes families with all members under 14 years of age.
[6]Excludes families with all members with health status unknown.

NOTE: Multiple-person families are families with average size 1.5 or greater.

Table VI

Sample size for 1-person families and standard errors for Tables 6, 16, and 26, by selected characteristics: United States, 1980

Characteristic	Sample size	Standard errors of mean					
		Table 6		Table 16		Table 26	
		All families	Families with discharges	All families	Families with care	All families	Families with visits
Total...........................	1,904	$13.3	$87.7	$3.6	$31.0	$3.4	$4.3
Sex							
Male...........................	837	13.3	105.6	5.0	61.0	2.8	4.5
Female.........................	1,067	21.5	125.1	4.5	28.4	5.5	6.4
Race and ethnicity[1]							
White..........................	1,657	11.6	77.2	3.3	28.9	3.8	4.7
Hispanic....................	63	136.4	*624.9	0.7	*8.1	5.3	*7.9
Non-Hispanic................	1,594	10.8	72.1	3.4	29.7	3.9	4.9
Black..........................	198	77.9	486.0	12.2	111.3	9.3	13.0
Other..........................	49	*106.9	*895.8	*51.1	*471.6	*19.6	*31.9
Family dynamics							
Unchanging, full year..........	1,445	10.9	74.3	3.9	33.9	3.3	4.2
Change in composition or existed less than full year..............	459	67.5	398.6	8.2	59.9	9.5	15.3
Poverty status in 1980							
Below 150 percent poverty level..........	730	31.0	159.9	6.1	45.4	7.3	9.3
Below poverty level..........	425	32.9	178.8	6.4	51.2	10.0	13.5
Poverty level to 149 percent..........	305	58.1	276.5	11.2	76.4	6.5	7.7
150-199 percent................	228	39.5	279.9	7.3	60.2	6.7	9.1
200-299 percent................	393	36.8	325.1	9.8	88.4	5.8	8.0
300-499 percent................	368	7.9	54.8	6.3	55.9	4.3	5.1
500 percent or more............	185	3.6	29.7	3.4	35.9	9.3	13.3
Family income in 1980[2]							
Less than $10,000..............	1,114	23.6	129.0	6.0	42.4	5.1	6.6
$10,000-$19,999................	568	25.9	242.2	3.8	43.4	3.9	4.9
$20,000-$34,999................	169	3.7	30.2	6.3	65.8	9.0	11.8
$35,000 or more................	53	4.5	40.1	6.3	60.1	18.7	25.9

243

Table VI—continued

Sample size for 1-person families and standard errors for Tables 6, 16, and 26, by selected characteristics: United States, 1980

| | | Standard errors of mean | | | | | |
| | | Table 6 | | Table 16 | | Table 26 | |
Characteristic	Sample size	All families	Families with discharges	All families	Families with care	All families	Families with visits
Education[3]							
None or elementary school	370	$21.2	$98.6	$9.3	$51.9	$10.7	$13.8
Some high school	323	72.7	410.1	10.8	84.7	4.3	5.8
High school graduate	537	30.8	220.2	4.9	43.6	5.5	6.9
Some college	337	9.5	74.1	3.9	37.9	5.4	6.6
College graduate or more	323	18.0	150.0	9.4	102.2	8.2	10.3
Employment status[4]							
Worked full year	691	4.5	60.5	1.5	29.1	3.8	4.8
Worked part year	530	50.4	341.1	9.1	75.5	5.2	6.9
Never worked	678	16.2	71.3	6.5	36.6	7.4	9.2
Perceived health status[5]							
Excellent	807	15.7	166.3	4.7	65.7	3.9	5.0
Good	698	34.0	258.4	6.3	65.7	6.5	8.2
Fair	275	18.5	67.1	9.9	42.4	10.1	11.3
Poor	116	73.6	200.3	16.0	50.8	10.3	12.2
Limitation in usual activity							
None	1,576	10.8	93.9	3.3	39.9	3.5	4.6
Some limitation	63	47.1	147.7	23.2	92.8	22.3	26.9
Cannot perform usual activity	265	76.0	226.4	13.8	48.8	10.6	13.1
Bed days[2]							
0	921	0.6	48.9	1.4	231.3	4.0	5.7
1-5	466	1.4	14.0	1.0	15.2	4.9	5.9
6-10	196	43.7	145.8	7.6	34.1	7.5	8.4
11-20	135	116.7	278.5	22.6	69.3	18.2	21.3
More than 20	186	94.7	149.3	26.2	52.6	12.2	13.8

Family health care coverage

All members covered full year................	1,504	12.4	74.9	3.8	31.0	4.0	4.8
Private insurance only.....................	728	8.4	92.9	4.2	56.5	4.1	5.6
Medicaid only.............................	19	*0.0	*0.0	*0.0	*0.0	*3.4	*6.2
Medicare only.............................	106	58.1	304.9	19.4	132.1	31.6	46.0
Medicare and other public programs........	83	22.5	78.8	9.5	53.1	26.1	31.8
Medicare and private insurance............	389	44.0	171.3	12.4	56.8	7.9	8.4
Other public and private mixes............	95	57.5	280.7	14.5	99.4	12.0	13.5
Other mixes of public programs............	11	*0.0	*0.0	*0.0	*0.0	*13.9	*23.9
Source unknown............................	73	32.2	99.5	1.8	10.2	9.8	12.5
All members covered, some part year.......	225	20.9	168.7	5.3	70.3	7.3	10.0
Some members not covered..................	2	*2501.5	*2501.5	*90.7	*0.0	*50.8	*50.8
All members not covered...................	173	114.3	1495.9	14.3	238.7	6.6	11.6

[1]There were too few Hispanic families of races other than white for separate tabulation.
[2]Annual rate.
[3]Includes only families with heads 17 years of age and over.
[4]Excludes families with all members under 14 years of age.
[5]Excludes families with all members with health status unknown.

NOTE: 1-person families are families with average size less than 1.5. For 1-person families with more than 1 distinct individual, characteristics are those of head or of family as in Table 1.

Table VII

Sample size for 1-person families under 65 years of age and standard errors for Tables 7, 17, and 27, by selected characteristics: United States, 1980

Characteristic	Sample size	Standard errors of mean					
		Table 7		Table 17		Table 27	
		All families	Families with discharges	All families	Families with care	All families	Families with visits
Total..........	1,274	$17.3	$149.6	$3.4	$42.9	$3.2	$4.2
Age							
Under 25 years.........	422	22.0	245.8	1.9	28.1	4.7	6.4
25–44 years.........	466	36.7	310.7	7.0	87.0	4.6	5.9
45–64 years.........	386	17.0	137.4	5.2	54.9	5.1	7.3
Sex							
Male.........	678	15.1	156.2	4.2	83.4	3.3	5.2
Female.........	596	33.1	242.1	5.4	44.3	5.0	6.1
Race and ethnicity[1]							
White.........	1,094	14.4	130.4	2.4	30.2	3.3	4.3
Hispanic.........	52	166.7	*992.0	0.9	*11.6	5.4	*8.5
Non-Hispanic.........	1,042	12.9	117.9	2.5	31.2	3.4	4.4
Black.........	141	99.6	598.2	15.4	143.4	11.6	16.5
Other.........	39	*126.7	*1045.0	*60.6	*499.6	*21.8	*36.6
Family dynamics							
Unchanging, full year.........	885	15.4	129.3	3.9	47.8	3.6	4.7
Change in composition or existed less than full year.........	389	71.9	832.2	8.3	91.3	7.2	12.4
Poverty status in 1980							
Below 150 percent.........	388	54.2	321.4	8.0	79.5	4.7	6.9
Below poverty level.........	244	60.2	315.0	11.3	97.6	4.7	6.9
Poverty level to 149 percent.........	144	101.7	785.2	10.7	141.5	7.5	10.5
150–199 percent.........	136	58.8	564.4	6.0	69.2	8.2	12.4
200–299 percent.........	287	20.6	239.6	9.7	131.2	7.5	10.4
300–499 percent.........	305	7.8	68.7	3.5	42.1	4.8	5.8
500 percent or more.........	158	3.7	37.5	3.1	46.7	9.9	14.1
Family income in 1980[2]							
Less than $10,000.........	605	38.1	249.3	7.2	70.5	4.4	6.4
$10,000–$19,999.........	474	5.3	66.7	1.3	21.9	4.3	5.5
$20,000–$34,999.........	156	3.8	32.9	6.5	74.8	8.5	11.1
$35,000 or more.........	39	*0.0	*0.0	*0.0	*0.0	*23.3	*32.8

Education[3]							
None or elementary school	116	7.3	48.3	11.8	124.8	6.4	9.2
Some high school	204	107.6	706.9	13.1	138.3	5.4	8.5
High school graduate	406	21.1	164.1	3.5	32.6	4.2	5.1
Some college	274	9.6	102.9	4.2	54.8	6.1	7.3
College graduate or more	260	20.4	247.2	9.0	166.4	10.4	13.7
Employment status[4]							
Worked full year	657	4.7	65.6	1.6	32.8	4.0	5.1
Worked part year	458	48.5	340.1	9.0	79.7	5.3	7.4
Never worked	154	40.6	198.3	8.5	65.5	5.4	8.9
Perceived health status[5]							
Excellent	624	19.3	266.1	3.4	68.3	3.1	4.4
Good	471	36.3	361.1	6.3	87.5	6.6	8.8
Fair	121	22.7	86.9	10.5	53.4	5.8	6.5
Poor	52	100.5	308.8	27.3	111.3	18.5	25.3
Limitation in usual activity							
None	1,171	13.3	134.3	3.3	47.5	3.1	4.2
Some limitation	17	*133.2	*0.0	*64.9	*0.0	*57.0	*66.6
Cannot perform usual activity	86	162.0	609.6	18.7	99.9	13.0	18.4
Bed days[2]							
0	571	0.3	22.6	0.0	0.0	4.2	6.6
1-5	396	0.9	12.3	0.9	22.0	5.7	6.9
6-10	142	56.9	251.4	8.5	44.1	8.8	10.1
11-20	77	176.2	517.4	33.6	138.8	13.8	16.9
More than 20	88	151.6	264.3	30.9	74.6	9.0	10.1
Family health care coverage							
All members covered full year	890	9.5	80.2	3.7	44.0	3.5	4.6
Private insurance only	727	8.4	94.1	4.2	57.4	4.2	5.6
Medicaid only	19	*0.0	*0.0	*0.0	*0.0	*3.4	*6.2
Medicare only	7	*175.6	*0.0	*0.0	*0.0	*33.0	*48.4
Medicare and other public programs	–	–	–	–	–	–	–
Medicare and private insurance	–	–	–	–	–	–	–
Other public and private mixes	95	57.5	280.7	14.5	99.4	12.0	13.5
Other mixes of public programs	11	*0.0	*0.0	*0.0	*0.0	*13.9	*23.9
Source unknown	31	*65.5	*132.1	*3.1	*11.7	*12.9	*14.5
All members covered, some part year	225	20.9	168.7	5.3	70.3	7.3	10.0
Some members not covered	–	–	–	–	–	–	–
All members not covered	159	122.9	1682.5	15.3	253.8	6.9	12.3

[1] There were too few Hispanic of races other than white families for separate tabulation.
[2] Annual rate.
[3] Includes only families with heads 17 years of age and over.
[4] Excludes families with all members under 14 years of age.
[5] Excludes families with all members with health status unknown.

NOTE: 1-person families are families with average size less than 1.5. For 1-person families with more than 1 distinct individual, characteristics are those of head or of family as in Table 2.

Table VIII

Sample size for 1-person families under 65 years of age with health care coverage all year and standard errors for Tables 8, 18, and 28, by selected characteristics: United States, 1980

Characteristic	Sample size	Standard errors of mean					
		Table 8		Table 18		Table 28	
		All families	Families with discharges	All families	Families with care	All families	Families with visits
Total...............	890	$9.5	$80.2	$3.7	$44.0	$3.5	$4.6
Age							
Under 25 years............	256	5.5	54.8	2.4	28.0	4.8	5.9
25-44 years...............	324	17.6	143.0	7.4	94.1	5.3	6.6
45-64 years...............	310	17.8	140.2	5.8	59.1	5.8	7.6
Sex							
Male......................	457	13.4	123.1	5.9	96.0	4.3	6.3
Female....................	433	13.5	101.5	4.2	33.4	4.6	5.5
Race and ethnicity[1]							
White.....................	772	8.5	75.3	1.7	20.4	3.5	4.6
Hispanic..................	28	*0.0	*0.0	*1.5	*0.0	*8.6	*12.3
Non-Hispanic..............	744	8.8	74.2	1.7	20.8	3.6	4.7
Black.....................	93	9.5	52.2	16.7	142.6	15.6	18.9
Other.....................	25	*199.0	*1045.0	*95.1	*499.6	*34.3	*50.0
Family dynamics							
Unchanging, full year.....	636	10.9	85.9	4.2	47.7	4.0	5.1
Change in composition or existed less than full year........	254	17.9	205.7	8.1	90.6	4.6	8.0
Poverty status in 1980							
Below 150 percent.........	212	31.2	165.9	6.8	61.6	4.7	6.3
Below poverty level.......	135	48.5	198.4	11.6	80.5	6.5	8.7
Poverty level to 149 percent...	77	29.7	230.3	2.0	25.9	6.6	8.7
150-199 percent...........	78	10.9	79.4	2.6	34.5	13.0	19.5
200-299 percent...........	207	27.5	264.1	13.6	146.5	7.4	9.6
300-499 percent...........	257	9.1	74.9	4.1	45.0	4.5	5.9
500 percent or more.......	136	3.3	38.1	3.0	43.1	11.6	16.1
Family income in 1980[2]							
Less than $10,000.........	343	24.6	145.6	9.3	82.4	4.8	7.2
$10,000-$19,999...........	380	6.6	66.7	1.7	21.9	4.3	5.6
$20,000-$34,999...........	132	3.4	37.6	7.4	89.9	10.0	12.8
$35,000 or more...........	35	*0.0	*0.0	*0.0	*0.0	*27.1	*37.0

248

Education[3]

None or elementary school	86	9.7	48.3	15.6	124.8	6.8	9.2
Some high school	130	55.6	388.4	3.4	30.6	5.0	6.9
High school graduate	281	5.1	41.4	2.8	28.6	4.5	5.4
Some college	192	6.5	56.9	5.6	59.4	5.5	6.8
College graduate or more	194	27.1	285.2	12.0	178.6	10.4	13.8

Employment status[4]

Worked full year	503	4.8	58.4	2.1	33.3	3.6	4.6
Worked part year	269	22.5	161.5	11.6	103.1	7.8	10.5
Never worked	117	49.8	198.9	10.7	66.6	6.6	9.6

Perceived health status[5]

Excellent	448	6.1	86.5	1.3	24.1	3.5	5.2
Good	308	18.0	164.5	8.7	109.3	7.7	9.9
Fair	91	3.2	13.1	4.9	26.8	5.2	5.5
Poor	37	*150.4	*327.9	*37.0	*111.3	*24.9	*31.3

Limitation in usual activity

None	806	7.6	74.1	3.8	51.4	3.6	4.9
Some limitation	12	*0.0	-	*0.0	-	*22.5	*23.0
Cannot perform usual activity	72	72.6	256.9	16.3	76.3	14.7	20.6

Bed days[2]

0	388	0.0	0.0	0.0	-	5.8	8.4
1-5	289	1.2	16.3	1.1	23.0	4.8	5.9
6-10	91	8.1	30.8	6.5	31.6	8.1	8.5
11-20	60	82.0	226.7	38.6	138.2	15.8	19.5
More than 20	62	104.6	172.8	28.9	66.1	10.4	11.0

Family health care coverage

Private insurance only	727	8.4	94.1	4.2	57.4	4.2	5.6
Medicaid only	19	*0.0	*0.0	*0.0	*0.0	*3.4	*6.2
Medicare only	7	*175.6	*0.0	*0.0	*0.0	*33.0	*48.4
Medicare and other public programs	-	-	-	-	-	-	-
Medicare and private insurance	-	-	-	-	-	-	-
Other public and private mixes	95	57.5	280.7	14.5	99.4	12.0	13.5
Other mixes of public programs	11	*0.0	*0.0	*0.0	*0.0	*0.0	*23.9
Source unknown	31	*65.5	*132.1	*3.1	*11.7	*12.9	*14.5

[1]There were too few Hispanic families of races other than white for separate tabulation.
[2]Annual rate.
[3]Includes only families with heads 17 years of age and over.
[4]Excludes families with all members under 14 years of age.
[5]Excludes families with all members with health status unknown.

NOTE: 1-person families are families with average size less than 1.5. For 1-person families with more than 1 distinct individual, characteristics are those of head or of family as in Table 2.

Table IX

Sample size for 1-person families under 65 years of age without health care coverage all year and standard errors for Tables 9, 19, and 29, by selected characteristics: United States, 1980

| | | Standard errors of mean | | | | | |
| | | Table 9 | | Table 19 | | Table 29 | |
Characteristic	Sample size	All families	Families with discharges	All families	Families with care	All families	Families with visits
Total.........	384	$53.5	$552.1	$7.3	$109.0	$5.4	$8.0
Age							
Under 25 years......	166	55.4	751.4	3.1	70.8	9.8	15.0
25–44 years......	142	110.3	1070.5	15.1	188.1	7.1	10.8
45–64 years......	76	46.7	349.9	12.2	102.9	9.4	16.9
Sex							
Male........	221	37.1	500.0	2.6	104.2	4.7	9.0
Female......	163	120.0	905.5	17.3	137.9	11.0	13.2
Race and ethnicity[1]							
White.......	322	43.4	444.5	7.0	105.9	6.1	8.5
Hispanic....	24	*388.1	*1474.6	*0.0	*0.0	*4.9	*9.3
Non-Hispanic..	298	38.3	428.8	7.5	112.3	6.4	8.8
Black.......	48	*308.5	*2450.2	*33.5	*392.1	*20.1	*34.4
Other.......	14	*0.0	–	*0.0	–	*5.9	*7.2
Family dynamics							
Unchanging, full year......	249	45.2	453.4	7.8	130.9	5.5	8.0
Change in composition or existed less than full year......	135	200.0	2020.9	17.9	184.0	15.2	26.0
Poverty status in 1980							
Below 150 percent......	176	112.8	872.8	15.3	177.1	7.4	11.8
Below poverty level......	109	118.1	923.8	20.4	244.1	6.8	10.9
Poverty level to 149 percent......	67	214.6	1583.8	22.3	241.7	14.4	21.1
150–199 percent......	58	138.2	*1450.8	13.8	*130.1	7.0	*10.5
200–299 percent......	80	20.5	526.9	1.8	55.6	18.2	27.8
300–499 percent......	48	*0.9	*8.5	*0.0	*0.0	*18.1	*22.8
500 percent or more......	22	*16.6	*95.7	*12.8	*0.0	*12.3	*15.4
Family income in 1980[2]							
Less than $10,000......	262	81.6	695.8	11.1	122.6	6.4	9.5
$10,000–$19,999......	94	0.0	–	0.0	–	12.2	16.9
$20,000–$34,999......	24	*14.9	*66.8	*11.5	*107.0	*10.9	*14.5
$35,000 or more......	4	*0.0	*0.0	*0.0	–	*10.7	*12.6

Education[3]						
None or elementary school	30	*0.0	–	*0.0	–	*10.1	*22.7
Some high school	74	257.5	*1526.2	32.3	*339.4	12.2	*22.8
High school graduate	125	70.2	485.5	9.6	75.3	7.3	10.3
Some college	82	29.6	404.2	9.2	172.2	17.6	22.7
College graduate or more	66	0.0	0.0	2.7	0.0	16.8	24.9
Employment status[4]						
Worked full year	154	12.8	294.5	0.0	0.0	11.4	17.8
Worked part year	189	108.7	714.7	14.6	114.2	5.4	7.7
Never worked	37	*61.0	*1083.0	*9.6	*0.0	*6.7	*18.9
Perceived health status[5]						
Excellent	176	66.1	689.3	11.3	198.8	5.1	8.1
Good	163	103.0	1334.6	7.7	160.2	12.2	19.6
Fair	30	*89.3	*305.1	*38.7	*127.1	*15.4	*18.4
Poor	15	*0.0	*0.0	*0.0	–	*16.9	*28.2
Limitation in usual activity						
None	365	38.2	405.5	6.1	100.8	5.7	8.3
Some limitation	5	*312.6	*0.0	*152.4	*0.0	*143.1	*173.7
Cannot perform usual activity	14	*1167.1	*7766.5	*95.9	*1118.8	*8.6	*13.0
Bed days[2]						
0	183	0.9	40.7	0.0	0.0	4.3	9.6
1–5	107	0.0	0.0	1.9	60.8	12.0	15.0
6–10	51	144.5	*781.8	19.6	*105.1	19.0	*24.5
11–20	17	*898.7	*3432.0	*76.7	*613.5	*23.1	*28.7
More than 20	26	*450.4	*853.5	*85.3	*225.0	*15.6	*18.0
Family health care coverage						
All members covered, some part year	225	20.9	168.7	5.3	70.3	7.3	10.0
Some members not covered	–	–	–	–	–	–	–
All members not covered	159	122.9	1682.5	15.3	253.8	6.9	12.3

[1] There were too few Hispanic families of races other than white for separate tabulation.
[2] Annual rate.
[3] Includes only families with heads 17 years of age and over.
[4] Excludes families with all members under 14 years of age.
[5] Excludes families with all members with health status unknown.

NOTE: 1-person families are families with average size less than 1.5. For 1-person families with more than 1 distinct individual, characteristics are those of head or of family as in Table 2.

Table X

Sample size for 1-person families 65 years of age and over and standard errors for Tables 10, 20, and 30, by selected characteristics: United States, 1980

Characteristic	Sample size	Standard errors of mean					
		Table 10		Table 20		Table 30	
		All families	Families with discharges	All families	Families with care	All families	Families with visits
Total...........	630	$20.3	$83.3	$7.6	$41.7	$9.0	$10.7
Sex							
Male...........	159	25.6	82.8	23.5	84.2	7.8	9.9
Female.........	471	25.3	113.7	6.9	40.4	11.4	13.4
Race and ethnicity[1]							
White..........	563	22.2	88.5	8.3	45.8	9.8	11.5
Hispanic.......	11	*0.0	*0.0	*0.0	*0.0	*12.3	*14.0
Non-Hispanic...	552	22.5	90.5	8.6	47.0	10.2	11.8
Black..........	57	4.4	*19.9	0.0	*0.0	6.6	*8.9
Other..........	10	*0.0	*0.0	*0.0	*0.0	*53.5	*84.7
Family dynamics							
Unchanging, full year.......	560	8.6	38.3	8.0	45.8	7.8	9.1
Change in composition or existed less than full year.......	70	217.2	395.7	30.4	90.8	38.3	48.0
Poverty status in 1980							
Below 150 percent poverty level.....	342	23.3	95.7	9.8	54.9	14.8	17.0
Below poverty level...........	181	16.1	92.3	2.0	14.2	21.9	26.3
Poverty level to 149 percent.....	161	46.6	143.9	19.5	85.1	10.9	11.5
150-199 percent.....	92	37.1	181.0	15.3	85.2	12.2	14.2
200-299 percent.....	106	160.7	697.2	25.8	132.1	8.4	11.2
300-499 percent.....	63	23.8	78.6	36.8	117.3	10.4	12.2
500 percent or more.....	27	*12.7	*40.7	*16.6	*43.6	*35.1	*42.0
Family income in 1980[2]							
Less than $10,000.....	509	18.2	76.9	8.3	49.1	10.5	12.5
$10,000-$19,999.....	94	177.0	639.2	25.1	96.5	9.3	10.6
$20,000-$34,999.....	13	*14.4	*54.5	*17.9	*62.2	*62.0	*88.1
$35,000 or more.....	14	*19.8	*54.5	*25.5	*55.9	*39.0	*41.6

Education

None or elementary school	254	33.0	127.1	12.4	59.2	16.6	19.1
Some high school	119	16.1	74.2	17.4	94.9	9.9	12.8
High school graduate	131	129.0	679.6	11.9	111.2	18.1	21.4
Some college	63	31.3	101.6	9.5	42.8	11.7	14.9
College graduate or more	63	18.3	59.5	20.4	74.7	14.3	15.1

Employment status

Worked full year	34	*8.6	*48.6	*1.8	*10.1	*15.9	*18.7
Worked part year	72	242.0	1163.1	30.7	174.5	14.4	17.6
Never worked	524	16.8	67.0	8.1	43.8	9.6	11.4

Perceived health status[3]

Excellent	183	8.4	46.8	17.6	114.1	12.8	15.9
Good	227	76.9	364.4	13.6	86.5	14.4	16.7
Fair	154	29.3	102.3	17.1	60.7	18.5	20.6
Poor	64	107.5	240.9	17.2	48.0	7.5	8.5

Limitation in usual activity

None	405	12.6	68.5	8.8	67.9	10.7	13.2
Some limitation	46	*41.8	*104.8	*18.1	*62.9	*21.0	*24.9
Cannot perform usual activity	179	70.2	172.0	18.3	56.2	15.1	17.7

Bed days[2]

0	350	1.7	98.2	4.1	317.5	8.7	11.0
1-5	70	8.7	28.5	4.4	20.3	8.8	9.4
6-10	54	32.5	67.3	11.0	37.7	13.6	14.4
11-20	58	83.7	138.9	20.2	40.4	42.0	43.2
More than 20	98	129.4	181.6	41.6	73.8	23.8	25.4

Family health care coverage

All members covered full year	614	29.7	122.2	7.6	42.1	9.1	10.8
Private insurance only	1	*0.0	*0.0	*0.0	*0.0	*0.0	*0.0
Medicaid only	-	-	-	-	-	-	-
Medicare only	99	60.6	324.2	20.9	143.1	34.4	49.3
Medicare and other public programs	83	22.5	78.8	9.5	53.1	26.1	31.8
Medicare and private insurance	389	44.0	171.3	12.4	56.8	7.9	8.4
Other public and private mixes	-	-	-	-	-	-	-
Other mixes of public programs	-	-	-	-	-	-	-
Source unknown	42	*5.6	*28.7	*2.1	*9.8	*13.0	*18.6
All members covered, some part year	-	-	-	-	-	-	-
Some members not covered	2	*2501.5	*2501.5	*90.7	*0.0	*50.8	*50.8
All members not covered	14	*97.5	*315.8	*15.4	*0.0	*8.5	*13.1

[1]There were too few Hispanic families of races other than white for separate tabulation.
[2]Annual rate.
[3]Excludes families with all members with health status unknown.

NOTE: 1-person families are families with average size less than 1.5. For 1-person families with more than 1 distinct individual, characteristics are those of head or of family as in Table 2.

Table XI

Standard errors for Tables 31, 41, 51, and 61, by selected characteristics: United States, 1980

Standard errors of mean

Characteristic	Table 31		Table 41		Table 51		Table 61	
	All families	Families with visits	All families	Families with visits	All families	Families with ac-quisitions	All families	Families using health care
Total............	$1.8	$2.8	$6.7	$8.3	$2.2	$2.3	$14.3	$14.3
Family size[1]								
2 persons........	2.2	4.3	7.7	11.3	3.3	3.5	22.2	22.8
3 persons........	2.7	4.3	8.2	11.0	3.3	3.4	17.3	17.4
4 persons........	5.9	8.8	14.8	17.4	3.5	3.6	23.0	23.0
5 or more persons......	4.3	5.2	19.1	21.9	3.9	4.1	40.8	40.9
Age of head								
Under 25 years.......	4.3	6.2	8.9	13.8	1.8	2.0	33.6	33.9
25-44 years..........	3.2	4.6	9.8	12.2	2.0	2.1	20.2	20.1
45-64 years..........	1.9	3.0	9.6	11.5	3.5	3.7	19.9	20.0
65 years and over....	4.4	8.8	10.4	15.9	6.2	6.4	39.3	40.3
Sex of head								
Male.................	1.7	2.6	8.2	10.1	2.2	2.3	17.2	17.3
Female...............	5.6	8.5	8.8	12.8	4.5	4.8	29.9	30.4
Race and ethnicity[2] of head								
White................	2.1	3.1	7.6	9.4	2.4	2.5	15.3	15.2
Hispanic.............	7.1	10.1	26.8	40.8	6.5	6.8	59.3	59.7
Non-Hispanic.........	2.3	3.5	7.9	9.6	2.6	2.7	15.1	15.1
Black................	4.5	6.3	10.4	16.7	4.2	4.7	37.9	38.6
Other................	9.6	15.5	38.9	50.5	4.7	5.2	71.3	71.8
Family structure								
Head and spouse present whole time......	1.8	2.6	8.8	10.9	2.1	2.2	17.9	17.9
Child under 17 years......	2.3	2.9	12.9	15.1	2.3	2.4	20.9	21.0
No child under 17 years...	2.2	4.3	9.2	12.9	3.1	3.2	23.2	23.4
Head only, no spouse at any time.....	5.1	8.0	8.3	12.8	4.3	4.8	36.3	37.0
Child under 17 years......	7.8	11.0	10.4	14.8	3.6	3.8	46.0	46.4
No child under 17 years...	3.9	7.5	12.1	21.3	7.7	8.8	49.2	51.0
Other................	14.4	19.5	26.0	36.0	14.5	14.6	88.1	88.6
Family dynamics								
Unchanging, full year.......	1.6	2.5	8.1	10.4	2.5	2.6	18.7	18.7
Change in composition or existed less than full year......	6.4	8.9	11.1	15.5	3.4	3.5	28.7	29.1

Family poverty status in 1980

Below 150 percent poverty level	3.3	4.9	8.6	13.2	4.4	5.0	25.3	26.0
Below poverty level	5.3	7.6	10.1	17.1	4.3	4.9	24.5	25.5
Poverty level to 149 percent	4.3	6.2	14.4	20.9	6.5	6.7	46.4	47.2
150-199 percent	10.6	17.6	13.8	20.6	6.9	7.3	69.9	70.4
200-299 percent	2.5	3.5	12.3	17.8	5.0	5.3	23.6	23.9
300-499 percent	2.5	3.9	12.5	15.1	2.8	2.9	18.8	19.2
500 percent or more	2.9	4.9	16.1	18.4	2.5	2.7	25.6	25.9

Family income in 1980[3]

Less than $10,000	3.5	5.5	7.3	13.7	5.7	6.3	31.1	31.9
$10,000-$19,999	4.2	7.1	8.1	12.4	4.0	4.0	27.9	28.1
$20,000-$34,999	2.5	3.7	9.1	11.3	2.4	2.6	18.2	18.3
$35,000 or more	3.6	5.3	17.5	19.1	2.8	2.9	28.4	28.2

Education of head[4]

None or elementary school	4.9	8.2	7.4	13.5	5.1	5.5	26.6	26.7
Some high school	7.9	12.1	9.3	13.7	4.6	4.8	37.9	38.0
High school graduate	2.1	3.1	9.6	12.1	2.9	3.1	19.4	19.5
Some college	3.1	4.6	20.0	23.6	3.6	3.8	27.4	27.4
College graduate or more	3.5	5.9	20.6	21.8	3.3	3.5	42.3	42.4

Family employment status[5]

2 or more persons worked full year	2.5	3.8	13.6	17.2	2.8	3.0	22.3	22.4
Only 1 person worked full year	3.5	5.9	8.7	11.3	2.2	2.3	22.7	22.9
Some part-year work	3.7	5.4	8.1	11.3	4.1	4.4	31.3	31.3
No person worked	2.7	4.8	11.5	19.5	7.0	7.4	41.8	42.9

Worst perceived health status of any family member[6]

Excellent	2.1	3.6	13.7	17.0	1.4	1.5	17.9	17.8
Good	2.0	3.1	8.7	11.2	2.5	2.6	19.7	19.8
Fair	6.7	9.6	8.9	12.8	4.7	4.9	31.6	31.9
Poor	6.4	8.3	14.7	22.0	8.8	9.1	70.0	70.9

Most severe limitation in usual activity of any family member

None	2.3	3.7	7.8	9.7	1.7	1.8	14.6	14.6
Some limitation	8.8	12.7	21.1	29.7	6.3	6.4	64.9	64.9
Cannot perform usual activity	3.6	4.8	11.0	15.9	6.9	7.1	39.1	39.5

Family's bed days[3]

0	2.1	5.3	12.7	18.0	3.5	4.2	16.0	16.3
1-5	1.9	3.4	8.1	11.6	2.3	2.4	12.7	13.0
6-10	3.6	5.3	15.3	19.3	3.5	3.7	23.5	23.3
11-20	2.9	4.1	14.1	18.6	2.8	2.9	29.9	30.0
More than 20	5.9	7.2	14.8	18.9	5.8	5.9	42.6	42.6

Table XI--continued

Standard errors for Tables 31, 41, 51, and 61, by selected characteristics: United States, 1980

Standard errors of mean

Characteristic	Table 31		Table 41		Table 51		Table 61	
	All families	Families with visits	All families	Families with visits	All families	Families with acquisitions	All families	Families using health care
Family health care coverage								
All members covered full year..........	$1.5	$2.2	$8.5	$10.3	$2.3	$2.5	$15.7	$15.9
Private insurance only.............	1.9	3.0	12.4	14.6	1.9	2.0	22.0	22.2
Medicaid only.....................	2.7	4.0	9.0	13.2	4.7	5.1	31.8	32.1
Medicare only....................	*5.6	*16.7	*11.8	*24.0	*14.2	*15.2	*45.2	*44.7
Medicare and other public programs....	*5.3	*8.3	*14.4	*38.0	*13.9	*14.3	*79.3	*79.3
Medicare and private insurance.......	4.0	7.3	13.6	20.1	7.2	7.2	33.0	32.9
Other public and private mixes........	3.7	4.9	15.5	19.4	4.9	5.1	31.5	31.8
Other mixes of public programs........	*1.9	*2.7	*57.2	*63.7	*16.6	*16.5	*89.9	*89.9
Source unknown...................	*8.5	*10.3	*12.5	*16.7	*15.1	*15.4	*177.5	*177.5
All members covered, some part year.....	3.9	6.2	11.9	16.5	4.6	4.8	30.0	30.0
Some members not covered.............	15.7	25.9	9.7	15.1	6.4	6.9	79.7	81.9
All members not covered.............	8.5	12.9	12.0	21.5	3.8	5.0	52.7	56.0

1 Average size during period of family's existence rounded to nearest integer; exactly half an integer rounded upward.
2 There were too few Hispanic families of races other than white for separate tabulation.
3 Annual rate.
4 Includes only families with heads 17 years of age and over.
5 Excludes families with all members under 14 years of age.
6 Excludes families with all members with health status unknown.

NOTE: Multiple-person families are families with average size 1.5 or greater.

Table XII

Standard errors for Tables 32, 42, 52, and 62, by selected characteristics: United States, 1980

| | Standard errors of mean | | | | | | | |
| | Table 32 | | Table 42 | | Table 52 | | Table 62 | |
Characteristic	All families	Families with visits	All families	Families with visits	All families	Families with ac-quisitions	All families	Families using health care
Total......	$2.0	$3.0	$7.3	$9.1	$1.7	$1.8	$15.3	$15.3
Family size[1]								
2 persons......	2.8	5.4	9.3	13.4	3.0	3.4	28.7	29.3
3 persons......	2.5	4.0	8.5	11.3	2.9	3.0	16.3	16.2
4 persons......	6.1	9.1	14.4	16.8	2.8	2.9	25.6	25.6
5 or more persons......	4.6	5.6	20.4	23.3	3.1	3.3	42.0	42.1
Age of head								
Under 25 years......	4.3	6.2	8.9	13.8	1.8	2.0	33.8	34.1
25-44 years......	3.2	4.7	10.0	12.4	1.9	2.1	20.4	20.4
45-64 years......	2.0	3.3	9.4	11.1	3.3	3.4	23.0	23.0
Sex of head								
Male......	2.0	3.0	9.2	11.0	1.9	1.9	16.4	16.4
Female......	6.3	9.1	10.3	14.8	2.8	3.1	34.4	35.0
Race and ethnicity[2] of head								
White......	2.3	3.4	8.4	10.3	1.8	1.9	16.0	16.0
Hispanic......	7.3	10.5	28.0	41.2	5.7	5.9	62.7	63.7
Non-Hispanic......	2.5	3.9	8.9	10.7	1.9	2.0	16.3	16.2
Black......	4.3	5.7	12.1	19.0	3.8	4.2	39.1	39.6
Other......	11.8	18.3	39.3	50.4	4.4	4.7	85.1	86.0
Family structure								
Head and spouse present whole time......	2.0	2.9	9.6	11.6	1.7	1.8	16.4	16.4
Child under 17 years......	2.3	2.9	13.2	15.5	1.9	2.1	21.0	21.2
No child under 17 years......	2.9	5.8	10.4	13.7	2.8	3.0	21.9	21.8
Head only, no spouse at any time......	6.2	9.3	9.5	14.2	3.3	3.7	42.8	43.6
Child under 17 years......	8.1	11.4	10.9	15.5	3.0	3.3	48.9	49.4
No child under 17 years......	5.9	11.0	19.3	32.3	8.0	9.1	70.3	73.8
Other......	11.2	16.2	21.8	26.8	14.3	14.3	82.2	82.2
Family dynamics								
Unchanging, full year......	1.7	2.7	9.2	11.5	1.8	1.9	17.8	17.8
Change in composition or existed less than full year......	7.0	9.8	9.2	12.7	3.3	3.4	30.9	31.1

257

Table XII—continued

Standard errors for Tables 32, 42, 52, and 62, by selected characteristics: United States, 1980

Standard errors of mean

Characteristic	Table 32		Table 42		Table 52		Table 62	
	All families	Families with visits	All families	Families with visits	All families	Families with ac-quisitions	All families	Families using health care
Family poverty status in 1980								
Below 150 percent poverty level......	$3.4	$4.9	$10.4	$14.8	$3.1	$3.4	$29.8	$30.1
Below poverty level.................	4.9	6.8	12.2	19.1	3.9	4.4	25.7	25.9
Poverty level to 149 percent........	5.2	7.1	17.5	23.4	4.3	4.5	56.5	57.1
150–199 percent.....................	13.9	21.7	17.8	25.3	5.3	5.6	71.5	72.1
200–299 percent.....................	2.7	3.5	14.6	20.1	4.3	4.6	24.5	24.9
300–499 percent.....................	2.8	4.2	13.3	15.8	2.5	2.6	20.1	20.5
500 percent or more.................	3.2	5.7	16.5	19.1	2.7	2.9	30.8	31.2
Family income in 1980[3]								
Less than $10,000...................	4.0	5.5	10.5	17.0	3.8	4.3	33.5	33.9
$10,000–$19,999.....................	5.3	8.4	9.8	14.9	3.4	3.6	33.1	33.4
$20,000–$34,999.....................	2.4	3.5	9.9	12.4	2.1	2.3	19.1	19.1
$35,000 or more.....................	3.7	5.5	18.9	20.7	2.9	3.0	30.6	30.7
Education of head[4]								
None or elementary school...........	5.9	8.9	11.9	20.4	3.6	3.9	32.0	32.3
Some high school....................	9.4	13.9	10.2	14.4	3.4	3.6	28.8	28.9
High school graduate................	2.2	3.2	9.7	12.6	2.8	2.9	21.4	21.3
Some college........................	3.6	5.2	20.7	24.3	2.8	3.0	26.3	26.2
College graduate or more............	3.5	5.5	21.3	22.6	3.0	3.1	47.6	47.7
Family employment status[5]								
2 or more persons worked full year...	2.6	4.0	14.8	18.5	2.2	2.3	23.8	24.0
Only 1 person worked full year......	4.0	6.5	8.6	11.1	2.3	2.4	22.7	22.9
Some part-year work.................	4.1	5.6	10.8	14.2	4.0	4.3	38.1	38.2
No person worked....................	4.8	7.1	23.7	36.1	5.6	6.1	52.1	52.3
Worst perceived health status of any family member[6]								
Excellent...........................	1.9	3.1	14.2	17.8	1.4	1.5	18.7	18.6
Good................................	2.2	3.4	8.9	11.3	2.2	2.3	21.3	21.5
Fair................................	9.0	12.2	11.0	14.8	4.0	4.1	43.6	43.7
Poor................................	7.5	8.7	16.8	21.7	10.4	10.5	83.9	83.9

Most severe limitation in usual activity of any family member

None..........................	2.4	3.8	8.1	10.0	1.6	1.7	15.9	15.9
Some limitation...............	7.2	9.7	24.7	34.4	7.4	7.5	75.7	75.7
Cannot perform usual activity.	5.3	6.3	15.7	21.0	8.1	8.3	52.1	52.4

Family's bed days[3]

0.............................	2.8	6.4	12.6	16.9	3.3	3.8	17.9	18.1
1-5...........................	2.2	3.7	9.1	12.4	2.1	2.1	14.4	14.6
6-10..........................	3.9	5.7	16.8	21.1	2.8	2.8	25.1	24.9
11-20.........................	2.6	3.7	14.5	18.6	2.9	3.1	33.6	33.8
More than 20..................	6.9	8.3	18.5	22.6	4.2	4.3	46.0	46.0

Family health care coverage

All members covered full year....	1.7	2.5	9.7	11.7	1.8	1.9	19.0	19.1
Private insurance only...........	1.9	2.9	12.6	14.8	1.8	1.9	22.1	22.2
Medicaid only....................	2.8	4.1	9.1	13.4	4.8	5.2	30.4	30.8
Medicare only....................	—	—	—	—	—	—	—	—
Medicare and other public programs....	*0.0	*0.0	*0.0	—	*0.0	*0.0	*0.0	*0.0
Medicare and private insurance....	*15.3	*27.8	*2.1	*4.9	*31.6	*31.6	*108.1	*108.1
Other public and private mixes....	3.7	5.0	15.5	19.5	4.7	4.8	33.3	33.3
Other mixes of public programs....	*1.9	*2.7	*57.2	*63.7	*16.6	*16.5	*89.9	*89.9
Source unknown....................	*9.9	*11.0	*14.9	*18.0	*13.1	*13.5	*214.0	*214.0
All members covered, some part year....	4.0	6.3	12.5	17.2	4.7	4.9	29.6	29.5
Some members not covered..........	19.4	30.1	12.9	19.1	6.4	7.0	75.5	76.8
All members not covered...........	8.8	12.9	12.5	22.2	3.9	4.9	40.2	42.6

[1] Average size during period of family's existence rounded to nearest integer; exactly half an integer rounded upward.
[2] There were too few Hispanic families of races other than white for separate tabulation.
[3] Annual rate.
[4] Includes only families with heads 17 years of age and over.
[5] Excludes families with all members under 14 years of age.
[6] Excludes families with all members with health status unknown.

NOTE: Multiple-person families are families with average size 1.5 or greater.

Table XIII

Standard errors for Tables 33, 43, 53, and 63, by selected characteristics: United States, 1980

	Standard errors of mean							
	Table 33		Table 43		Table 53		Table 63	
Characteristic	All families	Families with visits	All families	Families with visits	All families	Families with acquisitions	All families	Families using health care
Total	$1.7	$2.5	$9.7	$11.7	$1.8	$1.9	$19.0	$19.1
Family size[1]								
2 persons	3.1	5.9	12.1	16.7	3.8	4.2	35.7	36.4
3 persons	2.1	3.3	11.8	14.7	3.2	3.3	19.0	18.8
4 persons	2.9	4.1	17.3	19.8	3.0	3.0	31.1	31.2
5 or more persons	2.6	3.5	27.8	30.4	3.5	3.7	41.1	41.1
Age of head								
Under 25 years	3.6	4.9	9.6	13.6	2.3	2.4	45.3	45.6
25–44 years	2.3	3.3	13.8	16.0	1.6	1.7	25.6	25.7
45–64 years	2.1	3.7	11.8	14.3	4.0	4.2	25.2	25.1
Sex of head								
Male	1.9	3.0	11.2	13.2	2.0	2.1	20.5	20.6
Female	2.3	3.4	17.5	22.5	2.9	3.2	29.9	30.4
Race and ethnicity[2] of head								
White	1.8	2.7	10.7	12.8	1.9	2.0	19.4	19.5
Hispanic	6.8	11.2	41.0	56.5	6.9	7.1	101.1	101.4
Non-Hispanic	1.9	2.8	11.0	13.1	1.9	2.1	19.4	19.5
Black	3.4	4.7	18.7	26.2	4.5	5.1	56.9	57.7
Other	12.3	19.5	58.0	68.9	5.1	5.3	118.6	120.7
Family structure								
Head and spouse present whole time	2.0	3.0	11.8	13.9	1.9	2.0	19.6	19.6
Child under 17 years	2.1	2.8	16.2	18.3	1.8	1.9	24.8	24.8
No child under 17 years	3.1	6.0	12.8	16.5	3.7	4.0	25.9	25.9
Head only, no spouse at any time	2.2	3.3	16.5	21.7	3.6	4.1	52.8	53.8
Child under 17 years	2.9	4.1	17.7	22.8	3.5	3.8	52.7	53.4
No child under 17 years	3.6	6.2	35.7	51.8	10.6	12.3	143.6	149.2
Other	11.5	14.9	27.9	34.4	11.4	11.4	109.2	109.2
Family dynamics								
Unchanging, full year	1.7	2.7	11.3	13.6	1.9	2.1	20.3	20.4
Change in composition or existed less than full year	4.2	6.3	12.6	16.3	3.8	4.0	47.5	47.9

Family poverty status in 1980

Below 150 percent poverty level	3.2	4.5	16.7	21.3	3.9	4.2	54.0	54.6

Category								
Below 150 percent poverty level	3.2	4.5	16.7	21.3	3.9	4.2	54.0	54.6
Below poverty level	4.1	5.5	17.7	24.4	4.9	5.3	32.3	32.4
Poverty level to 149 percent	5.8	7.8	33.5	40.1	6.4	6.7	120.2	122.7
150-199 percent	4.5	6.8	30.5	42.4	7.4	7.9	84.5	84.9
200-299 percent	2.9	4.0	18.6	23.5	3.5	3.7	24.8	24.9
300-499 percent	2.5	3.7	15.9	18.9	2.5	2.7	22.6	23.0
500 percent or more	3.5	6.3	19.1	21.7	2.9	3.1	36.1	36.5

Family income in 1980[3]

Category								
Less than $10,000	3.6	5.1	15.8	22.2	5.3	5.8	61.9	62.7
$10,000-$19,999	3.4	5.4	14.3	20.5	3.9	4.1	35.1	35.3
$20,000-$34,999	2.0	2.9	11.9	14.9	2.1	2.3	19.5	19.6
$35,000 or more	3.6	5.7	22.7	24.1	3.0	3.0	37.6	37.6

Education of head[4]

Category								
None or elementary school	4.3	7.4	17.4	26.9	5.1	5.1	37.5	37.7
Some high school	4.1	6.1	14.3	18.3	4.0	4.3	27.3	27.3
High school graduate	1.9	2.9	12.9	15.8	2.8	2.9	21.9	21.9
Some college	3.1	4.6	26.2	30.3	3.2	3.5	32.1	32.1
College graduate or more	4.3	6.7	23.9	25.0	3.2	3.4	57.2	57.2

Family employment status[5]

Category								
2 or more persons worked full year	2.0	3.1	18.5	22.3	2.7	2.8	27.5	27.6
Only 1 person worked full year	2.6	4.0	11.1	13.8	2.4	2.6	27.2	27.5
Some part-year work	2.7	3.9	15.6	19.1	4.3	4.5	29.0	29.0
No person worked	4.2	6.4	31.8	45.5	6.6	7.0	69.5	69.5

Worst perceived health status of any family member[6]

Category								
Excellent	2.5	3.9	17.4	20.8	1.7	1.8	21.8	22.0
Good	1.8	2.8	11.3	13.9	2.2	2.3	21.4	21.4
Fair	3.5	4.7	15.2	19.5	4.9	5.1	57.6	57.8
Poor	9.7	11.9	31.0	41.6	12.9	13.4	116.4	116.4

Most severe limitation in usual activity of any family member

Category								
None	1.7	2.6	10.5	12.6	1.6	1.8	18.6	18.7
Some limitation	9.1	12.4	30.3	39.7	9.0	9.3	96.4	96.4
Cannot perform usual activity	6.2	8.0	22.7	29.9	9.4	9.7	63.6	63.9

Family's bed days[3]

Category								
0	1.9	4.0	15.9	20.6	4.0	4.6	21.9	21.7
1-5	2.1	3.6	11.6	14.7	2.4	2.5	18.0	18.3
6-10	2.7	4.0	21.0	25.1	2.7	2.8	28.3	28.2
11-20	2.9	3.8	17.9	22.7	3.9	4.1	27.0	27.1
More than 20	4.6	5.4	25.1	29.1	4.2	4.3	59.5	59.5

Table XIII--continued

Standard errors for Tables 33, 43, 53, and 63, by selected characteristics: United States, 1980

Standard errors of mean

Characteristic	Table 33		Table 43		Table 53		Table 63	
	All families	Families with visits	All families	Families with visits	All families	Families with acquisitions	All families	Families using health care
Family health care coverage								
Private insurance only................	$1.9	$2.9	$12.6	$14.8	$1.8	$1.9	$22.1	$22.2
Medicaid only........................	2.8	4.1	9.1	13.4	4.8	5.2	30.4	30.8
Medicare only........................	–	–	*0.0	–	*0.0	*0.0	–	–
Medicare and other public programs.....	*0.0	*27.8	*2.1	*4.9	*31.6	*31.6	*0.0	*0.0
Medicare and private insurance.........	*15.3	5.0	15.5	19.5	4.7	4.8	*108.1	*108.1
Other public and private mixes.........	3.7	*2.7	*57.2	*63.7	*16.6	*16.5	33.3	33.3
Other mixes of public programs.........	*1.9	*11.0	*14.9	*18.0	*13.1	*13.5	*89.9	*89.9
Source unknown.......................	*9.9						*214.0	*214.0

[1]Average size during period of family's existence rounded to nearest integer; exactly half an integer rounded upward.
[2]There were too few Hispanic families of races other than white for separate tabulation.
[3]Annual rate.
[4]Includes only families with heads 17 years of age and over.
[5]Excludes families with all members under 14 years of age.
[6]Excludes families with all members with health status unknown.

NOTE: Multiple-person families are families with average size 1.5 or greater.

Table XIV

Standard errors for Tables 34, 44, 54, and 64, by selected characteristics: United States, 1980

Characteristic	Table 34 All families	Table 34 Families with visits	Table 44 All families	Table 44 Families with visits	Standard errors of mean — Table 54 All families	Standard errors of mean — Table 54 Families with ac-quisitions	Standard errors of mean — Table 64 All families	Standard errors of mean — Table 64 Families using health care
Total............................	$5.8	$8.9	$7.3	$10.6	$3.5	$3.7	$25.8	$26.2
Family size[1]								
2 persons........................	6.4	10.9	8.0	14.4	5.4	6.2	33.6	34.2
3 persons........................	6.5	9.8	9.9	14.2	5.1	5.3	32.1	32.7
4 persons........................	22.3	33.3	17.5	23.4	6.1	6.3	49.8	49.8
5 or more persons................	10.7	12.0	24.5	30.2	8.0	8.6	89.0	89.7
Age of head								
Under 25 years...................	8.6	13.6	18.8	38.0	2.5	2.7	54.3	55.2
25-44 years......................	11.9	17.5	8.6	12.8	5.0	5.4	38.2	38.6
45-64 years......................	4.3	5.9	15.5	21.6	6.1	6.7	49.1	50.0
Sex of head								
Male.............................	4.2	6.7	10.9	15.1	4.7	5.0	26.9	27.2
Female...........................	14.9	21.6	8.8	13.5	5.2	5.7	66.6	68.0
Race and ethnicity[2] of head								
White............................	6.9	10.7	8.9	12.2	3.9	4.2	30.9	31.5
Hispanic.........................	17.1	22.2	20.4	35.1	8.1	9.1	76.3	80.7
Non-Hispanic.....................	7.7	12.0	9.5	12.9	4.2	4.5	33.8	34.2
Black............................	7.9	10.0	13.5	23.4	6.4	7.0	47.5	47.3
Other............................	*22.6	*38.0	*27.8	*42.1	*7.8	*9.6	*72.4	*73.3
Family structure								
Head and spouse present whole time......	4.3	6.8	12.1	16.5	4.4	4.7	29.3	29.6
Child under 17 years.............	6.0	7.8	17.8	23.1	5.8	6.2	40.4	41.2
No child under 17 years..........	6.9	12.9	12.0	19.2	5.4	5.8	27.5	27.7
Head only, no spouse at any time........	14.9	21.6	9.0	13.9	5.9	6.7	64.1	65.8
Child under 17 years.............	21.1	28.3	10.4	14.8	5.1	5.9	90.4	91.5
No child under 17 years..........	10.0	19.0	15.3	28.0	12.3	14.2	42.8	44.2
Other............................	*21.3	*32.6	*38.8	*51.2	*31.8	*31.8	*108.4	*108.4
Family dynamics								
Unchanging, full year............	4.0	6.4	9.6	14.5	3.7	4.1	32.7	33.4
Change in composition or existed less than full year...........	15.9	22.5	14.3	22.4	5.7	5.8	42.4	43.4

Table XIV--continued

Standard errors for Tables 34, 44, 54, and 64, by selected characteristics: United States, 1980

Standard errors of mean

Characteristic	Table 34		Table 44		Table 54		Table 64	
	All families	Families with visits	All families	Families with visits	All families	Families with acquisitions	All families	Families using health care
Family poverty status in 1980								
Below 150 percent poverty level......	$6.1	$8.9	$11.0	$19.6	$4.9	$5.6	$31.0	$31.0
Below poverty level..........	9.6	14.0	17.3	33.1	7.0	8.1	44.0	44.4
Poverty level to 149 percent........	8.5	12.3	11.6	19.0	5.6	6.3	44.3	43.0
150-199 percent................	30.1	49.2	13.1	20.0	6.0	6.4	127.2	128.7
200-299 percent................	8.1	11.2	18.0	29.2	11.6	13.0	63.6	66.3
300-499 percent................	9.1	13.5	19.8	24.8	5.9	6.4	47.0	47.5
500 percent or more..............	6.3	10.3	35.2	43.7	6.6	6.8	53.2	54.0
Family income in 1980[3]								
Less than $10,000................	6.9	10.1	11.3	22.8	5.7	6.7	31.3	31.7
$10,000-$19,999................	14.2	22.6	9.6	15.7	5.9	6.5	59.1	60.4
$20,000-$34,999................	7.9	11.7	14.4	18.2	8.6	9.3	58.2	58.2
$35,000 or more................	11.0	15.4	31.3	39.4	7.6	8.0	52.3	53.5
Education of head[4]								
None or elementary school........	10.1	14.5	14.2	26.8	5.9	6.4	43.4	43.1
Some high school................	23.6	34.1	12.2	21.4	5.6	6.0	60.3	61.9
High school graduate............	6.6	9.9	13.4	20.3	7.1	8.2	62.9	63.7
Some college..................	9.5	13.6	23.8	33.2	3.9	4.0	46.7	46.8
College graduate or more........	5.7	11.0	27.7	37.3	5.2	5.4	48.9	49.8
Family employment status[5]								
2 or more persons worked full year...	8.5	12.5	23.3	31.7	4.4	4.9	44.2	45.3
Only 1 person worked full year......	13.8	22.6	10.3	14.2	4.5	4.7	36.0	36.6
Some part-year work..............	7.1	9.2	8.7	14.3	7.1	7.8	76.0	76.7
No person worked................	*13.1	*17.7	*27.4	*49.7	*13.4	*15.7	*70.8	*71.8
Worst perceived health status of any family member[6]								
Excellent....................	3.5	5.9	15.4	22.9	2.3	2.5	27.5	27.8
Good......................	5.2	8.3	11.8	17.0	4.0	4.3	47.3	48.1
Fair......................	24.4	31.8	16.9	26.1	6.4	6.7	73.8	74.0
Poor......................	12.5	13.8	21.6	27.4	17.6	17.6	114.8	114.8

Most severe limitation in usual activity
of any family member

None..................................	7.1	11.5	8.7	13.3	3.1	3.3	29.7	30.1
Some limitation.......................	9.5	12.5	28.2	48.5	9.2	9.1	68.3	68.3
Cannot perform usual activity.........	11.1	12.2	20.8	29.3	17.9	18.3	96.5	98.1

Family's bed days[3]

0.....................................	9.2	21.0	17.8	32.7	4.3	5.0	26.6	28.4
1-5...................................	4.9	8.4	12.9	19.0	3.6	3.8	29.6	30.1
6-10..................................	12.0	17.5	19.6	28.1	6.4	6.8	48.1	48.3
11-20.................................	5.2	7.6	20.8	29.8	3.9	4.2	89.4	90.4
More than 20..........................	21.3	26.2	19.6	29.6	9.6	9.9	76.2	76.2

Family health care coverage

All members covered, some part year....	4.0	6.3	12.5	17.2	4.7	4.9	29.6	29.5
Some members not covered...............	19.4	30.1	12.9	19.1	6.4	7.0	75.5	76.8
All members not covered................	8.8	12.9	12.5	22.2	3.9	4.9	40.2	42.6

[1]Average size during period of family's existence rounded to nearest integer; exactly half an integer rounded upward.
[2]There were too few Hispanic families of races other than white for separate tabulation.
[3]Annual rate.
[4]Includes only families with heads 17 years of age and over.
[5]Excludes families with all members under 14 years of age.
[6]Excludes families with all members with health status unknown.

NOTE: Multiple-person families are families with average size 1.5 or greater.

Table XV

Standard errors for Tables 35, 45, 55, and 65, by selected characteristics: United States, 1980

	Standard errors of mean							
	Table 35		Table 45		Table 55		Table 65	
Characteristic	All families	Families with visits	All families	Families with visits	All families	Families with acquisitions	All families	Families using health care
Total.................	$3.6	$6.5	$11.9	$17.9	$6.5	$6.7	$33.7	$34.6
Family size[1]								
2 persons...............	3.4	7.3	9.5	16.1	6.7	6.8	34.3	35.3
3 persons...............	13.5	25.8	25.8	37.8	14.0	14.6	99.3	97.9
4 persons...............	15.8	22.5	90.5	120.9	31.8	32.0	138.4	138.4
5 or more persons.......	7.7	8.7	44.5	51.3	20.1	20.3	131.1	131.1
Family age								
All members 65 years and over.........	2.3	5.0	15.0	26.1	9.6	9.8	77.9	79.6
Some members under 65........	5.0	8.4	16.5	23.4	8.3	8.7	38.6	39.1
Sex of head								
Male...................	2.8	5.6	14.5	22.2	6.7	6.7	45.0	46.1
Female.................	11.6	20.6	10.7	18.8	14.4	15.6	60.1	61.7
Race and ethnicity[2] of head								
White..................	4.0	7.1	13.1	19.4	7.0	7.2	38.4	39.0
Hispanic.............	*2.3	*5.5	*60.8	*112.3	*24.6	*25.4	*132.2	*136.8
Non-Hispanic.........	4.2	7.2	13.4	19.7	7.2	7.3	40.4	41.1
Black..................	15.6	32.7	11.5	23.1	12.8	13.4	138.7	142.9
Other..................	*2.8	*7.1	*77.1	*101.9	*23.9	*27.0	*121.4	*121.4
Family structure								
Head and spouse present whole time......	2.6	5.0	16.1	24.6	6.6	6.6	45.3	46.4
Child under 17 years.....	13.8	17.0	58.6	66.4	21.8	21.8	106.2	106.2
No child under 17 years......	3.6	7.6	15.6	25.2	6.4	6.5	48.6	49.8
Head only, no spouse at any time......	5.0	9.1	9.6	17.8	12.0	13.4	51.7	53.4
Child under 17 years......	*14.9	*17.9	*13.3	*20.9	*35.4	*35.5	*117.3	*117.3
No child under 17 years......	4.7	9.5	11.2	19.8	12.3	14.0	56.1	58.0
Other..................	*41.8	*51.3	*88.0	*127.2	*39.5	*40.3	*282.8	*285.9
Family dynamics								
Unchanging, full year......	2.5	4.8	11.0	16.3	7.3	7.7	39.5	40.5
Change in composition or existed less than full year......	16.8	23.0	49.2	71.4	13.6	13.2	115.5	116.1

266

Family poverty status in 1980

Below 150 percent poverty level	10.5	18.9	5.1	12.0	12.7	15.1	59.9	64.6
Below poverty level	22.0	41.1	9.3	21.1	13.3	15.0	66.1	72.6
Poverty level to 149 percent	5.7	10.4	7.3	19.4	19.2	20.3	96.6	99.1
150-199 percent	9.2	16.8	15.4	27.7	23.4	23.5	160.3	160.3
200-299 percent	4.1	8.0	14.9	23.7	13.0	13.7	47.4	47.8
300-499 percent	4.1	7.5	26.3	36.4	11.1	11.6	64.9	65.6
500 percent or more	10.9	20.6	50.9	57.5	10.9	11.3	84.0	84.8

Family income in 1980[3]

Less than $10,000	8.0	15.7	7.1	16.5	12.8	14.0	72.0	75.3
$10,000-$19,999	3.5	6.7	14.6	23.7	9.7	10.1	45.6	45.9
$20,000-$34,999	9.5	17.8	23.9	28.4	9.8	10.2	55.8	56.4
$35,000 or more	8.5	13.4	70.1	78.7	14.1	13.4	127.8	127.8

Education of head[4]

None or elementary school	8.5	16.5	8.3	16.5	9.7	10.1	45.4	45.4
Some high school	7.5	11.9	23.0	42.1	17.4	18.1	142.8	145.4
High school graduate	4.5	8.1	27.9	35.9	9.0	9.1	61.5	62.6
Some college	5.1	10.0	44.1	49.1	14.9	15.6	105.1	105.2
College graduate or more	8.4	19.9	69.9	82.6	15.6	16.1	100.3	100.3

Family employment status[5]

2 or more persons worked full year	8.0	12.0	52.7	61.9	27.3	27.6	96.8	96.8
Only 1 person worked full year	6.6	12.9	31.3	43.9	10.3	11.4	74.3	77.3
Some part-year work	8.6	15.1	15.6	31.9	10.3	11.1	43.1	44.0
No person worked	3.4	6.7	11.1	19.1	9.5	9.7	49.7	50.8

Worst perceived health status of any family member[6]

Excellent	13.3	38.1	30.3	38.6	6.6	8.4	77.7	78.3
Good	2.3	4.1	19.2	27.3	9.2	9.4	37.9	37.6
Fair	3.4	5.5	15.6	27.1	11.1	11.6	38.5	39.7
Poor	11.5	18.0	27.5	52.4	14.3	15.9	99.8	103.3

Most severe limitation in usual activity of any family member

None	4.5	9.8	19.6	28.4	7.3	7.3	34.4	35.1
Some limitation	28.4	58.5	27.9	38.8	12.2	12.4	114.0	114.5
Cannot perform usual activity	5.3	8.8	14.8	24.1	10.2	10.4	51.6	52.2

Family's bed days[3]

0	2.0	6.1	19.6	33.9	7.8	9.1	26.7	28.2
1-5	5.0	10.9	18.6	29.6	8.9	9.0	41.8	42.3
6-10	9.2	16.6	29.5	49.1	15.8	16.1	46.9	47.2
11-20	16.5	25.4	30.8	47.7	13.4	13.2	100.3	100.3
More than 20	6.7	8.3	26.4	41.6	16.9	16.9	95.0	94.3

Table XV--continued

Standard errors for Tables 35, 45, 55, and 65, by selected characteristics: United States, 1980

Standard errors of mean

Characteristic	Table 35		Table 45		Table 55		Table 65	
	All families	Families with visits	All families	Families with visits	All families	Families with acquisitions	All families	Families using health care
Family health care coverage								
All members covered full year.........	$3.1	$5.7	$13.5	$20.4	$7.1	$7.1	$28.8	$29.3
Private insurance only...............	*22.9	*30.2	*235.6	*334.1	*48.6	*51.2	*264.4	*270.0
Medicaid only.......................	*0.0	*0.0	*0.0	*0.0	*0.0	*0.0	*0.0	*0.0
Medicare only.......................	*5.6	*16.7	*11.8	*24.0	*14.2	*15.2	*45.2	*44.7
Medicare and other public programs....	*5.4	*8.3	*14.8	*38.0	*14.0	*14.4	*81.4	*81.4
Medicare and private insurance........	4.0	7.4	13.8	20.3	7.4	7.4	33.6	33.5
Other public and private mixes........	*4.9	*6.3	*102.8	*178.4	*93.3	*99.5	*166.4	*172.1
Other mixes of public programs........	–	–	–	–	–	–	–	–
Source unknown......................	*14.2	*28.6	*15.6	*33.8	*56.6	*56.6	*151.7	*151.7
All members covered, some part year....	11.8	22.2	44.6	62.2	22.4	22.7	188.1	195.6
Some members not covered.............	19.8	34.7	16.1	32.2	16.3	17.9	219.3	232.0
All members not covered..............	*0.0	*0.0	*15.1	*19.1	*41.4	*41.3	*983.5	*983.5

1Average size during period of family's existence rounded to nearest integer; exactly half an integer rounded upward.
2There were too few Hispanic families of races other than white for separate tabulation.
3Annual rate.
4Includes only families with heads 17 years of age and over.
5Excludes families with all members under 14 years of age.
6Excludes families with all members with health status unknown.

NOTE: Multiple-person families are families with average size 1.5 or greater.

Table XVI

Standard errors for Tables 36, 46, 56, and 66, by selected characteristics: United States, 1980

Standard errors of mean

Characteristic	Table 36		Table 46		Table 56		Table 66	
	All families	Families with visits	All families	Families with visits	All families	Families with acquisitions	All families	Families using health care
Total......................	$1.1	$3.0	$5.7	$11.6	$1.8	$2.4	$18.1	$19.8
Sex								
Male.......................	1.2	3.5	8.4	18.0	1.4	2.4	22.7	26.6
Female.....................	1.8	4.3	6.7	13.1	3.0	3.5	27.0	27.8
Race and ethnicity[1]								
White......................	1.2	3.1	5.6	10.9	1.6	2.2	16.2	17.4
Hispanic...................	4.5	*9.8	23.8	*59.9	3.3	*4.9	157.5	*183.5
Non-Hispanic...............	1.2	3.2	5.6	11.0	1.6	2.3	15.4	16.7
Black......................	4.4	10.6	9.5	34.6	8.0	10.5	85.9	99.1
Other......................	*4.1	*9.8	*80.4	*141.1	*2.1	*2.8	*256.2	*286.5
Family dynamics								
Unchanging, full year......	1.2	3.0	6.4	12.6	2.0	2.6	18.1	19.6
Change in composition or existed less than full year......	3.0	10.1	9.6	28.4	3.5	5.9	74.9	90.8
Poverty status in 1980								
Below 150 percent poverty level....	1.9	4.7	3.2	9.6	3.4	4.2	37.2	40.4
Below poverty level........	2.4	5.9	6.3	19.7	4.8	6.3	43.8	49.5
Poverty level to 149 percent....	2.8	7.3	7.2	17.3	4.9	6.0	64.4	69.3
150-199 percent............	1.4	3.9	9.0	23.2	5.3	8.0	48.6	54.8
200-299 percent............	2.5	6.4	14.0	29.6	3.0	4.3	50.1	56.2
300-499 percent............	2.4	5.5	11.1	18.1	3.6	4.8	19.7	21.4
500 percent or more........	2.3	7.8	14.9	21.8	3.9	5.1	33.2	35.0
Family income in 1980[2]								
Less than $10,000..........	1.5	3.9	5.9	16.1	2.4	3.3	31.9	35.4
$10,000-$19,999............	2.1	4.8	8.8	15.9	3.1	4.1	28.9	31.9
$20,000-$34,999............	2.8	8.0	15.9	27.1	4.2	5.3	32.5	33.2
$35,000 or more............	2.1	9.7	28.1	37.9	5.5	8.6	67.4	69.7

269

Table XVI—continued

Standard errors for Tables 36, 46, 56, and 66, by selected characteristics: United States, 1980

Standard errors of mean

Characteristic	Table 36		Table 46		Table 56		Table 66	
	All families	Families with visits	All families	Families with visits	All families	Families with acquisitions	All families	Families using health care
Education[3]								
None or elementary school	$2.5	$6.7	$6.6	$28.2	$4.9	$5.8	$35.5	$39.5
Some high school	3.3	9.1	5.4	15.9	4.3	6.9	84.8	103.2
High school graduate	2.0	5.3	5.2	11.3	3.3	4.5	35.4	37.0
Some college	2.3	5.8	11.2	19.1	2.6	3.4	18.2	18.8
College graduate or more	2.3	6.1	17.4	27.5	4.1	5.4	44.8	48.7
Employment status[4]								
Work full year	1.5	4.5	8.4	14.3	1.6	2.3	12.1	13.2
Worked part time	1.9	5.1	11.3	24.8	3.6	5.0	60.4	69.1
Never worked	2.0	5.0	6.0	14.0	3.3	4.1	26.2	28.5
Perceived health status[5]								
Excellent	1.4	4.2	6.1	12.2	1.4	2.1	20.2	22.8
Good	1.4	3.9	10.6	19.8	3.6	4.4	43.5	47.2
Fair	3.9	8.3	7.3	19.3	5.4	6.2	40.8	41.6
Poor	6.5	11.5	6.0	21.2	12.8	13.8	84.4	88.3
Limitation in usual activity								
None	1.1	3.3	6.5	12.9	1.8	2.5	17.3	19.2
Some limitation	10.3	18.9	20.5	49.1	10.9	12.4	87.2	95.3
Cannot perform usual activity	2.7	5.0	7.9	20.4	6.4	7.9	89.5	95.8
Bed days[2]								
0	1.3	5.0	5.1	11.2	1.8	2.6	10.8	11.8
1-5	1.9	5.7	14.6	27.9	2.8	3.5	19.6	20.5
6-10	2.8	5.3	12.2	23.6	5.8	6.6	54.5	55.6
11-20	5.2	9.5	28.0	55.3	8.1	9.5	147.6	148.9
More than 20	5.3	8.3	8.2	20.4	7.8	8.3	114.4	116.9

Family health care coverage

All members covered full year..........	1.1	2.9	5.0	10.1	2.0	2.6	18.2	19.5
Private insurance only.................	1.5	4.2	7.6	12.9	2.2	3.0	19.9	22.1
Medicaid only.........................	*0.0	*0.0	*1.9	*6.0	*1.8	*2.4	*8.3	*10.3
Medicare only.........................	3.8	11.8	19.6	75.5	11.2	12.8	88.5	105.7
Medicare and other public programs....	1.6	3.5	11.2	43.2	5.1	6.0	45.2	47.3
Medicare and private insurance........	2.5	6.6	7.7	16.7	4.8	5.3	50.6	52.1
Other public and private mixes........	3.8	7.7	17.1	36.9	10.6	12.4	78.5	83.5
Other mixes of public programs........	*0.0	*0.0	*60.5	*85.8	*4.4	*4.2	*77.8	*71.5
Source unknown.......................	2.2	4.1	11.8	32.0	10.8	11.6	41.3	42.2
All members covered, some part year....	2.3	5.4	15.6	36.4	5.1	7.8	31.2	35.1
Some members not covered...............	*10.1	*10.1	*0.0	—	*74.2	*74.2	*2236.4	*2236.4
All members not covered...............	5.0	19.0	18.1	45.3	2.6	4.0	131.4	160.7

1There were too few Hispanic families of races other than white for separate tabulation.
2Annual rate.
3Includes only families with heads 17 years of age and over.
4Excludes families with all members under 14 years of age.
5Excludes families with all members with health status unknown.

NOTE: 1-person families are families with average size less than 1.5. For 1-person families with more than 1 distinct individual, characteristics are those of head or of family as in Table 1.

271

Table XVII

Standard errors for Tables 37, 47, 57, and 67, by selected characteristics: United States, 1980

Standard errors of mean

Characteristic	Table 37		Table 47		Table 57		Table 67	
	All families	Families with visits	All families	Families with visits	All families	Families with ac-quisitions	All families	Families using health care
Total	$1.3	$3.4	$7.4	$13.9	$2.2	$3.1	$22.3	$25.1
Age								
Under 25 years	2.3	5.1	7.9	16.6	1.7	2.4	27.8	31.4
25–44 years	1.5	4.4	16.3	27.9	2.5	3.2	48.7	53.5
45–64 years	2.5	7.2	7.8	16.8	5.4	7.3	25.9	28.8
Sex								
Male	1.2	3.4	9.1	18.1	1.4	2.3	25.1	29.3
Female	2.3	5.7	10.3	18.3	4.1	4.9	39.2	40.6
Race and ethnicity[1]								
White	1.3	3.5	7.6	13.5	1.8	2.5	19.3	21.4
Hispanic	5.5	*12.3	28.9	*75.4	3.7	*6.3	189.9	*225.5
Non-Hispanic	1.3	3.5	7.6	13.4	1.9	2.6	17.7	19.8
Black	6.0	13.5	11.9	40.7	9.6	12.6	109.7	128.2
Other	*4.6	*10.9	*82.4	*144.1	*2.2	*3.2	*283.9	*324.8
Family dynamics								
Unchanging, full year	1.4	3.5	8.6	15.4	2.5	3.4	23.1	25.3
Change in composition or existed less than full year	2.7	10.4	9.5	28.1	2.9	6.3	80.1	102.8
Poverty status in 1980								
Below 150 percent	2.7	6.8	5.5	16.0	4.4	6.4	62.1	71.2
Below poverty level	3.4	8.6	10.1	30.4	5.6	8.7	74.0	87.5
Poverty level to 149 percent	4.2	17.4	13.8	28.1	5.5	7.4	112.7	125.2
150–199 percent	1.9	5.6	8.9	22.1	4.9	8.1	69.3	81.8
200–299 percent	2.3	6.1	17.5	38.0	3.5	5.2	47.8	54.0
300–499 percent	2.8	6.3	12.7	20.3	3.8	5.2	20.0	21.8
500 percent or more	2.1	7.9	16.6	24.5	3.8	5.0	37.5	39.8
Family income in 1980[2]								
Less than $10,000	1.9	5.2	8.2	21.8	2.9	4.6	46.9	54.3
$10,000–$19,999	2.2	5.2	10.2	17.9	3.4	4.8	16.3	18.5
$20,000–$34,999	2.6	7.5	16.4	27.5	4.2	5.4	32.8	33.6
$35,000 or more	*2.6	*14.9	*34.1	*44.7	*2.7	*5.3	*84.1	*87.1

Education[3]

None or elementary school	5.3	14.9	11.8	44.7	7.1	9.7	30.8	36.0
Some high school	3.6	10.2	8.1	20.1	5.0	8.8	122.2	154.2
High school graduate	2.1	5.3	6.6	14.1	3.5	4.9	27.9	30.2
Some college	2.4	5.9	12.9	22.2	2.3	3.0	18.9	19.6
College graduate or more	2.5	7.6	19.9	32.5	4.6	6.5	51.4	56.3

Employment status[4]

Worked full year	1.5	4.7	8.8	14.7	1.7	2.4	12.6	13.8
Worked part year	1.9	4.9	12.3	26.2	3.9	5.6	61.0	70.1
Never worked	4.9	11.0	14.0	36.0	7.9	10.9	55.4	61.2

Perceived health status[5]

Excellent	1.5	4.3	7.4	14.1	1.4	2.1	24.0	27.2
Good	1.9	5.5	12.8	22.4	4.5	6.0	48.5	53.6
Fair	6.2	12.7	12.4	27.6	6.5	7.5	43.3	46.0
Poor	5.4	9.2	10.0	41.9	17.9	20.8	124.9	126.8

Limitation in usual activity

None	*1.3	3.6	*7.9	14.6	*1.9	*2.8	*19.9	*22.4
Some limitation	*11.4	*22.4	*18.1	*35.5	*30.7	*36.3	*252.3	*275.4
Cannot perform usual activity	5.5	9.1	12.7	33.6	10.5	14.1	180.6	200.5

Bed days[2]

0	1.7	6.4	6.8	13.8	1.8	3.0	13.7	15.8
1-5	2.2	6.6	16.6	31.2	2.6	3.5	22.8	24.1
6-10	3.4	7.5	16.1	28.3	7.0	8.0	70.0	71.3
11-20	5.4	9.9	43.2	69.6	9.2	10.7	218.8	221.8
More than 20	6.5	10.0	12.2	28.1	10.8	12.4	185.3	192.3

Family health care coverage

All members covered full year	1.3	3.4	6.3	11.1	2.5	3.4	18.3	20.2
Private insurance only	1.5	4.3	7.6	12.9	2.2	3.0	19.9	22.1
Medicaid only	*0.0	*0.0	*1.9	*6.0	*1.8	*2.4	*8.3	*10.3
Medicare only	*21.9	*49.1	*1.8	*0.0	*55.8	*87.6	*240.4	*276.1
Medicare and other public programs	—	—	—	—	—	—	—	—
Medicare and private insurance	—	—	—	—	—	—	—	—
Other public and private mixes	3.8	7.7	17.1	36.9	10.6	12.4	78.5	83.5
Other mixes of public programs	*0.0	*0.0	*60.5	*85.8	*4.4	*4.2	*77.8	*71.5
Source unknown	*2.5	*3.2	*5.2	*18.7	*15.2	*16.0	*72.0	*72.0
All members covered, some part year	2.3	5.4	15.6	36.4	5.1	7.8	31.2	35.1
Some members not covered	—	—	—	—	—	—	—	—
All members not covered	4.6	20.0	19.3	46.6	2.4	3.4	141.0	172.7

[1]There were too few Hispanic of races other than white families for separate tabulation.
[2]Annual rate.
[3]Includes only families with heads 17 years of age and over.
[4]Excludes families with all members under 14 years of age.
[5]Excludes families with all members with health status unknown.

NOTE: 1-person families are families with average size less than 1.5. For 1-person families with more than 1 distinct individual, characteristics are those of head or of family as in Table 2.

273

Table XVIII

Standard errors for Tables 38, 48, 58, and 68, by selected characteristics: United States, 1980

Standard errors of mean

Characteristic	Table 38		Table 48		Table 58		Table 68	
	All families	Families with visits	All families	Families with visits	All families	Families with ac-quisitions	All families	Families using health care
Total..............	$1.3	$3.4	$6.3	$11.1	$2.5	$3.4	$18.3	$20.2
Age								
Under 25 years.........	2.9	6.8	9.8	19.3	2.5	3.8	14.0	15.0
25-44 years...........	1.9	4.9	13.6	22.0	2.1	2.4	38.6	41.2
45-64 years...........	2.2	5.9	9.4	18.4	6.0	7.6	30.3	32.8
Sex								
Male.................	1.3	3.7	11.0	21.7	1.2	1.8	29.6	34.0
Female...............	2.6	5.9	7.7	11.7	4.9	5.7	21.9	22.8
Race and ethnicity[1]								
White................	1.4	3.6	6.0	9.6	2.0	2.8	13.4	14.6
Hispanic...........	*5.9	*11.3	*21.8	*53.0	*5.1	*8.1	*39.9	*44.9
Non-Hispanic.......	1.5	3.8	6.0	9.6	2.0	2.8	13.2	14.4
Black................	5.7	13.1	17.3	49.9	13.7	17.2	55.8	59.9
Other................	*2.6	*6.3	*123.5	*199.7	*2.1	*3.5	*450.1	*509.3
Family dynamics								
Unchanging, full year...........	1.4	3.5	7.2	12.3	2.9	3.6	21.7	23.1
Change in composition or existed less than full year...........	3.8	13.4	7.9	24.8	2.8	5.6	25.2	32.1
Poverty status in 1980								
Below 150 percent...........	2.3	6.3	6.1	16.6	6.9	9.2	41.6	46.6
Below poverty level.........	3.5	8.5	13.0	38.6	10.0	13.6	65.7	74.7
Poverty level to 149 percent.....	2.7	8.3	23.4	48.0	8.4	11.1	40.7	44.3
150-199 percent...........	2.5	6.2	10.7	25.1	7.9	11.7	25.1	29.0
200-299 percent...........	2.6	6.5	20.7	42.7	5.1	7.1	64.1	69.8
300-499 percent...........	3.2	6.8	7.9	11.7	2.3	3.0	14.7	15.4
500 percent or more...........	2.4	9.0	14.7	22.1	3.7	4.8	41.8	44.6
Family income in 1980[2]								
Less than $10,000...........	2.0	5.1	12.2	28.7	4.5	6.3	44.5	51.7
$10,000-$19,999...........	2.6	5.8	7.3	12.7	3.1	3.9	13.2	14.2
$20,000-$34,999...........	2.8	8.2	14.1	23.8	4.3	5.4	35.3	36.2
$35,000 or more...........	*2.9	*20.4	*38.1	*50.3	*3.1	*5.8	*97.8	*101.9

Education[3]								
None or elementary school	2.4	6.3	15.8	51.2	9.3	12.0	39.7	43.8
Some high school	2.9	8.2	7.6	22.6	7.3	10.6	68.5	79.6
High school graduate	2.4	5.8	7.5	13.7	3.6	4.8	12.8	13.3
Some college	3.2	7.8	10.1	17.0	3.3	4.3	18.9	20.7
College graduate or more	3.1	9.5	19.5	29.9	4.7	6.3	61.0	66.8
Employment status[4]								
Worked full year	1.9	5.6	6.8	10.8	2.0	2.7	10.9	12.0
Worked part year	2.4	5.7	18.4	36.6	4.3	6.3	54.6	62.0
Never worked	3.9	7.4	14.7	34.6	9.6	12.1	67.5	73.8
Perceived health status[5]								
Excellent	1.8	5.4	6.5	10.5	1.9	2.6	12.2	13.6
Good	2.1	5.9	13.4	23.7	4.7	6.0	43.2	46.4
Fair	5.7	11.7	16.1	33.4	5.1	5.8	25.5	26.7
Poor	*4.9	*7.4	*0.6	*2.3	*25.1	*28.5	*189.0	*189.0
Limitation in usual activity								
None	*1.4	3.7	*6.8	11.8	2.3	3.3	17.8	19.6
Some limitation	*17.8	*32.4	*25.3	*45.2	*16.4	*16.9	*77.6	*79.2
Cannot perform usual activity	5.7	9.1	14.5	37.6	11.6	15.5	94.7	110.2
Bed days[2]								
0	1.8	6.3	7.1	12.7	2.1	3.4	18.0	20.1
1-5	2.9	8.3	11.0	19.3	2.9	4.0	17.2	18.2
6-10	3.8	7.8	14.8	24.9	9.5	10.1	34.3	34.6
11-20	5.3	9.6	51.6	85.6	10.0	11.3	183.4	186.1
More than 20	5.9	9.0	16.7	37.3	14.5	15.1	135.5	136.3
Family health care coverage								
Private insurance only	1.5	4.3	7.6	12.9	2.2	3.0	19.9	22.1
Medicaid only	*0.0	*0.0	*1.9	*6.0	*1.8	*2.4	*8.3	*10.3
Medicare only	*21.9	*49.1	*1.8	*0.0	*55.8	*87.6	*240.4	*276.1
Medicare and other public programs	-	-	-	-	-	-	-	-
Medicare and private insurance	-	-	-	-	-	-	-	-
Other public and private mixes	3.8	7.7	17.1	36.9	10.6	12.4	78.5	83.5
Other mixes of public programs	*0.0	*0.0	*60.5	*85.8	*4.4	*4.2	*77.8	*71.5
Source unknown	*2.5	*3.2	*5.2	*18.7	*15.2	*16.0	*72.0	*72.0

[1]There were too few Hispanic families of races other than white for separate tabulation.
[2]Annual rate.
[3]Includes only families with heads 17 years of age and over.
[4]Excludes families with all members under 14 years of age.
[5]Excludes families with all members with health status unknown.

NOTE: 1-person families are families with average size less than 1.5. For 1-person families with more than 1 distinct individual, characteristics are those of head or of family as in Table 2.

Table XIX

Standard errors for Tables 39, 49, 59, and 69, by selected characteristics: United States, 1980

Standard errors of mean

Characteristic	Table 39		Table 49		Table 59		Table 69	
	All families	Families with visits	All families	Families with visits	All families	Families with acquisitions	All families	Families using health care
Total	$2.3	$6.9	$15.7	$36.3	$3.3	$5.1	$62.1	$72.6
Age								
Under 25 years	3.4	8.6	13.7	33.7	1.6	2.3	68.2	80.6
25-44 years	2.9	8.9	33.3	71.7	4.9	7.6	127.2	146.2
45-64 years	7.7	27.6	9.2	35.1	10.0	18.6	60.9	72.1
Sex								
Male	2.1	6.2	9.7	22.4	3.0	6.5	42.2	54.1
Female	4.7	13.6	28.7	65.0	5.4	6.6	140.1	148.1
Race and ethnicity[1]								
White	1.9	6.7	16.4	35.0	3.8	6.0	56.3	64.0
Hispanic	*11.0	*25.4	*64.8	*138.9	*3.6	*7.4	*440.8	*534.4
Non-Hispanic	1.9	6.7	16.5	35.2	4.0	6.2	51.6	58.9
Black	*12.0	*24.1	*8.2	*33.2	*12.0	*19.2	*336.4	*413.0
Other	*10.2	*15.4	*81.3	*174.6	*4.0	*6.1	*80.0	*105.0
Family dynamics								
Unchanging, full year	2.7	7.8	18.8	41.9	3.8	5.7	56.3	64.3
Change in composition or existed less than full year	3.8	15.6	22.8	71.0	6.8	13.8	220.7	281.5
Poverty status in 1980								
Below 150 percent	4.6	11.8	10.8	32.6	3.9	6.5	128.9	154.1
Below poverty level	5.6	16.7	16.3	51.7	2.8	4.8	141.5	174.2
Poverty level to 149 percent	8.5	20.6	14.4	34.1	8.6	11.3	237.5	271.2
150-199 percent	3.3	*10.9	16.0	*42.5	3.5	*4.5	159.8	*192.9
200-299 percent	3.3	11.9	25.5	64.5	2.5	3.5	41.5	50.5
300-499 percent	*3.7	*8.3	*63.4	*108.4	*18.5	*28.4	*105.1	*114.2
500 percent or more	*5.0	*13.1	*36.6	*56.4	*15.4	*30.3	*64.1	*67.0
Family income in 1980[2]								
Less than $10,000	3.2	8.9	10.7	30.7	2.9	4.7	92.6	109.6
$10,000-$19,999	2.0	6.8	33.4	69.7	9.1	16.1	55.5	67.1
$20,000-$34,999	*5.6	*15.2	*33.3	*61.7	*14.0	*25.7	*56.0	*58.1
$35,000 or more	*5.7	*11.2	*8.6	*10.5	*5.7	*8.5	*106.6	*106.6

Education[3]

None or elementary school	*16.9	*62.2	*17.9	*102.6	*6.4	*8.3	*28.5	*39.6
Some high school	7.0	*20.3	15.7	*48.0	6.3	*12.3	292.3	*395.7
High school graduate	2.9	8.6	14.3	38.1	6.6	10.1	87.8	98.8
Some college	3.6	6.9	36.0	67.2	2.6	3.6	46.5	45.8
College graduate or more	3.0	9.8	36.7	78.2	7.5	14.7	61.8	72.5

Employment status[4]

Worked full year	1.8	5.5	28.9	57.3	3.2	5.7	35.0	42.3
Worked part year	3.1	8.4	10.6	29.8	5.0	6.9	123.3	143.9
Never worked	*14.8	*77.8	*38.4	*109.2	*9.5	*20.9	*94.7	*107.4

Perceived health status[5]

Excellent	2.8	7.7	20.5	50.1	1.9	3.8	79.5	96.0
Good	3.3	10.3	19.5	40.5	6.6	10.1	114.8	135.6
Fair	*19.0	*40.9	*7.3	*16.6	*19.3	*23.6	*149.9	*156.4
Poor	*12.0	*32.6	*34.2	*97.1	*8.2	*7.6	*36.8	*38.2

Limitation in usual activity

None	2.3	7.0	16.3	37.5	3.2	4.9	48.0	56.3
Some limitation	*7.8	*16.6	*24.1	*54.4	*73.7	*97.8	*608.3	*734.3
Cannot perform usual activity	*15.2	*38.2	*0.0	*0.0	*22.3	*28.9	*1268.0	*1373.6

Bed days[2]

0	3.3	14.9	12.8	33.5	3.5	8.2	18.8	23.8
1-5	2.9	7.8	37.1	81.0	4.6	5.4	45.2	48.2
6-10	6.8	*16.9	35.2	*69.1	9.4	*12.3	165.5	*170.4
11-20	*15.2	*25.0	*42.9	*59.1	*22.7	*29.3	*976.5	*990.2
More than 20	*16.5	*26.5	*5.4	*16.5	*13.3	*17.4	*554.4	*614.8

Family health care coverage

All members covered, some part year	2.3	5.4	15.6	36.4	5.1	7.8	31.2	35.1
Some members not covered	—	—	—	—	—	—	—	—
All members not covered	4.6	20.0	19.3	46.6	2.4	3.4	141.0	172.7

[1]There were too few Hispanic families of races other than white for separate tabulation.
[2]Annual rate.
[3]Includes only families with heads 17 years of age and over.
[4]Excludes families with all members under 14 years of age.
[5]Excludes families with all members with health status unknown.

NOTE: 1-person families are families with average size less than 1.5. For 1-person families with more than 1 distinct individual, characteristics are those of head or of family as in Table 2.

Table XX

Standard errors for Tables 40, 50, 60, and 70, by selected characteristics: United States, 1980

| | Standard errors of mean | | | | | | | |
| | Table 40 | | Table 50 | | Table 60 | | Table 70 | |
Characteristic	All families	Families with visits	All families	Families with visits	All families	Families with acquisitions	All families	Families using health care
Total...................	$1.9	$4.7	$6.5	$15.7	$3.5	$4.0	$30.2	$32.0
Sex								
Male...................	4.1	10.7	12.1	46.9	6.2	7.8	49.2	55.1
Female.................	2.2	5.5	7.5	16.8	3.7	4.5	33.2	35.1
Race and ethnicity[1]								
White..................	2.0	5.2	6.9	16.6	3.5	4.1	32.3	34.3
Hispanic...............	*1.6	*3.3	*18.3	*28.8	*7.3	*7.3	*21.6	*21.5
Non-Hispanic...........	2.1	5.3	7.0	17.1	3.5	4.1	32.9	35.0
Black..................	3.4	*7.0	7.1	*26.7	12.2	*15.0	21.9	*23.3
Other..................	*7.9	*20.3	*81.1	*173.6	*4.5	*4.8	*121.3	*121.3
Family dynamics								
Unchanging, full year..	1.8	4.6	6.5	15.2	3.8	4.4	25.3	27.0
Change in composition or existed less than full year...	11.1	21.5	26.8	90.3	12.0	12.5	215.6	220.8
Poverty status in 1980								
Below 150 percent poverty level........	2.4	5.8	4.4	11.8	5.5	6.3	36.8	37.4
Below poverty level....	2.7	7.0	6.9	21.2	7.6	8.8	37.9	39.8
Poverty level to 149 percent...	4.0	9.7	4.5	11.0	9.0	10.7	56.1	57.8
150-199 percent........	2.4	5.2	21.3	57.6	11.2	13.4	55.3	58.4
200-299 percent........	7.2	19.4	19.5	40.3	5.8	6.6	168.1	186.5
300-499 percent........	2.2	5.2	21.6	35.6	10.5	12.2	67.6	70.3
500 percent or more....	*11.4	*27.3	*46.7	*79.3	*13.3	*14.0	*91.2	*94.1
Family income in 1980[2]								
Less than $10,000......	2.0	5.0	6.8	18.1	4.2	5.0	31.8	33.0
$10,000-$19,999........	6.1	14.0	17.0	26.2	7.5	8.3	177.4	184.5
$20,000-$34,999........	*24.3	*49.9	*76.4	*191.9	*21.3	*23.8	*144.5	*164.5
$35,000 or more........	*0.0	*0.0	*58.2	*77.3	*16.7	*16.7	*118.9	*118.9
Education								
None or elementary school...	2.5	6.3	8.5	34.8	7.1	7.7	50.3	52.5
Some high school.......	5.1	15.4	8.9	29.5	7.1	8.7	39.2	42.8
High school graduate...	4.3	14.0	8.0	13.8	7.3	9.6	134.8	140.8
Some college...........	5.0	15.5	21.9	41.3	9.4	11.2	55.9	58.2
College graduate or more...	6.8	10.7	32.9	48.3	9.8	9.7	57.5	58.4

Employment status

	Col 1	Col 2	Col 3	Col 4	Col 5	Col 6	Col 7	Col 8
Worked full year	*4.6	*15.6	*11.6	*22.3	*9.9	*12.1	*30.5	*30.9
Worked part year	7.0	20.1	25.7	83.1	9.0	10.0	244.3	272.9
Never worked	2.0	4.9	7.0	16.0	3.8	4.5	30.3	32.0

Perceived health status[3]

	Col 1	Col 2	Col 3	Col 4	Col 5	Col 6	Col 7	Col 8
Excellent	2.8	9.8	11.6	26.1	3.3	4.2	30.5	34.4
Good	1.2	3.2	12.2	29.6	5.3	6.4	83.1	90.5
Fair	4.6	9.7	7.4	22.9	8.9	9.2	62.7	64.6
Poor	11.8	22.1	6.3	16.4	18.3	19.1	114.9	118.2

Limitation in usual activity

	Col 1	Col 2	Col 3	Col 4	Col 5	Col 6	Col 7	Col 8
None	2.3	7.2	8.1	19.5	4.2	4.7	27.4	29.6
Some limitation	*13.5	*23.4	*27.6	*70.6	*8.9	*10.0	*72.5	*79.9
Cannot perform usual activity	2.4	4.5	8.2	21.5	8.4	8.9	90.6	93.1

Bed days[2]

	Col 1	Col 2	Col 3	Col 4	Col 5	Col 6	Col 7	Col 8
0	1.7	6.5	8.1	18.9	3.3	4.3	19.9	21.4
1-5	3.2	7.2	28.5	63.6	14.1	15.7	40.4	41.2
6-10	5.6	7.9	9.3	24.5	7.9	8.8	48.4	48.6
11-20	10.0	18.7	24.3	71.4	18.0	19.4	117.3	117.3
More than 20	8.0	13.6	10.5	27.5	10.5	10.5	147.2	149.1

Family health care coverage

	Col 1	Col 2	Col 3	Col 4	Col 5	Col 6	Col 7	Col 8
All members covered full year	1.8	4.7	6.7	15.9	3.5	4.0	37.0	39.3
Private insurance only	*0.0	*0.0	*0.0	—	*0.0	*0.0	*0.0	*0.0
Medicaid only	—	—	—	—	—	—	—	—
Medicare only	3.5	11.6	21.2	77.1	10.9	12.7	91.7	108.3
Medicare and other public programs	1.6	3.5	11.2	43.2	5.1	6.0	45.2	47.3
Medicare and private insurance	2.5	6.6	7.7	16.7	4.8	5.3	50.6	52.1
Other public and private mixes	—	—	—	—	—	—	—	—
Other mixes of public programs	—	—	—	—	—	—	—	—
Source unknown	*4.0	11.4	*21.5	*46.1	*12.6	*13.4	*40.2	*41.2
All members covered, some part year	—	—	—	—	—	—	—	—
Some members not covered	*10.1	*10.1	*0.0	—	*74.2	*19.8	*119.3	*144.2

[1]There were too few Hispanic families of races other than white for separate tabulation.
[2]Annual rate.
[3]Excludes families with all members with health status unknown.

NOTE: 1-person families are families with average size less than 1.5. For 1-person families with more than 1 distinct individual, characteristics are those of head or of family as in Table 2.

279

Table XXI

Standard errors for the percent of multiple-person families that use health care services, by type of service and selected characteristics: United States, 1980

Characteristic	Hospital inpatient care	Physician inpatient care	Ambulatory physician visits	Hospital outpatient and emergency visits	Dental visits	Prescription acquisitions	All health care services[1]
Total	0.8	0.7	0.5	1.2	0.8	0.3	0.2
Family size[2]							
2 persons	1.0	1.0	1.0	1.6	1.3	0.8	0.4
3 persons	1.6	1.4	0.7	1.8	1.3	0.8	0.3
4 persons	1.6	1.4	0.6	2.1	1.4	0.6	0.0
5 or more persons	1.8	1.5	0.7	1.6	1.5	0.7	0.2
Age of head							
Under 25 years	2.6	2.3	1.3	2.5	2.8	1.3	0.5
25-44 years	1.2	1.0	0.7	1.4	1.0	0.5	0.2
45-64 years	1.4	1.2	0.7	1.5	1.2	0.7	0.2
65 years and over	2.0	1.9	1.3	2.2	2.1	1.0	0.7
Sex of head							
Male	0.8	0.8	0.4	1.3	0.8	0.4	0.2
Female	2.0	1.6	1.3	1.7	1.8	1.0	0.5
Race and ethnicity[3] of head							
White	0.8	0.7	0.5	1.3	0.8	0.4	0.2
Hispanic	3.0	2.7	1.7	3.3	3.8	1.5	0.8
Non-Hispanic	0.8	0.8	0.6	1.4	0.8	0.4	0.2
Black	2.6	2.0	1.7	2.7	3.1	1.5	0.9
Other	5.6	3.9	4.2	4.9	4.7	4.3	0.9
Family structure							
Head and spouse present whole time	0.8	0.8	0.4	1.3	0.8	0.4	0.2
Child under 17 years	1.3	1.1	0.4	1.6	1.0	0.4	0.1
No child under 17 years	0.9	1.0	0.7	1.5	1.2	0.8	0.3
Head only, no spouse at any time	1.8	1.6	1.1	1.8	1.7	1.0	0.5
Child under 17 years	2.4	2.0	1.1	1.9	1.6	1.0	0.4
No child under 17 years	2.6	2.4	2.0	3.2	2.9	1.7	1.2
Other	4.8	3.9	2.5	4.4	4.4	0.7	0.6
Family dynamics							
Unchanging, full year	0.8	0.7	0.5	1.3	0.8	0.4	0.2
Change in composition or existed less than full year	1.9	1.8	0.9	1.6	1.4	0.8	0.3

Family poverty status in 1980							
Below 150 percent poverty level	1.9	1.7	1.0	2.0	2.2	1.0	0.6
Below poverty level	2.6	2.0	1.4	2.4	2.6	1.6	0.6
Poverty level to 149 percent	2.6	2.6	1.4	3.0	3.0	1.5	1.0
150-199 percent	2.3	1.9	1.5	2.8	2.8	1.1	0.4
200-299 percent	1.6	1.5	0.8	1.9	1.7	1.0	0.3
300-499 percent	1.2	1.2	0.7	1.7	1.2	0.8	0.3
500 percent or more	1.4	1.4	0.9	2.0	1.4	0.7	0.4
Family income in 1980[4]							
Less than $10,000	1.7	1.5	1.2	2.2	2.1	1.1	0.6
$10,000-$19,999	1.2	1.1	1.0	1.6	1.5	0.8	0.3
$20,000-$34,999	1.3	1.3	0.6	1.6	1.1	0.6	0.3
$35,000 or more	1.5	1.4	0.6	1.9	1.0	0.8	0.1
Education of head[5]							
None or elementary school	1.7	1.6	1.1	2.2	1.7	0.8	0.6
Some high school	2.1	1.8	1.0	2.3	1.9	1.1	0.5
High school graduate	1.2	1.1	0.9	1.5	1.1	0.6	0.3
Some college	1.9	1.6	1.1	1.8	1.5	0.8	0.2
College graduate or more	1.7	1.5	0.6	2.2	1.3	0.9	0.2
Family employment status[6]							
2 or more persons worked full year	1.5	1.4	0.7	1.9	1.2	0.8	0.2
Only 1 person worked full year	1.1	1.0	0.6	1.5	1.1	0.6	0.3
Some part-year work	1.9	1.9	1.0	2.1	2.0	1.0	0.4
No person worked	2.1	2.2	1.2	2.3	2.3	1.2	0.6
Worst perceived health status of any family member[7]							
Excellent	1.1	0.9	1.1	1.8	1.5	0.9	0.3
Good	1.2	1.2	0.6	1.6	1.0	0.5	0.3
Fair	1.9	1.7	0.9	1.9	1.7	0.7	0.3
Poor	2.8	2.8	0.9	2.4	2.1	0.7	0.5
Most severe limitation in usual activity of any family member							
None	0.9	0.8	0.6	1.2	0.8	0.4	0.2
Some limitation	3.1	2.9	1.0	3.0	3.4	1.2	0.3
Cannot perform usual activity	1.7	1.8	0.9	2.0	1.6	0.7	0.4
Family's bed days[4]							
0	0.4	0.3	1.2	2.2	1.9	1.3	0.8
1-5	1.3	1.2	1.1	1.8	1.4	0.8	0.3
6-10	1.8	1.7	0.8	2.1	1.7	0.8	0.2
11-20	1.9	1.5	0.7	1.8	1.7	0.7	0.2
More than 20	1.7	1.9	0.5	1.4	1.5	0.4	0.1

Table XXI—continued

Standard errors for the percent of multiple-person families that use health care services, by type of service and selected characteristic: United States, 1980

Characteristic	Hospital inpatient care	Physician inpatient care	Ambulatory physician visits	Hospital outpatient and emergency visits	Dental visits	Prescription acquisitions	All health care services [1]
Family health care coverage							
All members covered full year...........	0.8	0.7	0.5	1.3	0.8	0.4	0.2
Private insurance only...............	1.0	0.9	0.5	1.4	0.9	0.5	0.2
Medicaid only.......................	6.0	3.6	2.4	5.2	4.9	3.0	1.1
Medicare only.......................	*5.8	*5.6	*5.1	*6.1	*7.2	*3.9	*2.7
Medicare and other public programs....	*9.4	*6.8	*3.1	*8.6	*9.6	*4.0	*0.0
Medicare and private insurance.......	2.0	1.9	1.5	2.3	2.1	1.0	0.6
Other public and private mixes.......	2.4	2.1	1.2	2.2	1.7	1.0	0.2
Other mixes of public programs.......	*11.8	*11.8	*8.6	*14.3	*12.8	*1.1	*0.0
Source unknown......................	*8.2	*8.1	*4.2	*4.8	*7.0	*2.3	*0.0
All members covered, some part year....	2.3	1.9	1.2	2.2	1.8	0.9	0.5
Some members not covered.............	2.6	2.4	1.6	2.5	2.5	1.4	0.9
All members not covered..............	2.2	1.8	2.9	4.8	4.5	3.2	1.7

1Includes use of other medical providers and other medical expenditures not shown separately or included in any other service in this table.
2Average size during period of family's existence rounded to nearest integer; exactly half an integer rounded upward.
3There were too few Hispanic families of races other than white for separate tabulation.
4Annual rate.
5Includes only families with heads 17 years of age and over.
6Excludes families with all members under 14 years of age.
7Excludes families with all members with health status unknown.

NOTE: Multiple-person families are families with average size 1.5 or greater.

Table XXII

Standard errors for the percent of multiple-person families with all members under 65 years of age that use health care services, by type of service and selected characteristic: United States, 1980

Characteristic	Hospital inpatient care	Physician inpatient care	Ambulatory physician visits	Hospital outpatient and emergency visits	Dental visits	Prescription acquisitions	All health care services [1]
Total.............................	0.9	0.8	0.5	1.2	0.8	0.4	0.2
Family size [2]							
2 persons..........	1.3	1.1	1.1	1.8	1.3	1.0	0.4
3 persons..........	1.5	1.3	0.7	1.8	1.3	0.8	0.2
4 persons..........	1.6	1.5	0.6	2.1	1.5	0.6	0.0
5 or more persons..........	1.9	1.6	0.8	1.7	1.6	0.8	0.2
Age of head							
Under 25 years..........	2.5	2.3	1.3	2.5	2.9	1.3	0.5
25-44 years..........	1.2	1.0	0.7	1.4	1.0	0.5	0.2
45-64 years..........	1.4	1.3	0.8	1.5	1.3	0.7	0.3
Sex of head							
Male..........	0.8	0.8	0.4	1.4	0.9	0.4	0.1
Female..........	2.2	1.8	1.3	1.8	1.8	1.0	0.5
Race and ethnicity [3] of head							
White..........	0.9	0.8	0.5	1.3	0.9	0.4	0.2
Hispanic..........	3.5	2.8	1.8	3.4	4.0	1.8	0.8
Non-Hispanic..........	0.9	0.8	0.5	1.4	0.9	0.4	0.1
Black..........	3.0	2.2	1.8	2.7	3.2	1.4	0.8
Other..........	5.6	3.8	5.1	5.9	4.8	4.4	1.1
Family structure							
Head and spouse present whole time......	0.9	0.9	0.4	1.4	0.9	0.4	0.1
Child under 17 years..........	1.3	1.1	0.4	1.6	1.1	0.4	0.1
No child under 17 years..........	1.3	1.3	0.8	1.7	1.2	1.0	0.3
Head only, no spouse at any time........	1.9	1.7	1.3	1.8	1.7	1.2	0.6
Child under 17 years..........	2.5	2.1	1.1	2.0	1.7	1.1	0.4
No child under 17 years..........	2.5	2.4	3.0	4.0	3.7	2.6	1.6
Other..........	5.4	4.2	3.1	5.1	5.7	0.3	0.0
Family dynamics							
Unchanging, full year...........	0.9	0.8	0.5	1.3	0.9	0.5	0.2
Change in composition or existed less than full year..........	2.1	2.0	1.0	1.9	1.6	0.9	0.4

283

Table XXII—continued

Standard errors for the percent of multiple-person families with all members under 65 years of age that use health care services, by type of service and selected characteristic: United States, 1980

Characteristic	Hospital inpatient care	Physician inpatient care	Ambulatory physician visits	Hospital outpatient and emergency visits	Dental visits	Prescription acquisitions	All health care services[1]
Family poverty status in 1980							
Below 150 percent poverty level	2.3	1.9	1.3	2.3	2.3	1.1	0.5
Below poverty level	2.9	2.2	1.5	2.5	2.6	1.5	0.4
Poverty level to 149 percent	3.1	2.9	1.7	3.6	3.3	1.8	1.0
150–199 percent	2.8	2.3	1.8	2.8	2.9	1.3	0.5
200–299 percent	1.8	1.6	0.9	2.0	1.9	1.1	0.4
300–499 percent	1.3	1.2	0.6	1.7	1.3	0.8	0.3
500 percent or more	1.7	1.5	0.9	2.1	1.4	0.8	0.3
Family income in 1980[4]							
Less than $10,000	2.1	1.9	1.5	2.4	2.2	1.4	0.6
$10,000–$19,999	1.5	1.3	1.1	1.7	1.8	0.9	0.4
$20,000–$34,999	1.3	1.2	0.5	1.7	1.1	0.6	0.3
$35,000 or more	1.7	1.5	0.7	2.0	1.0	0.8	0.2
Education of head[5]							
None or elementary school	2.5	2.0	1.4	2.5	2.1	1.3	0.9
Some high school	2.1	1.8	1.0	2.3	2.2	1.1	0.4
High school graduate	1.3	1.2	1.0	1.5	1.1	0.7	0.3
Some college	2.0	1.7	1.1	2.0	1.6	0.9	0.3
College graduate or more	1.9	1.6	0.6	2.4	1.5	1.0	0.2
Family employment status[6]							
2 or more persons worked full year	1.6	1.4	0.8	1.9	1.2	0.8	0.2
Only 1 person worked full year	1.1	1.0	0.6	1.5	1.2	0.6	0.3
Some part-year work	2.2	1.9	1.0	2.3	2.2	1.0	0.5
No person worked	3.3	2.9	1.9	3.0	3.4	2.0	0.4
Worst perceived health status of any family member[7]							
Excellent	1.2	1.0	1.1	1.8	1.5	0.9	0.3
Good	1.3	1.2.	0.6	1.7	1.0	0.5	0.3
Fair	2.2	2.1	1.0	2.0	1.9	0.8	0.2
Poor	3.6	3.4	1.0	2.6	2.6	0.7	0.0
Most severe limitation in usual activity of any family member							
None	0.9	0.8	0.6	1.3	0.8	0.4	0.2
Some limitation	3.5	3.4	1.0	3.2	3.9	1.6	0.0
Cannot perform usual activity	2.8	2.8	0.8	2.6	2.4	0.9	0.5

Family's bed days[4]

0...	0.5	0.4	1.3	2.4	2.0	1.7	0.9
1-5...	1.3	1.0	1.2	2.0	1.4	0.9	0.3
6-10..	1.7	1.5	0.8	2.4	1.8	0.9	0.2
11-20...	2.1	1.5	0.8	1.9	1.7	0.8	0.3
More than 20..................................	1.9	2.1	0.4	1.5	1.7	0.3	0.0

Family health care coverage

All members covered full year.................	0.9	0.7	0.4	1.3	0.8	0.4	0.2
Private insurance only........................	1.0	0.9	0.5	1.5	0.9	0.5	0.2
Medicaid only.................................	5.8	3.5	2.4	5.3	5.0	3.0	1.1
Medicare only.................................	–	–	–	–	–	–	–
Medicare and other public programs...........	*0.0	*0.0	*0.0	*0.0	*0.0	*0.0	*0.0
Medicare and private insurance...............	*15.2	*15.2	*15.1	*15.5	*14.9	*0.0	*0.0
Other public and private mixes...............	2.4	2.1	1.2	2.2	1.7	1.0	0.0
Other mixes of public programs...............	*11.8	*11.8	*8.6	*14.3	*12.8	*1.1	*0.0
Source unknown................................	*9.1	*8.6	*3.4	*4.9	*7.0	*2.9	*0.0
All members covered, some part year..........	2.4	2.0	1.3	2.2	2.0	0.9	0.5
Some members not covered......................	2.8	2.6	1.8	2.9	2.9	1.8	0.8
All members not covered.......................	2.2	1.8	2.9	5.0	4.5	3.4	1.8

[1] Includes use of other medical providers and other medical expenditures not shown separately or included in any other service in this table.
[2] Average size during period of family's existence rounded to nearest integer; exactly half an integer rounded upward.
[3] There were too few Hispanic families of races other than white for separate tabulation.
[4] Annual rate.
[5] Includes only families with heads 17 years of age and over.
[6] Excludes families with all members under 14 years of age.
[7] Excludes families with all members with health status unknown.

NOTE: Multiple-person families are families with average size 1.5 or greater.

Table XXIII

Standard errors for the percent of multiple-person families with all members under 65 years of age and all members with health care coverage all year that use health care services, by type of service and selected characteristics: United States, 1980

Characteristic	Hospital inpatient care	Physician inpatient care	Ambulatory physician visits	Hospital outpatient and emergency visits	Dental visits	Prescription acquisitions	All health care services[1]
Total	0.9	0.7	0.4	1.3	0.8	0.4	0.2
Family size[2]							
2 persons	1.5	1.3	0.8	2.1	1.5	1.1	0.5
3 persons	1.9	1.5	0.9	1.9	1.6	0.8	0.1
4 persons	1.9	1.7	0.7	2.4	1.4	0.8	0.0
5 or more persons	2.3	1.8	0.8	2.0	1.4	0.8	0.0
Age of head							
Under 25 years	3.2	2.9	1.6	3.3	3.9	1.7	0.3
25-44 years	1.2	0.9	0.6	1.6	1.1	0.6	0.2
45-64 years	1.6	1.3	0.7	1.8	1.2	0.8	0.2
Sex of head							
Male	1.0	0.8	0.4	1.4	0.8	0.4	0.2
Female	2.5	1.9	1.3	2.6	2.3	1.3	0.5
Race and ethnicity[3] of head							
White	0.9	0.8	0.4	1.4	0.9	0.4	0.1
Hispanic	5.1	4.7	2.0	5.1	5.2	1.7	0.5
Non-Hispanic	0.9	0.8	0.4	1.5	0.9	0.4	0.2
Black	3.4	2.0	2.2	3.4	3.7	1.7	0.8
Other	8.4	5.9	5.9	8.6	5.0	5.0	1.2
Family structure							
Head and spouse present whole time	1.0	0.9	0.4	1.5	0.8	0.5	0.1
Child under 17 years	1.4	1.1	0.5	1.7	1.0	0.5	0.0
No child under 17 years	1.5	1.4	0.7	1.9	1.3	0.9	0.3
Head only, no spouse at any time	2.3	1.8	1.4	2.7	2.3	1.5	0.7
Child under 17 years	2.9	2.1	1.4	2.7	2.4	1.4	0.6
No child under 17 years	4.1	4.2	3.5	6.1	5.6	3.8	2.0
Other	7.5	5.9	3.4	6.0	6.3	0.5	0.0
Family dynamics							
Unchanging, full year	1.0	0.8	0.4	1.5	0.9	0.5	0.2
Change in composition or existed less than full year	2.5	2.4	1.1	2.3	1.9	1.0	0.4

Family poverty status in 1980

Below 150 percent poverty level	2.7	2.3	1.5	2.8	2.9	1.3	0.6
Below poverty level	3.6	2.7	1.9	3.4	3.4	1.8	0.5
Poverty level to 149 percent	4.5	4.5	2.6	4.4	3.8	2.3	1.4
150–199 percent	3.8	3.1	1.6	3.8	4.0	1.8	0.4
200–299 percent	1.8	1.6	0.9	2.3	1.8	1.1	0.2
300–499 percent	1.5	1.4	0.6	1.9	1.4	0.7	
500 percent or more	1.8	1.6	1.0	2.3	1.6	0.9	0.3

Family income in 1980[4]

Less than $10,000	2.8	2.4	1.6	3.0	2.9	1.5	0.7
$10,000–$19,999	1.9	1.6	1.1	2.1	2.0	1.1	0.3
$20,000–$34,999	1.5	1.4	0.6	1.8	1.2	0.7	0.3
$35,000 or more	1.9	1.6	0.8	2.1	1.3	0.9	0.0

Education of head[5]

None or elementary school	3.0	2.5	1.6	3.2	3.0	1.7	0.6
Some high school	2.3	2.0	1.3	2.8	2.6	1.2	0.2
High school graduate	1.4	1.1	0.8	1.7	1.1	0.8	0.3
Some college	2.1	1.8	1.1	2.3	1.7	1.0	0.3
College graduate or more	2.1	1.7	0.6	2.6	1.5	1.1	0.1

Family employment status[6]

2 or more persons worked full year	1.7	1.4	0.7	1.9	1.4	0.8	0.2
Only 1 person worked full year	1.2	1.1	0.6	1.8	1.2	0.7	0.3
Some part-year work	2.6	2.3	1.2	2.5	2.3	1.2	0.4
No person worked	3.4	3.0	2.0	3.7	3.7	2.2	0.0

Worst perceived health status of any family member[7]

Excellent	1.4	1.0	0.8	2.0	1.3	1.0	0.3
Good	1.5	1.3	0.7	1.8	1.0	0.6	0.2
Fair	2.4	2.2	0.9	2.5	2.1	0.8	0.2
Poor	3.5	3.8	1.5	3.5	3.3	1.0	0.0

Most severe limitation in usual activity of any family member

None	1.0	0.8	0.5	1.4	0.8	0.5	0.2
Some limitation	4.5	4.5	1.1	4.1	3.5	1.7	0.0
Cannot perform usual activity	3.0	3.2	1.1	3.1	2.8	1.1	0.6

Family's bed days[4]

0	0.5	0.5	1.3	2.1	2.9	1.8	0.7
1–5	1.3	1.1	1.2	1.4	2.3	0.9	0.4
6–10	2.1	1.7	0.6	1.8	2.6	1.0	0.2
11–20	2.3	1.8	0.8	2.0	2.2	0.7	0.2
More than 20	2.0	2.3	0.4	1.8	1.8	0.3	0.0

Table XXIII—continued

Standard errors for the percent of multiple-person families with all members under 65 years of age and all members with health care coverage all year that use health care services, by type of service and selected characteristics: United States, 1980

Characteristic	Hospital inpatient care	Physician inpatient care	Ambulatory physician visits	Hospital outpatient and emergency visits	Dental visits	Prescription acquisitions	All health care services [1]
Family health care coverage							
Private insurance only...............	1.0	0.9	0.5	1.5	0.9	0.5	0.2
Medicaid only.......................	5.8	3.5	2.4	5.3	5.0	3.0	1.1
Medicare only.......................	-	-	-	-	-	-	-
Medicare and other public programs.....	*0.0	*0.0	*0.0	*0.0	*0.0	*0.0	*0.0
Medicare and private insurance.........	*15.2	*15.2	*15.1	*15.5	*14.9	*0.0	*0.0
Other public and private mixes.........	2.4	2.1	1.2	2.2	1.7	1.0	0.0
Other mixes of public programs.........	*11.8	*11.8	*8.6	*14.3	*12.8	*1.1	*0.0
Source unknown......................	*9.1	*8.6	*3.4	*4.9	*7.0	*2.9	*0.0

[1]Includes use of other medical providers and other medical expenditures not shown separately or included in any other service in this table.
[2]Average size during period of family's existence rounded to nearest integer; exactly half an integer rounded upward.
[3]There were too few Hispanic families of races other than white for separate tabulation.
[4]Annual rate.
[5]Includes only families with heads 17 years of age and over.
[6]Excludes families with all members under 14 years of age.
[7]Excludes families with all members with health status unknown.

NOTE: Multiple-person families are families with average size 1.5 or greater.

Table XXIV

Standard errors for the percent of multiple-person families with all members under 65 years of age and some members without health care coverage all year that use health care services, by type of service and selected characteristics: United States, 1980

Characteristic	Hospital inpatient care	Physician inpatient care	Ambulatory physician visits	Hospital outpatient and emergency visits	Dental visits	Prescription acquisitions	All health care services[1]
Total..............	1.7	1.6	1.1	1.9	1.5	1.0	0.5
Family size[2]							
2 persons................	2.4	2.0	3.0	3.0	3.1	2.4	1.2
3 persons................	2.8	2.8	1.3	3.3	2.9	1.5	0.8
4 persons................	2.8	2.7	0.9	3.5	3.0	1.4	0.0
5 or more persons........	3.7	3.2	1.6	3.1	3.1	1.6	0.6
Age of head							
Under 25 years...........	4.1	3.7	2.2	5.0	4.3	2.4	1.0
25-44 years..............	2.3	2.3	1.5	2.5	2.1	1.1	0.5
45-64 years..............	2.4	2.3	1.9	2.6	2.5	1.8	0.7
Sex of head							
Male.....................	1.7	1.6	1.0	2.1	2.0	1.1	0.5
Female...................	3.6	3.2	2.4	2.8	3.2	1.7	0.8
Race and ethnicity[3] of head							
White....................	1.8	1.5	1.1	2.1	1.7	1.0	0.4
Hispanic.................	4.7	2.9	2.5	5.0	5.4	3.6	1.8
Non-Hispanic.............	1.9	1.6	1.1	2.2	1.8	1.2	0.5
Black....................	4.4	4.6	2.7	4.2	4.4	2.5	1.4
Other....................	*11.7	*7.8	*7.9	*10.3	*10.4	*7.0	*2.1
Family structure							
Head and spouse present whole time......	1.7	1.7	0.9	2.2	2.0	1.1	0.5
Child under 17 years.....	2.4	2.2	0.8	2.8	2.4	1.1	0.4
No child under 17 years..	2.3	2.2	2.2	3.1	3.3	2.4	1.0
Head only, no spouse at any time.........	3.2	3.0	2.3	2.8	2.9	1.8	0.9
Child under 17 years.....	4.1	4.0	2.1	3.6	3.3	1.9	0.6
No child under 17 years..	3.6	3.3	4.8	4.9	4.8	3.6	2.3
Other....................	*8.2	*4.6	*5.6	*7.8	*9.3	*0.0	*0.0
Family dynamics							
Unchanging, full year....	1.8	1.6	1.2	2.1	1.8	1.3	0.5
Change in composition or existed less than full year..........	3.3	3.1	1.6	2.9	2.3	1.4	0.7

Table XXIV—continued

Standard errors for the percent of multiple-person families with all members under 65 years of age and some members without health care coverage all year that use health care services, by type of service and selected characteristics: United States, 1980

Characteristic	Hospital inpatient care	Physician inpatient care	Ambulatory physician visits	Hospital outpatient and emergency visits	Dental visits	Prescription acquisitions	All health care services[1]
Family poverty status in 1980							
Below 150 percent poverty level	3.4	2.8	2.0	3.2	2.8	1.9	0.9
Below poverty level	4.1	3.6	2.3	3.9	4.0	2.8	0.8
Poverty level to 149 percent	4.1	3.5	2.8	4.9	4.4	3.0	1.6
150–199 percent	3.7	3.6	3.2	4.0	3.9	2.3	0.9
200–299 percent	3.6	2.9	1.7	3.3	3.9	2.2	1.1
300–499 percent	2.7	2.7	2.0	3.4	2.7	2.3	0.8
500 percent or more	3.3	3.6	2.4	4.8	3.7	2.3	1.1
Family income in 1980[4]							
Less than $10,000	3.1	2.9	2.3	3.3	3.3	2.5	1.0
$10,000–$19,999	2.6	2.5	2.1	2.7	2.6	1.6	0.9
$20,000–$34,999	2.5	2.0	1.4	3.2	2.6	1.4	0.3
$35,000 or more	3.7	3.7	1.8	4.2	2.9	2.0	0.8
Education of head[5]							
None or elementary school	3.8	3.1	2.8	3.6	3.1	2.4	2.0
Some high school	3.9	3.4	1.6	3.7	3.3	2.0	0.9
High school graduate	2.7	2.6	2.0	2.5	2.7	1.6	0.4
Some college	3.9	3.0	2.9	4.1	3.3	2.2	0.6
College graduate or more	3.8	3.6	2.1	4.5	3.5	2.2	1.0
Family employment status[6]							
2 or more persons worked full year	2.8	2.7	1.9	3.5	2.7	2.1	0.8
Only 1 person worked full year	2.4	2.3	1.4	2.7	2.3	1.5	0.6
Some part-year work	2.9	2.3	1.9	3.7	3.1	1.9	0.9
No person worked	*8.0	*7.5	*5.0	*7.3	*7.3	*4.6	*1.6
Worst perceived health status of any family member[7]							
Excellent	2.8	2.6	2.5	3.3	3.7	2.2	1.1
Good	2.6	2.2	1.3	2.6	2.2	1.3	0.7
Fair	3.9	4.1	2.4	3.3	3.5	1.5	0.4
Poor	5.7	5.0	1.1	3.9	4.4	0.9	0.0
Most severe limitation in usual activity of any family member							
None	1.8	1.6	1.4	2.1	1.7	1.1	0.5
Some limitation	5.4	5.2	2.3	6.0	7.8	2.0	0.0
Cannot perform usual activity	4.6	4.6	1.2	3.8	4.3	1.3	0.9

Family's bed days[4]

0............................	1.0	3.7	3.5	4.1	3.8	2.5
1-5..........................	2.6	2.1	2.9	2.8	2.0	0.6
6-10.........................	3.5	2.5	4.8	3.9	1.8	0.5
11-20........................	4.3	1.7	4.0	3.0	1.6	0.7
More than 20.................	3.2	1.0	2.3	3.0	1.0	0.0
Family health care coverage						
All members covered, some part year.....	2.4	1.3	2.2	2.0	0.9	0.5
Some members not covered.............	2.8	1.8	2.9	2.9	1.8	0.8
All members not covered.............	2.2	2.9	5.0	4.5	3.4	1.8

[1]Includes use of other medical providers and other medical expenditures not shown separately or included in any other service in this table.
[2]Average size during period of family's existence rounded to nearest integer; exactly half an integer rounded upward.
[3]There were too few Hispanic families of races other than white for separate tabulation.
[4]Annual rate.
[5]Includes only families with heads 17 years of age and over.
[6]Excludes families with all members under 14 years of age.
[7]Excludes families with all members with health status unknown.

NOTE: Multiple-person families are families with average size 1.5 or greater.

Table XXV

Standard errors for the percent of multiple-person families with members 65 years of age and over that use health care services, by type of service and selected characteristics: United States, 1980

Characteristic	Hospital inpatient care	Physician inpatient care	Ambulatory physician visits	Hospital outpatient and emergency visits	Dental visits	Prescription acquisitions	All health care services[1]
Total.............................	1.8	1.7	1.2	2.0	1.8	0.9	0.6
Family size[2]							
2 persons........................	2.0	1.8	1.5	2.1	1.9	1.0	0.6
3 persons........................	5.4	5.9	3.0	4.8	5.3	2.9	2.4
4 persons........................	6.8	6.5	4.6	6.9	5.3	1.2	0.0
5 or more persons................	6.2	5.9	1.3	5.1	4.5	1.6	0.0
Family age							
All members 65 years and over....	2.5	2.4	1.9	2.5	3.1	1.4	0.9
Some members under 65............	2.6	2.4	1.5	2.5	2.6	1.1	0.8
Sex of head							
Male.............................	1.7	1.7	1.1	2.0	1.8	1.1	0.6
Female...........................	5.1	4.6	3.1	4.2	4.8	2.1	1.7
Race and ethnicity[3] of head							
White............................	1.8	1.7	1.3	2.1	1.9	0.9	0.6
Hispanic.........................	*6.8	*5.8	*3.4	*7.8	*9.7	*2.9	*2.9
Non-Hispanic.....................	1.9	1.8	1.3	2.1	2.0	0.9	0.6
Black............................	5.4	4.2	5.1	7.1	6.5	4.1	3.2
Other............................	*15.8	*10.8	*10.3	*16.2	*11.8	*11.0	*0.0
Family structure							
Head and spouse present whole time.....	1.6	1.6	1.1	2.0	1.8	1.1	0.5
Child under 17 years.............	5.7	5.6	2.6	6.5	4.3	2.8	0.0
No child under 17 years..........	1.7	1.7	1.2	1.9	2.0	1.2	0.6
Head only, no spouse at any time.........	4.4	3.9	2.8	3.9	4.0	2.3	1.6
Child under 17 years.............	*10.6	*10.6	*0.0	*8.9	*11.0	*0.6	*0.0
No child under 17 years..........	4.7	4.2	3.3	4.3	4.4	2.6	1.9
Other............................	*5.5	*8.6	*3.7	*7.6	*7.9	*2.5	*2.5
Family dynamics							
Unchanging, full year............	1.8	1.7	1.4	2.1	1.9	0.9	0.7
Change in composition or existed less than full year..............	4.6	4.8	2.4	3.9	4.5	2.0	0.7

292

Family poverty status in 1980

Below 150 percent poverty level	4.0	3.4	2.7	4.2	3.6	2.4	2.2
Below poverty level	6.4	4.8	5.2	7.4	6.2	4.5	4.1
Poverty level to 149 percent	5.0	5.1	3.7	4.8	4.2	3.3	2.5
150-199 percent	3.9	3.6	2.6	5.7	4.7	1.6	0.0
200-299 percent	3.6	3.4	2.0	4.1	3.3	1.9	0.7
300-499 percent	3.3	2.9	2.2	3.4	2.8	1.8	0.9
500 percent or more	4.4	4.8	3.0	4.1	4.5	1.6	1.7

Family income in 1980[4]

Less than $10,000	3.4	2.8	1.9	4.0	3.5	1.8	1.5
$10,000-$19,999	2.7	2.8	1.7	3.1	2.4	1.5	0.7
$20,000-$34,999	3.9	3.9	2.5	3.7	3.4	1.9	1.3
$35,000 or more	6.3	6.3	1.0	4.8	3.8	4.1	0.0

Education of head[5]

None or elementary school	2.7	2.6	2.0	3.4	2.5	1.2	1.0
Some high school	4.7	4.2	3.0	4.7	4.9	2.9	1.9
High school graduate	3.8	3.3	1.4	3.7	2.8	1.5	1.0
Some college	5.1	4.8	4.3	5.9	5.1	3.3	0.1
College graduate or more	5.1	4.9	2.3	5.2	4.7	3.4	0.0

Family employment status[6]

2 or more persons worked full year	6.2	5.9	3.7	6.2	3.9	2.8	0.0
Only 1 person worked full year	3.4	2.9	2.2	3.8	3.1	1.8	1.5
Some part-year work	4.1	4.5	2.7	4.0	4.0	2.2	1.0
No person worked	2.7	2.7	1.6	2.6	2.8	1.2	0.9

Worst perceived health status
of any family member[7]

Excellent	3.6	3.4	4.1	5.2	4.6	3.7	2.0
Good	3.2	3.1	1.5	3.1	2.7	1.3	0.6
Fair	3.5	3.1	2.2	3.1	3.0	1.3	0.9
Poor	3.9	3.6	1.6	4.2	3.5	1.5	1.3

Most severe limitation in usual activity
of any family member

None	2.7	2.5	2.1	3.0	2.7	2.0	1.1
Some limitation	6.1	5.5	2.7	6.0	5.7	1.6	1.3
Cannot perform usual activity	2.5	2.3	1.2	2.5	2.3	0.8	0.6

Family's bed days[4]

0	0.7	0.5	2.6	3.3	2.8	1.8	1.5
1-5	3.6	3.9	2.1	4.4	3.8	1.6	0.9
6-10	5.1	5.4	2.0	4.7	4.6	1.9	0.9
11-20	4.4	4.9	1.5	5.4	5.4	1.8	0.0
More than 20	3.0	3.2	1.9	3.4	3.5	1.2	0.4

Table XXV—continued

Standard errors for the percent of multiple-person families with members 65 years of age and over that use health care services, by type of service and selected characteristics: United States, 1980

Characteristic	Hospital inpatient care	Physician inpatient care	Ambulatory physician visits	Hospital outpatient and emergency visits	Dental visits	Prescription acquisitions	All health care services [1]
Family health care coverage							
All members covered full year............	2.0	1.8	1.3	2.1	2.0	1.0	0.5
Private insurance only..............	*11.5	*11.5	*4.8	*11.0	*10.5	*6.7	*4.8
Medicaid only.....................	*0.0	*0.0	*0.0	*0.0	*0.0	*0.0	*0.0
Medicare only.....................	*5.8	*5.6	*5.1	*6.1	*7.2	*3.9	*2.7
Medicare and other public programs.....	*9.6	*6.9	*3.2	*8.6	*9.7	*4.1	*0.0
Medicare and private insurance.....	2.0	2.0	1.5	2.3	2.1	1.0	0.6
Other public and private mixes......	*20.7	*12.1	*10.9	*15.8	*20.1	*10.9	*10.9
Other mixes of public programs.........	–	–	–	–	–	–	–
Source unknown.....................	*15.4	*15.4	*15.4	*15.6	*15.0	*0.0	*0.0
All members covered, some part year.....	7.0	6.9	4.6	8.4	7.1	3.4	3.6
Some members not covered............	7.1	6.4	4.7	6.0	6.7	3.3	3.0
All members not covered.............	*12.7	*12.7	*20.2	*12.7	*20.7	*21.0	*0.0

[1]Includes use of other medical providers and other medical expenditures not shown separately or included in any other service in this table.
[2]Average size during period of family's existence rounded to nearest integer; exactly half an integer rounded upward.
[3]There were too few Hispanic families of races other than white for separate tabulation.
[4]Annual rate.
[5]Includes only families with heads 17 years of age and over.
[6]Excludes families with all members under 14 years of age.
[7]Excludes families with all members with health status unknown.

NOTE: Multiple-person families are families with average size 1.5 or greater.

294

Table XXVI

Standard errors for the percent of 1-person families that use health care services, by type of service and selected characteristics: United States, 1980

Characteristic	Hospital inpatient care	Physician inpatient care	Ambulatory physician visits	Hospital outpatient and emergency visits	Dental visits	Prescription acquisitions	All health care services [1]
Total..........	0.9	0.8	1.1	1.2	1.3	1.1	0.8
Sex							
Male..........	1.3	1.0	1.9	1.9	2.2	2.1	1.4
Female........	1.4	1.3	1.2	1.7	1.4	1.3	0.8
Race and ethnicity[2]							
White.........	1.0	0.8	1.3	1.3	1.4	1.1	0.9
Hispanic......	6.2	3.7	6.0	7.0	6.6	6.1	3.9
Non-Hispanic..	1.0	0.9	1.3	1.3	1.4	1.1	0.8
Black.........	2.6	2.2	4.6	3.3	3.6	3.7	2.5
Other.........	*4.1	*4.0	*7.8	*8.3	*9.7	*6.1	*4.7
Family dynamics							
Unchanging, full year....	1.0	0.8	1.1	1.3	1.5	1.1	0.8
Change in composition or existed less than full year......	2.1	1.8	3.0	2.1	2.6	2.7	2.3
Poverty status in 1980							
Below 150 percent poverty level.....	1.6	1.4	1.8	2.0	1.5	1.6	1.4
Below poverty level.........	2.1	1.7	2.2	2.7	2.0	2.4	1.7
Poverty level to 149 percent......	2.5	2.2	3.0	2.9	2.7	2.7	1.8
150-199 percent...........	2.4	2.1	3.0	4.0	3.2	3.1	2.2
200-299 percent...........	1.4	1.5	2.4	2.9	2.8	2.6	1.7
300-499 percent...........	2.0	1.8	2.5	2.8	3.1	2.4	1.2
500 percent or more.......	2.2	1.9	3.4	2.7	4.4	3.7	2.4
Family income in 1980[3]							
Less than $10,000.........	1.3	1.1	1.4	1.6	1.3	1.4	1.2
$10,000-$19,999...........	1.5	1.3	2.1	2.5	2.4	2.0	1.5
$20,000-$34,999...........	2.4	2.3	3.7	3.9	4.0	4.0	2.4
$35,000 or more...........	4.1	3.8	6.2	5.5	7.5	7.2	2.5
Education[4]							
None or elementary school....	2.2	1.9	2.2	2.8	2.2	1.8	1.6
Some high school.....	2.3	2.1	3.0	3.1	2.5	2.9	2.2
High school graduate.....	1.5	1.3	2.1	2.2	1.9	2.3	1.2
Some college.....	1.8	1.4	2.7	2.9	2.9	2.8	1.8
College graduate or more.....	1.9	1.6	2.7	2.8	3.0	2.6	1.6

295

Table XXVI—continued

Standard errors for the percent of 1-person families that use health care services, by type of service and selected characteristics: United States, 1980

Characteristic	Hospital inpatient care	Physician inpatient care	Ambulatory physician visits	Hospital outpatient and emergency visits	Dental visits	Prescription acquisitions	All health care services[1]
Employment status[5]							
Worked full year	1.3	0.9	1.8	1.8	2.1	1.7	1.1
Worked part year	1.8	1.6	2.2	2.0	2.6	2.2	1.6
Never worked	1.7	1.5	1.7	2.1	2.1	1.5	0.9
Perceived health status[6]							
Excellent	1.1	0.9	1.9	1.8	1.8	1.6	1.2
Good	1.4	1.1	1.9	1.9	2.8	2.2	1.6
Fair	3.0	2.6	2.6	3.5	2.8	2.3	1.5
Poor	4.3	4.0	4.5	5.4	4.6	2.8	1.3
Limitation in usual activity							
None	0.9	0.7	1.3	1.2	1.5	1.2	0.9
Some limitation	5.4	4.6	5.5	6.8	5.7	5.7	3.4
Cannot perform usual activity	3.2	2.7	2.6	3.0	2.9	2.6	1.8
Bed days[3]							
0	0.5	0.3	1.7	1.6	2.0	1.6	1.5
1–5	1.6	1.2	2.3	1.9	2.4	2.4	1.3
6–10	3.6	2.8	2.0	4.0	3.7	2.3	0.9
11–20	4.4	4.2	3.3	5.0	3.9	2.6	0.6
More than 20	3.0	3.9	2.2	3.9	3.9	1.7	1.0
Family health care coverage							
All members covered full year	0.9	0.8	1.3	1.4	1.5	1.2	0.9
Private insurance only	1.2	1.0	2.1	2.0	2.4	2.1	1.2
Medicaid only	*13.2	*6.6	*13.9	*13.3	*13.0	*8.9	*6.9
Medicare only	3.9	3.7	4.6	4.6	4.8	4.6	4.3
Medicare and other public programs	5.2	4.3	4.6	6.0	4.5	4.0	2.2
Medicare and private insurance	2.3	2.1	1.8	2.2	2.8	2.1	1.0
Other public and private mixes	4.5	4.1	4.8	5.1	5.8	3.8	2.8
Other mixes of public programs	*9.4	*9.4	*13.6	*12.3	*5.8	*14.2	*9.3
Source unknown	5.5	4.6	5.1	6.4	5.4	3.7	1.7
All members covered, some part year	2.6	2.0	2.9	3.3	3.6	3.4	1.8
Some members not covered	*0.0	*35.0	*0.0	*0.0	*0.0	*0.0	*0.0
All members not covered	2.2	1.7	4.1	2.9	4.4	3.8	3.4

[1]Includes use of other medical providers and other medical expenditures not shown separately or included in any other service in this table.
[2]There were too few Hispanic families of races other than white for separate tabulation.
[3]Annual rate.
[4]Includes only families with heads 17 years of age and over.
[5]Excludes families with all members under 14 years of age.
[6]Excludes families with all members with health status unknown.

NOTE: 1-person families are families with average size less than 1.5. For 1-person families with more than 1 distinct individual, characteristics are those of head or of family as in Table 1.

Table XXVII

Standard errors for the percent of 1-person families under 65 years of age that use health care services, by type of service and selected characteristics: United States, 1980

Characteristic	Hospital inpatient care	Physician inpatient care	Ambulatory physician visits	Hospital outpatient and emergency visits	Dental visits	Prescription acquisitions	All health care services[1]
Total	1.1	0.9	1.5	1.4	1.7	1.4	0.9
Age							
Under 25 years	1.8	1.5	2.6	2.7	2.8	2.8	2.0
25-44 years	1.8	1.2	2.6	2.2	3.2	3.1	1.7
45-64 years	1.7	1.5	2.2	2.7	2.8	2.3	1.5
Sex							
Male	1.3	1.0	2.3	2.0	2.4	2.4	1.4
Female	1.9	1.7	1.8	2.5	1.8	1.9	1.0
Race and ethnicity[2]							
White	1.2	0.9	1.7	1.7	1.8	1.5	1.0
Hispanic	6.5	3.6	6.5	7.7	7.4	7.3	4.1
Non-Hispanic	1.2	1.0	1.7	1.7	1.9	1.5	1.0
Black	3.2	2.6	4.8	3.9	4.1	3.9	2.9
Other	*4.4	*4.4	*8.5	*9.5	*10.2	*6.8	*5.3
Family dynamics							
Unchanging, full year	1.3	1.0	1.4	1.6	2.0	1.6	0.9
Change in composition or existed less than full year	2.0	1.8	3.1	2.4	3.1	3.0	2.7
Poverty status in 1980							
Below 150 percent	2.0	1.6	2.3	2.7	2.4	2.2	1.8
Below poverty level	2.8	2.5	3.3	3.9	3.1	3.3	2.5
Poverty level to 149 percent	2.9	2.2	3.8	4.3	4.5	3.9	2.6
150-199 percent	2.8	2.3	4.2	5.0	4.2	4.5	3.2
200-299 percent	1.5	1.5	2.8	3.5	3.6	3.0	2.0
300-499 percent	1.9	1.7	2.9	3.1	3.4	2.8	1.3
500 percent or more	2.2	1.8	3.8	3.0	4.6	4.1	2.5
Family income in 1980[3]							
Less than $10,000	1.6	1.4	1.9	2.2	1.9	2.0	1.5
$10,000-$19,999	1.4	1.2	2.3	2.9	2.7	2.4	1.7
$20,000-$34,999	2.4	2.3	3.9	4.0	4.1	4.2	2.4
$35,000 or more	*3.2	*2.2	*7.7	*6.0	*8.7	*8.8	*3.1

Education[4]

None or elementary school	3.2	2.4	4.0	6.3	4.1	4.0	3.4
Some high school	3.0	2.7	3.3	3.4	3.5	3.7	2.6
High school graduate	1.9	1.6	2.6	2.7	2.3	2.8	1.5
Some college	1.9	1.5	3.1	3.2	3.3	3.1	2.1
College graduate or more	1.8	1.5	3.2	3.1	3.4	3.1	1.9

Employment status[5]

Worked full year	1.3	0.9	1.9	1.8	2.2	1.8	1.1
Worked part year	2.0	1.7	2.4	2.2	2.9	2.4	1.7
Never worked	3.2	2.7	3.8	4.3	4.8	3.6	2.2

Perceived health status[6]

Excellent	1.3	1.1	2.1	2.0	2.1	1.9	1.3
Good	1.7	1.2	2.1	2.3	3.2	2.8	1.8
Fair	4.2	3.8	4.2	4.5	4.8	3.9	2.4
Poor	6.5	5.3	7.9	7.9	6.8	4.7	1.7

Limitation in usual activity

None	1.1	0.9	1.5	1.5	1.8	1.6	0.9
Some limitation	*9.8	*9.8	*10.0	*14.9	*12.8	*14.0	*7.7
Cannot perform usual activity	5.2	4.1	4.8	5.3	6.1	4.5	3.3

Bed days[3]

0	0.6	0.3	2.1	1.9	2.6	2.2	1.7
1–5	1.7	1.2	2.6	2.1	2.7	2.5	1.5
6–10	3.9	3.5	2.6	5.0	4.4	2.8	0.7
11–20	6.2	5.0	5.1	6.6	5.9	3.7	0.9
More than 20	4.7	5.8	3.6	5.7	5.8	2.8	1.7

Family health care coverage

All members covered full year	1.2	0.9	1.7	1.8	2.1	1.8	1.1
Private insurance only	1.2	1.0	2.1	2.0	2.4	2.1	1.2
Medicaid only	*13.2	*6.6	*13.9	*13.3	*13.0	*8.9	*6.9
Medicare only	*12.1	*12.1	*19.1	*18.2	*12.1	*19.1	*14.3
Medicare and other public programs	–	–	–	–	–	–	–
Medicare and private insurance	–	–	–	–	–	–	–
Other public and private mixes	4.5	4.1	4.8	5.1	5.8	3.8	2.8
Other mixes of public programs	*9.4	*9.4	*13.6	*12.3	*5.8	*14.2	*9.3
Source unknown	*9.2	*8.1	*5.9	*8.5	*7.2	*4.1	*0.0
All members covered, some part year	2.6	2.0	2.9	3.3	3.6	3.4	1.8
Some members not covered	–	–	–	–	–	–	–
All members not covered	2.4	1.8	4.4	2.8	4.2	3.9	3.8

[1]Includes use of other medical providers and other medical expenditures not shown separately or included in any other service in this table.
[2]There were too few Hispanic families of races other than white for separate tabulation.
[3]Annual rate.
[4]Includes only families with heads 17 years of age and over.
[5]Excludes families with all members under 14 years of age.
[6]Excludes families with all members with health status unknown.

NOTE: 1-person families are families with average size less than 1.5. For 1-person families with more than 1 distinct individual, characteristics are those of head or of family as in Table 2.

299

Table XXVIII

Standard errors for the percent of 1-person families under 65 years of age with health care coverage all year that use health care services, by type of service and selected characteristics: United States, 1980

Characteristic	Hospital inpatient care	Physician inpatient care	Ambulatory physician visits	Hospital outpatient and emergency visits	Dental visits	Prescription acquisitions	All health care services[1]
Total..........................	1.2	0.9	1.7	1.8	2.1	1.8	1.1
Age							
Under 25 years..............	1.9	1.8	3.3	3.0	3.5	3.3	2.0
25-44 years.................	2.0	1.4	3.1	2.9	3.9	3.3	1.7
45-64 years.................	1.9	1.7	2.4	3.2	3.1	2.2	1.5
Sex							
Male........................	1.7	1.4	2.9	2.1	3.0	3.0	1.9
Female......................	2.1	1.8	1.8	2.9	2.4	2.0	1.0
Race and ethnicity[2]							
White.......................	1.3	1.0	1.8	2.0	2.2	1.8	1.2
Hispanic....................	*8.9	*4.5	*9.0	*9.8	*9.7	*8.3	*5.7
Non-Hispanic................	1.3	1.0	1.8	2.0	2.3	1.9	1.1
Black.......................	3.7	3.1	5.8	4.5	4.9	4.6	2.8
Other.......................	*6.7	*6.7	*8.5	*10.2	*13.1	*7.1	*7.1
Family dynamics							
Unchanging, full year.......	1.3	1.1	1.7	2.0	2.3	1.9	1.0
Change in composition or existed less than full year...	2.2	2.2	3.7	3.4	3.3	4.0	3.3
Poverty status in 1980							
Below 150 percent..........	2.5	2.1	3.6	4.0	3.5	3.1	2.4
Below poverty level........	3.9	3.5	4.2	5.9	4.2	4.2	3.1
Poverty level to 149 percent...	3.9	2.9	5.7	5.6	6.5	5.4	3.4
150-199 percent............	3.9	2.8	6.0	6.3	5.3	6.3	4.2
200-299 percent............	2.2	2.2	3.2	4.0	4.1	3.4	2.0
300-499 percent............	2.2	1.9	2.8	3.3	3.9	2.9	1.3
500 percent or more........	2.2	2.1	3.7	3.4	4.7	4.2	2.7
Family income in 1980[3]							
Less than $10,000..........	2.0	1.7	2.8	3.0	2.7	2.7	1.9
$10,000-$19,999............	1.8	1.5	2.5	2.9	2.9	2.3	1.2
$20,000-$34,999............	2.4	2.3	4.3	4.2	4.8	4.5	2.7
$35,000 or more............	*2.4	*2.4	*8.3	*5.1	*8.7	*9.2	*3.5

Education[4]						
None or elementary school	4.1	3.0	4.3	7.5	5.1	4.7	3.6
Some high school	4.0	3.5	4.5	4.1	3.9	4.6	3.2
High school graduate	2.0	1.7	3.1	3.1	3.1	3.3	1.8
Some college	2.4	2.0	3.8	3.6	3.5	3.9	2.6
College graduate or more	2.2	1.9	3.3	3.4	4.4	3.5	2.0
Employment status[5]						
Worked full year	1.4	1.1	2.2	1.9	2.7	2.3	1.2
Worked part year	2.3	2.0	3.0	3.1	4.0	2.8	2.2
Never worked	4.0	3.5	4.4	5.3	5.4	3.8	2.5
Perceived health status[6]						
Excellent	1.5	1.2	2.7	2.4	2.6	2.5	1.7
Good	2.0	1.5	2.5	2.5	3.8	3.0	1.7
Fair	4.5	4.3	4.8	5.3	5.3	4.3	2.9
Poor	*8.4	*7.3	*9.1	*10.1	*8.0	*5.0	*0.0
Limitation in usual activity						
None	1.3	0.9	1.8	1.8	2.3	2.0	1.1
Some limitation	*0.0	*0.0	*9.0	*18.1	*18.0	*3.7	*3.6
Cannot perform usual activity	6.0	4.6	4.6	5.5	6.7	4.9	3.7
Bed days[3]						
0	0.7	0.0	2.8	2.3	3.0	2.6	1.9
1–5	1.7	1.4	3.1	2.3	3.2	3.0	1.6
6–10	5.0	4.5	3.3	5.9	5.5	2.2	0.6
11–20	6.5	6.1	5.2	6.8	6.4	4.2	1.1
More than 20	5.8	6.8	3.5	6.1	7.2	2.1	0.4
Family health care coverage						
Private insurance only	1.2	1.0	2.1	2.0	2.4	2.1	1.2
Medicaid only	*13.2	*6.6	*13.9	*13.3	*13.0	*8.9	*6.9
Medicare only	*12.1	*12.1	*19.1	*18.2	*12.1	*19.1	*14.3
Medicare and other public programs	—	—	—	—	—	—	—
Medicare and private insurance	—	—	—	—	—	—	—
Other public and private mixes	4.5	4.1	4.8	5.1	5.8	3.8	2.8
Other mixes of public programs	*9.4	*9.4	*13.6	*12.3	*5.8	*14.2	*9.3
Source unknown	*9.2	*8.1	*5.9	*8.5	*7.2	*4.1	*0.0

[1] Includes use of other medical providers and other medical expenditures not shown separately or included in any other service in this table.
[2] There were too few Hispanic families of races other than white for separate tabulation.
[3] Annual rate.
[4] Includes only families with heads 17 years of age and over.
[5] Excludes families with all members under 14 years of age.
[6] Excludes families with all members with health status unknown.

NOTE: 1-person families are families with average size less than 1.5. For 1-person families with more than 1 distinct individual, characteristics are those of head or of family as in Table 2.

Table XXIX

Standard errors for the percent of 1-person families under 65 years of age without health care coverage all year that use health care services, by type of service and selected characteristics: United States, 1980

Characteristic	Hospital inpatient care	Physician inpatient care	Ambulatory physician visits	Hospital outpatient and emergency visits	Dental visits	Prescription acquisitions	All health care services [1]
Total	1.9	1.5	2.8	2.3	2.8	2.6	1.9
Age							
Under 25 years	2.5	2.1	4.0	3.8	4.3	4.8	3.0
25–44 years	3.2	2.4	4.3	3.9	4.7	4.8	3.5
45–64 years	3.9	2.9	6.5	5.1	4.7	6.5	4.4
Sex							
Male	1.9	1.1	3.4	3.7	3.6	3.4	2.6
Female	3.4	3.1	3.6	3.5	3.5	4.3	2.0
Race and ethnicity[2]							
White	1.9	1.6	3.3	2.6	3.0	3.0	2.2
Hispanic	*9.2	*5.8	*11.5	*12.3	*11.1	*12.2	*6.9
Non-Hispanic	1.8	1.7	3.4	2.7	3.1	3.0	2.4
Black	*7.1	*4.5	*7.8	*7.0	*5.4	*6.0	*5.6
Other	*0.0	*0.0	*12.3	*13.3	*11.1	*12.3	*10.3
Family dynamics							
Unchanging, full year	2.1	1.6	3.1	2.7	3.4	3.0	2.4
Change in composition or existed less than full year	3.4	3.1	5.2	3.6	5.0	5.4	3.5
Poverty status in 1980							
Below 150 percent	3.2	2.5	4.1	3.9	3.3	3.8	2.9
Below poverty level	4.1	3.4	5.8	5.2	4.5	5.1	3.9
Poverty level to 149 percent	4.6	3.3	6.8	6.9	6.1	7.0	4.8
150–199 percent	3.9	3.9	7.0	6.3	7.0	8.4	5.3
200–299 percent	2.0	1.7	5.6	5.3	6.5	5.8	4.6
300–499 percent	*4.4	*3.6	*7.1	*6.3	*9.0	*7.8	*3.9
500 percent or more	*7.8	*3.8	*11.2	*11.1	*13.2	*12.6	*4.3
Family income in 1980[3]							
Less than $10,000	2.6	2.0	3.0	3.0	2.7	3.1	2.2
$10,000–$19,999	0.0	0.0	5.8	4.2	6.0	6.1	5.3
$20,000–$34,999	*8.8	*6.9	*9.0	*11.9	*12.8	*11.9	*3.9
$35,000 or more	*20.9	*0.0	*17.8	*24.5	*23.6	*24.5	*0.0

Education[4]

Category	1	2	3	4	5	6	7
None or elementary school	*0.0	*0.0	*8.9	*8.4	*6.5	*8.3	*9.3
Some high school	4.8	3.8	5.4	5.6	5.8	6.6	5.0
High school graduate	3.7	3.4	3.8	4.6	4.6	5.1	2.8
Some college	2.8	2.0	6.0	5.6	7.2	5.2	3.0
College graduate or more	2.5	1.3	6.0	6.9	5.3	6.2	4.0

Employment status[5]

Category	1	2	3	4	5	6	7
Worked full year	1.9	0.7	3.3	4.2	4.4	3.3	3.0
Worked part year	3.4	2.8	4.2	3.4	3.5	4.0	3.0
Never worked	*3.5	*1.8	*7.4	*6.1	*8.5	*8.6	*6.1

Perceived health status[6]

Category	1	2	3	4	5	6	7
Excellent	2.4	1.9	4.2	4.1	4.0	3.8	3.5
Good	2.6	1.9	3.8	3.6	4.5	4.5	3.4
Fair	*9.2	*7.2	*8.6	*10.8	*9.4	*8.2	*3.8
Poor	*6.5	*0.0	*13.3	*11.9	*11.8	*11.0	*5.9

Limitation in usual activity

Category	1	2	3	4	5	6	7
None	*1.8	*1.5	2.8	2.4	2.9	2.6	2.0
Some limitation	*23.1	*23.1	*17.5	*25.4	*16.6	*25.4	*18.5
Cannot perform usual activity	*9.7	*5.4	*13.8	*13.2	*13.3	*13.0	*7.1

Bed days[3]

Category	1	2	3	4	5	6	7
0	1.2	1.0	3.7	3.1	4.0	4.0	3.5
1-5	3.4	2.3	3.8	5.3	6.2	5.0	3.1
6-10	5.8	5.5	5.6	7.1	7.5	5.6	1.4
11-20	*11.2	*6.9	*10.5	*14.7	*12.2	*11.5	*1.0
More than 20	*11.8	*10.7	*9.5	*11.3	*9.9	*8.6	*6.3

Family health care coverage

Category	1	2	3	4	5	6	7
All members covered, some part year	2.6	2.0	2.9	3.3	3.6	3.4	1.8
Some members not covered	-	-	-	-	-	-	-
All members not covered	2.4	1.8	4.4	2.8	4.2	3.9	3.8

[1] Includes use of other medical providers and other medical expenditures not shown separately or included in any other service in this table.
[2] There were too few Hispanic families of races other than white for separate tabulation.
[3] Annual rate.
[4] Includes only families with heads 17 years of age and over.
[5] Excludes families with all members under 14 years of age.
[6] Excludes families with all members with health status unknown.

NOTE: 1-person families are families with average size less than 1.5. For 1-person families with more than 1 distinct individual, characteristics are those of head or of family as in Table 2.

Table XXX

Standard errors for the percent of 1-person families 65 years of age and over that use health care services, by type of service and selected characteristics: United States, 1980

Characteristic	Hospital inpatient care	Physician inpatient care	Ambulatory physician visits	Hospital outpatient and emergency visits	Dental visits	Prescription acquisitions	All health care services[1]
Total........................	1.8	1.6	1.7	1.8	2.1	1.4	1.1
Sex							
Male........................	4.0	3.5	4.3	4.3	3.5	3.8	3.3
Female......................	1.9	1.8	1.8	2.1	2.3	1.6	0.9
Race and ethnicity[2]							
White.......................	1.9	1.7	1.5	1.8	2.2	1.4	1.2
Hispanic....................	*15.0	*13.0	*10.1	*14.9	*15.4	*10.1	*8.1
Non-Hispanic................	2.0	1.7	1.6	1.9	2.2	1.4	1.1
Black.......................	5.1	4.3	7.5	6.7	5.2	6.4	3.8
Other.......................	*13.7	*10.3	*16.2	*14.8	*16.0	*14.3	*0.0
Family dynamics							
Unchanging, full year.......	1.7	1.6	1.8	1.8	2.3	1.5	1.2
Change in composition or existed less than full year....	6.3	5.4	6.9	7.3	6.0	3.2	1.1
Poverty status in 1980							
Below 150 percent poverty level....	2.5	2.2	2.7	2.7	2.6	2.1	1.7
Below poverty level.........	2.7	2.3	3.3	3.8	3.2	2.8	2.1
Poverty level to 149 percent....	3.7	3.6	3.9	3.7	3.3	3.5	1.9
150-199 percent.............	4.0	3.6	3.7	5.6	4.6	3.4	2.3
200-299 percent.............	3.4	2.9	4.3	5.2	4.8	3.8	3.3
300-499 percent.............	5.3	5.1	4.7	5.6	6.8	4.5	2.6
500 percent or more.........	*8.6	*8.6	*8.3	*9.1	*10.0	*7.6	*5.6
Family income in 1980[3]							
Less than $10,000...........	1.9	1.8	2.0	2.1	2.3	1.6	1.3
$10,000-$19,999.............	4.5	4.3	3.3	5.2	5.3	3.4	2.0
$20,000-$34,999.............	*11.9	*11.9	*14.3	*14.4	*14.1	*14.3	*11.7
$35,000 or more.............	*12.3	*12.3	*7.8	*12.3	*11.8	*0.1	*0.0
Education							
None or elementary school...	2.9	2.6	2.9	2.8	2.9	2.2	1.7
Some high school............	3.5	3.3	4.9	4.9	3.7	4.0	3.1
High school graduate........	3.3	2.5	2.9	4.1	3.9	3.2	2.1
Some college................	5.3	4.9	6.2	5.5	6.3	5.5	3.1
College graduate or more....	5.5	5.4	3.0	7.2	6.1	2.9	1.6

Employment status

	1	2	3	4	5	6	7
Worked full year...	*6.7	*6.7	*7.4	*8.0	*9.0	*6.5	*5.1
Worked part year...	4.8	4.3	5.7	5.7	4.6	5.5	4.4
Never worked...	2.0	1.8	1.8	2.2	2.4	1.4	1.0

Perceived health status[4]

	1	2	3	4	5	6	7
Excellent...	2.6	2.2	3.4	2.9	3.1	2.8	2.1
Good...	2.8	2.3	3.1	3.3	4.0	2.8	1.9
Fair...	4.0	3.7	2.8	4.6	3.9	2.4	1.6
Poor...	7.1	6.0	5.2	6.8	6.1	3.2	2.1

Limitation in usual activity

	1	2	3	4	5	6	7
None...	2.0	1.8	2.1	2.1	2.6	1.9	1.6
Some limitation...	*6.6	*6.0	*6.4	*7.8	*6.4	*5.1	*3.6
Cannot perform usual activity...	3.7	3.6	3.1	3.6	3.4	2.6	1.5

Bed days[3]

	1	2	3	4	5	6	7
0...	0.6	0.5	2.5	2.3	3.2	2.1	1.9
1-5...	5.0	4.5	4.8	5.6	5.1	4.7	2.1
6-10...	6.9	5.4	3.1	6.6	6.5	3.9	2.4
11-20...	6.2	6.4	2.1	6.5	6.1	3.1	0.0
More than 20...	4.5	4.8	3.1	5.3	4.7	1.7	1.2

Family health care coverage

	1	2	3	4	5	6	7
All members covered full year...	1.8	1.6	1.6	1.8	2.2	1.3	1.2
Private insurance only...	*0.0	*0.0	*0.0	*0.0	*0.0	*0.0	*0.0
Medicaid only...	-	-	-	-	-	-	-
Medicare only...	3.9	3.7	4.6	4.6	5.1	4.4	4.5
Medicare and other public programs...	5.2	4.3	4.6	6.0	4.5	4.0	2.2
Medicare and private insurance...	2.3	2.1	1.8	2.2	2.8	2.1	1.0
Other public and private mixes...	-	-	-	-	-	-	-
Other mixes of public programs...	-	-	-	-	-	-	-
Source unknown...	*5.5	*4.2	*8.0	*7.9	*8.3	*6.0	*3.1
All members covered, some part year...	-	-	-	-	-	-	-
Some members not covered...	*0.0	*35.0	*0.0	*0.0	*0.0	*0.0	*0.0
All members not covered...	*8.5	*4.1	*11.1	*16.3	*10.3	*11.5	*9.1

[1]Includes use of other medical providers and other medical expenditures not shown separately or included in any other service in this table.
[2]There were too few Hispanic families of races other than white for separate tabulation.
[3]Annual rate.
[4]Excludes families with all members with health status unknown.

NOTE: 1-person families are families with average size less than 1.5. For 1-person families with more than 1 distinct individual, characteristics are those of head or of family as in Table 2.

305

Appendix II.
Definitions of Terms

Age of family head—Age is as of January 1, 1980.

Ambulatory physician visit—A visit by a patient to a physician's office, clinic, or similar place is an ambulatory physician visit. Visits are counted whether a physician or only a member of the physician's staff is seen. House calls and visits to school or workplace clinics are also included. Family visits are the sum of all visits by family members during the time they were in the family.

Bed days—Bed days are days spent in bed by a family member because of illness or injury. Family bed days are the sum of all bed days of family members during the time they were in the survey, prorated to the time they were in the family.

Civilian noninstitutionalized family—This refers to families in which all members are members of the civilian noninstitutionalized population. Families whose heads are members of the military are defined as not being civilian families and are excluded in their entirety from this report, although they were included in the sample and the weighting. In the sample, there were 49 such families (about 0.7 percent). Family members other than the head who were in the military were excluded from the survey even if they resided with the family.

Dental visit—A visit to a dentist's office is a dental visit. A dentist or a member of the dentist's office staff may have provided services. Family visits are the sum of all visits by family members during the time they were in the family.

Education of family head—The years of school completed by family heads 17 years of age and over constitute the education of family heads. Only years completed in regular schools, where persons are given a formal education, are included. A "regular" school is one that advances a person toward an elementary or high school diploma or a college, university, or professional school degree. Thus, education in vocational, trade, or business schools outside the regular school system was not counted in determining the highest grade of school completed.

Employment status of family—Family employment status was measured by an index dividing families into four categories: Two or more family members worked a full year (48–52 weeks); only one family member worked a full year; some family members worked part year (less than 48 weeks) but none worked a full year; and no family members worked. If they worked, family members in the survey less than a full year were coded as having worked less than a full year. Family members under 14 years of age were assumed not to have worked.

Ethnicity of family head—The ethnicity of family heads 17 years of age and over is as reported by the family respondent. The ethnicity of family heads under 17 was imputed. Ethnicity is classified as (1) Hispanic, which includes Puerto Rican, Cuban, Mexican, Mexicano, Mexican American, Chicano, other Latin American, and other Spanish or (2) non-Hispanic.

Family—A family is a group of people who share a common housing unit and are related to each other by blood, marriage, adoption, or a foster care relationship. An unmarried student 17–22 years of age living away from home is also considered part of a family even though his or her residence was in a different location. The group of people who compose the family may change composition over time, causing the family to take on one or a combination of the following time-related states: existing over time without change in membership; existing over time with change in membership; going out of existence before the end of the survey; coming into existence after the beginning of the survey; or existing for the whole survey. For more detail, see Appendix I.

Family dynamics—A family is considered unchanging, or static, if it existed for the whole of 1980 and its membership was unchanged. Families that had changes in membership and/or did not exist for the whole of 1980 are considered changing, or dynamic, families.

Family income in 1980—For each person in the family, data were collected on 12 categories of income. These included income from employment for persons 14 years of age and over; income from various government programs; income from pensions; alimony or child support; interest income; and net rental income. When information was missing, income was imputed. The total income of persons who were members of more than one family was allocated to each family they were in, in proportion to the amount of time they were in that family. Person-level incomes in each family were summed to create a family-level total. If a family did not exist for an entire year, the family income was adjusted to an annual basis by dividing actual income by the proportion of the year the family existed.

Family size—The time-weighted average number of

persons in a family determines the size. Family size was computed by (1) summing the number of days in the family for each person who was ever a family member and (2) dividing this sum by the number of days the family was in existence. For example, if a family existed for 200 days and had two persons who were members throughout its existence and one person who was a member for 80 days, the family size is 2.4. In all tables, the time-weighted average family size is rounded to the nearest integer.

Family structure—Family structure refers to the presence or absence of family head, spouse, and children under 17, and whether these persons were present for the family's entire duration or part of its duration.

Family years—Family years refers to the length of time that a family, or a collection of families, existed as a unit of analysis in (were eligible for) the survey, as measured in units of a year or fractions of such units.

For an individual longitudinal family in the NMCUES sample, the number of family years equals the number of days the family was eligible for the NMCUES sample divided by 366, the number of days in 1980 (the NMCUES sample period). For such a family weighted to represent a group of families in the NMCUES universe, the number of family years is AWEIGHT(j), which is equal to FWEIGHT(j), the basic adjusted weight, times $PE(j)$, the proportion of the year the family was eligible for the sample. For a group of sample families, the associated number of family years is the sum of the AWEIGHT's. For further details and fuller definitions of variables, see the section on estimators in Appendix I.

Group quarters—This is a structure occupied by five or more unrelated people who lived or ate together, or for whom there was neither direct access from the outside or through a common hall nor complete kitchen facilities. Only noninstitutional group quarters were included in the NMCUES sample frame. Each unrelated person in a group-quarter household was considered a separate one-person family, unless he (or she) was a student away from home. (See definition of family.)

Head of family—A person was designated as the family head by the respondent at the time of the first interview. If no head was designated or this information was missing, a family head was imputed. Among families in which the person designated as head changed over time, the characteristics of the person who was designated head the longest were used for all head-of-family variables.

Health care coverage—Health care coverage refers to the situation in which a public health care coverage program (Medicare, Medicaid, and so forth) or private health insurance can be used to pay all or part of the health care expenditures of a family's members. "Full-year coverage" refers to coverage for the whole time the family or family member was eligible for the survey. "Without health care coverage all year" includes coverage

for less than the time the family or family member was eligible for the survey and the complete absence of coverage.

For this report, a family was coded as having a particular type of health care coverage (such as private insurance, Medicare, Medicaid, or a particular combination of coverages) on the basis of the known coverage of family members. Only when the type of coverage was unknown, or not assignable, for all family members was the family coded as having an unknown type of coverage. The coding categories for individuals, however, upon which the family health care coverage coding in this report were based are different from the categories used in a previous family report (Dicker, 1983a) that dealt with only a part of the survey year. As a result, there may be differences in coverage estimates between the reports.

Hospital admission—Hospital admission is the formal acceptance by a hospital of a patient who is provided room, board, and regular nursing care in a unit of the hospital, including patients admitted for childbirth. A patient admitted to the hospital and discharged on the same day is included as a hospital admission. A hospital stay resulting from an emergency department visit is also included. Family hospital admissions are the sum of all admissions of family members during the time they were in the family.

Hospital day—A day is spent in a hospital by a person who has been admitted and discharged. Persons admitted and discharged on the same day are counted as having zero hospital days. Others are counted by the number of nights spent in the hospital. For example, a person admitted on Monday and discharged on the following Wednesday would be counted as having two hospital days, not three. Because patients admitted and discharged on the same day are counted as having zero hospital days, some families that experience hospital discharges nonetheless have zero hospital days.

Hospital discharge—A hospital discharge is the formal release by a hospital of a patient who was provided room, board, and regular nursing care in a unit of the hospital. A patient admitted to the hospital and discharged on the same day is included as a hospital discharge. A hospital stay resulting from an emergency room visit and subsequent admission of the patient is also included. Family hospital discharges are the sum of all discharges by family members during the time they were in the family.

Hospital emergency room—The emergency room is a facility within a hospital organized to provide medical services to people needing immediate medical or surgical intervention. People receiving care in the emergency room may be admitted to a hospital.

Hospital emergency room visit—This is a face-to-face encounter between a patient (not necessarily ambulatory) and a medical person in the hospital emergency room. Encounters by patients transported to the emergency room by police or the emergency medical service, are included. The visit may result in a hospital admission. Family emergency room visits are the sum of all emergency room visits by family members during the time they were in the family.

Hospital outpatient department—This is a hospital-based ambulatory care facility organized to provide non-emergency medical services. Persons receiving services do not receive inpatient nursing care. Examples of outpatient departments or clinics are pediatrics, obstetrics and gynecology, eye, and psychiatric.

Hospital outpatient department visit—This is a face-to-face encounter between an ambulatory patient and a medical person in a hospital outpatient department. The patient comes to a hospital-based ambulatory care facility to receive services and departs on the same day. If more than one department or clinic was visited on a single trip, each department or clinic visited was counted as a separate visit. Family outpatient department visits are the sum of all hospital outpatient department visits by family members during the time they were in the family.

Household—This refers to occupants of a housing unit or group quarters included in the sample. A household can be one person, a family of related people, a number of unrelated people, or a combination of related and unrelated people. Therefore, a household can contain more than one family. (See definition of family.)

Housing unit—A housing unit is a group of rooms or a single room occupied or intended for occupancy as separate living quarters. This means that (1) the occupants do not live and eat with any other persons in the structure, and (2) there is either direct access from the outside or through a common hall or complete kitchen facilities for the use of the occupants only.

Inpatient hospital care—This is health care provided to a patient by a hospital during the period from the patient's admission to the patient's discharge. This includes admissions for deliveries of babies.

Inpatient physician care—This care is provided to a patient by a physician (or a physician's staff) during the period from the patient's admission to a hospital to the time of the patient's discharge from the hospital.

Institution—An institution is a place providing room, board, and certain other services for residents or patients. Correctional institutions, military barracks, and orphanages were always considered institutions in NMCUES. Places that provide long term health care were also identified as institutions if they provide either nursing or personal care services. Certain other facilities licensed, registered, or certified by a State agency or affiliated with a Federal, State, or local government agency were also defined as institutions. People residing in institutions were not included in the household sample.

Key person—See the discussion under "Sample Design" in Appendix I.

Limitation in major activity—Four categories were developed for classifying limitation in major activity:

1. Cannot perform usual major activity (such as working, going to school, or keeping house).

2. Can perform usual major activity but limited in kind or amount.

3. Can perform usual major activity but limited in kind or amount of other activity.

4. Not limited.

People 6 years of age and over were classified into any of the categories; children 1–5 years of age were classified into categories 1, 2, and 4; and children under 1 year of age were classified into categories 1 and 4. In this report, categories 2 and 3 are combined into the category "some limitation."

Longitudinal family—A longitudinal family is a family identified as the same family over a time period. It may or may not have had changes in family membership during the time period. (See the definition of family.)

Marital status—Marital status for each person 17 years of age and over is as indicated by the household respondent.

Multiple-person family—A family with an average size of 1.5 members or more is a multiple-person family.

National household component—One component of NMCUES, this consists of multiple household interviews with an area probability sample of people in the noninstitutionalized population of the United States in 1980.

Nonkey person—See the discussion under "Sample Design" in Appendix I.

Number of families—This refers to the average number of families with a given set of characteristics that would have been found at a randomly chosen point in time in 1980. This is equal to the number of family years experienced during 1980 by families with the given characteristics. It is, in general, less than the cumulative total number of distinct longitudinal families with the given characteristics that ever existed at any time in 1980, some of which existed for only part of the year.

One-person family—A family with average size less than 1.5 is a one-person family. More than one distinct individual may be involved.

Out-of-pocket expenditures—Amounts paid by a family that are not reimbursed by insurance or other health care payment programs constitute out-of-pocket expenditures.

Out-of-pocket expenditures for all health care combined—This term refers to the sum of out-of-pocket expenditures for all types of health care recorded in NMCUES. In addition to types of expenses reported in the detailed tables of this report, the sum includes the following expenditures: those on other independent medical providers, such as chiropractors, speech therapists, faith healers, and psychologists. (However, if such providers are working as part of a physician's staff, their services and related expenses are counted as physicians' care); and those on other health care supplies, including eyeglasses, orthopedic items, hearing aids, ambulance services, and diabetic items. Expenses for nonprescription medicines, and for nursing home care and other long-term care institutions, are excluded from the report (and generally also from NMCUES data collection).

Perceived health status—This is the family respondent's rating on a 4-point scale of the health of a family member compared with the health of other persons of the same age, as reported at the time of the first interview. The categories are "excellent," "good," "fair," and "poor." When a family consisted of only one member, this was a self-rating.

Point-interval family—A point-interval family is a family with exactly the same family membership over a time period. A change in family membership ends one point-interval family and begins another.

Poverty status of family—The poverty status in 1980 was calculated by dividing the family's income in 1980 by the appropriate 1980 poverty level threshold and converting it to a percent. For example, a family with income between two and three times the poverty level threshold that corresponds to its size and other characteristics would be classified in the 200–299 percent category. The poverty level thresholds, as used by the U.S. Bureau of Census, are determined by the age and sex of the family head and the average number of persons in the family. In 1980, average poverty level thresholds by family size (weighted for the mix of families by sex and age of head) were: 1-person, $4,190; 2-person, $5,368; 3-person, $6,565; 4-person, $8,414; 5-person, $9,966; 6-person, $11,269, 7-person, $12,761; 8-person, $14,199; 9-person and larger, $16,896.

Prescription acquisition—This describes the obtaining of a medication by a family member requiring a prescription from a doctor or dentist. Both initial fillings of prescriptions and refills are counted as acquisitions. Family prescription acquisitions are the sum of all acquisitions by family members during the time they were in the family.

Principal respondent—This is the member of the reporting unit who provided most of the information for the people in the reporting unit.

Proxy respondent—As used in this survey, a proxy respondent was a person who provided information for people in the reporting unit but who was not a member of the reporting unit. A proxy respondent was used only when no member of the reporting unit could supply the information because of physical or mental incapacity.

Race of family head—The race of the family head is as reported by the family respondent or imputed. Race is classified as "white," "black," or "other." The "other" race category includes American Indians, Alaskan Natives, Asians, Pacific Islanders, and people not identified by race. The category "all other" includes the categories "black" and "other."

Rate per family year—Amount of care used or dollars expended by a family or group of families is divided by the number of family years experienced by these families while eligible for the NMCUES sample. All data on use of care in this report are presented in terms of rate of use of care per family year. For a given family, the rate per family year equals $Y(j)/PE(j)$,

where $Y(j)$ = use of care during family's period of eligibility for NMCUES sample, and

$PE(j)$ = proportion of year family was eligible for the NMCUES sample.

The section on estimators in Appendix I presents more details of calculations.

Reporting unit (RU)—A reporting unit is the basic unit for collecting data in the household components of NMCUES at the time of each interview. A reporting unit consisted of all related people residing in the same housing unit or group quarters during the reference period covered by a particular interview. One person could give information for all members of the reporting unit.

Ref. date—The reference date was the date of the previous interview in most cases. For the first interview, however, it was January 1, 1980. For new persons, it was the date they joined the reporting unit. For the final interview, it spanned the time between the next-to-last interview and December 31, 1980.

Secondary reporting unit—Unmarried students 17–22 years of age usually living in a sampled household but away from home as full-time students were considered secondary reporting units. Also, in a household with multiple families, the reporting unit with the largest number of individuals was usually designated the primary reporting unit, and all other families were designated secondary reporting units.

Sex—Sex was recorded by the interviewer in the initial NMCUES interview.

Worked full year—"Worked full year" refers to 48 or more weeks of work during the year.

Worked part year—"Worked part year" refers to less than 48 weeks of work during the year.

Department of Health and Human Services
Otis R. Bowen, M.D., Secretary

Health Care Financing Administration
William L. Roper, M.D., Administrator

Office of Research and Demonstrations
Joseph R. Antos, Ph.D., Director

Office of Research
J. Michael Fitzmaurice, Acting Director

Division of Program Studies
Carl Josephson, Director

Surveys Studies Branch
Herbert A. Silverman, Ph.D., Chief

Public Health Service
Robert E. Windom, M.D.,
Assistant Secretary for Health

National Center for Health Statistics
Manning Feinleib, M.D., Dr.P.H., Director

Office of Interview and Examination Statistics Program
Peter L. Hurley, Acting Associate Director

Division of Health Interview Statistics
Owen T. Thornberry, Jr., Ph.D., Director

Utilization and Expenditure Statistics Branch
Robert A. Wright, Chief

www.ingramcontent.com/pod-product-compliance
Lightning Source LLC
Chambersburg PA
CBHW081058290526
45795CB00006B/1904